Clinical Anatomy of the Lumbar Spine.

Clinical Anatomy of
the Lumbar Spine

Nikolai Bogduk BSc(Med) MBBS PhD
Dip Anat HonFACRM
Associate Professor, Faculty of Medicine,
University of Newcastle, Newcastle, New South Wales

Lance T. Twomey BAppSc BSc(Hons) PhD
Deputy Vice Chancellor
Professor of Physiotherapy
Curtin University, Perth, Western Australia

SECOND EDITION

CHURCHILL LIVINGSTONE
MELBOURNE EDINBURGH LONDON NEW YORK AND TOKYO 1991

CHURCHILL LIVINGSTONE
Medical Division of Longman Group UK Limited

Distributed in Australia by Longman Cheshire Pty
Limited, Longman House, Kings Gardens, 95 Coventry
Street, South Melbourne 3205, and by associated
companied, branches and representatives throughout the
world.

First edition 1987
Second edition 1991
Reprinted 1992 (twice)
Reprinted 1994

ISBN 0-443-04339 6

National Library of Australia Cataloguing in Publication
Data

Bogduk, Nikolai.
    Clinical anatomy of the lumbar spine.

    2nd ed.
    Bibliography.
    Includes index.
    ISBN 0 443 04339 6.

    1. Vertebrae, Lumbar – Anatomyl. I. Twomey, Lance. T.
II. Title.   II. Title.

611.711

A Library of Congress Catalog record is available for this title.

Produced by Churchill Livingstone in Melbourne
Printed in Singapore

Preface to the second edition

In preparing the second edition we have attended to minor errors in the text and in some of the figures that appeared in the first edition. We have also taken the opportunity to incorporate several references that were available at the time that the first edition was being prepared but which had not been included. However, the overriding reason for producing this second edition has been the large amount of new data on the lumbar spine that has appeared since the first edition was published. This has allowed certain sections of the text to be elaborated on to include new details; new sections have been added, and others have been totally revised.

Overall, the theme of the text remains the same. The reader is taken through the basic structure of the lumbar spine, its movements and mechanics, its muscles, nerves and blood supply, its development and ageing. These topics form the foundation finally for a consideration of lumbar spinal pain and its common causes.

In revising the text, Chapters 1 and 3 on the morphology of the vertebrae and the zygapophysial joints remain essentially unchanged, but new details on the biochemistry of the disc are introduced in Chapter 2. Chapter 4, on the lumbar ligaments, has been modified to incorporate new interpretations of the significance of certain ligaments. Chapter 5 remains the same, but Chapter 6 on biomechanics has been revised to include a new section on forces and moments. New details on lumbar movements have been added to Chapter 7. Chapter 8 on muscles has been revised; former views on the mechanism of lifting have been refuted and replaced with current theories and new conjectures. Further details on the dorsal rami have been added to Chapter 9 together with striking new findings on the microscopic innervation of the lumbar vertebral bodies and discs. Chapter 10 remains unchanged, but the development and age changes of the zygapophysial joints have been elaborated on in Chapters 11 and 12. New information on dural pain appears in Chapter 13.

The greatest changes appear in Chapter 14 in response to increasing amounts of new data on the pathology of low-back pain. Concepts that in the first edition had been raised only cautiously have now been largely vindicated, necessitating a major revision of Chapter 14. The pathology of disc herniation has been de-emphasised in accordance with its relatively low prevalence as a cause of back pain. Instead, emphasis is laid on the mechanical causes of low-back pain which are discussed systematically in terms of flexion, extension, rotation and compression injuries, drawing together concepts and data outlined in earlier chapters, demonstrating how back injuries and pain can be understood in terms of excessive forces having been applied to an otherwise normal lumbar spine.

Nikolai Bogduk
Lance Twomey
1991

Preface to the first edition

Low-back pain is a major problem in medicine and can constitute more than 60% of consultations in private physiotherapy practice. Yet, the emphasis given to spinal anatomy in conventional courses in anatomy for medical students and physiotherapists is not commensurate with the magnitude of the problem of spinal pain in clinical practice. The anatomy of the lumbar spine usually constitutes only a small component of such courses.

Having been involved in spinal research and in teaching medical students and physiotherapists both at undergraduate and postgraduate levels, we have become conscious of how little of the basic sciences relating to the lumbar spine is taught to students, and how difficult it can be to obtain information which is available but scattered through a diversity of textbooks and journal articles. Therefore, we have composed this textbook in order to collate that material which we consider fundamental to the understanding of the structure, function and common disorders of the lumbar spine.

We see the text as one which can be used as a companion to other textbooks in introductory courses in anatomy, and which can also remain as source throughout later years of undergraduate and postgraduate education in physiotherapy and physical medicine. In this regard, references are made throughout the text to contemporary and major earlier research papers so that the reader may consult the original literature upon which descriptions, interpretations and points of view are based. Moreover, the reference list has been made extensive in order to provide students seeking to undertake research projects on some aspect

of the lumbar spine with a suitable starting point in their search through the literature.

Chapters 1–4 outline the structure of the individual components of the lumbar spine, and the intact spine is described in Chapter 5. In describing the lumbar vertebrae and their joints, we have gone beyond the usual scope of textbooks of anatomy by endeavouring to explain why the vertebrae and their components are constructed the way they are.

Chapter 6 summarises some basic principles of biomechanics in preparation for the study of the movements of the lumbar spine which is dealt with in Chapter 7. Chapter 8 provides an account of the lumbar back muscles which are described in exhaustive detail because of the increasing contemporary interest amongst physiotherapists and others in physical medicine in the biomechanical functions and so-called dysfunctional states of the back muscles.

Chapters 9 and 10 describe the nerves and blood supply of the lumbar spine, and its embryology and development is described in Chapter 11. This leads to a description of the age changes of the lumbar spine in Chapter 12. The theme developed through Chapters 11 and 12 is that the lumbar spine is not a constant stereotyped structure as described in conventional textbooks, but one that continually changes in form and functional capacity throughout life. Any concept of normality must be modified according to the age of the patient or subject.

The final two chapters provide a bridge between basic anatomy and the clinical problem of lumbar pain syndromes. Chapter 13 outlines the possible mechanisms of lumbar pain in terms of the innervation of the lumbar spine and the relations of the lumbar spinal nerves and nerve roots, thereby providing an anatomical foundation for the appreciation of patho- logical conditions that can cause spinal pain.

Chapter 14 deals with pathological anatomy. Traditional topics like congenital disorders, fractures, dislocations and tumours are not covered, although the reader is directed to the pertinent literature on these topics. Instead, the scope is restricted to conditions which clinically are interpreted as mechanical disorders. The aetiology and pathology of these conditions is described in terms of the structural and biomechanical principles developed in earlier chapters, with the view to providing a rational basis for the interpretation and treatment of a group of otherwise poorly understood conditions which account for the majority of presentations of low-back pain syndromes.

We anticipate that the detail and extent of our account of the clinical anatomy of the lumbar spine will be perceived as far in excess of what is conventionally taught. However, we believe that our text is not simply an expression of a personal interest of the authors, but rather is an embodiment of what we consider the essential knowledge of basic sciences for anyone seeking to be trained to deal with disorders of the lumbar spine.

Nikolai Bogduk
Lance Twomey
1987

Contents

1. The lumbar vertebrae

The lumbar vertebral column consists of five separate vertebrae, which are named according to their location in the intact column. From above downwards, they are named as the first, second, third, fourth and fifth lumbar vertebrae (Fig. 1.1). Although there are certain features that typify each lumbar vertebra, and enable each to be individually identified and numbered, at an early stage of study it is not necessary for students to be able to do so. Indeed, to learn to do so would be both impractical and burdensome. Many of the distinguishing features are better appreciated and more easily understood once the whole structure of the lumbar vertebral column and its mechanics have been studied. To this end, a description of the features of individual lumbar vertebrae is provided in Appendix 1, and it is recommended that this be studied after Chapter 7.

What is appropriate at this stage is to consider those features common to all lumbar vertebrae, and to appreciate how typical lumbar vertebrae are designed to subserve their functional roles. Accordingly, the following description is divided into parts. In the first part, the features of a typical lumbar vertebra are described. This section serves either as an introduction for students commencing their study of the lumbar vertebral column, or as a revision for students already familiar with the essentials of vertebral anatomy. The second section deals with particular details germane to the appreciation of the function of the lumbar vertebrae, and is a foundation for later chapters.

It is strongly recommended that these sections be read with specimens of the lumbar vertebrae at the reader's disposal, for not only will visual inspection reinforce the written information, but tactile examination of a specimen will enhance the three-dimensional perception of structure.

A TYPICAL LUMBAR VERTEBRA

The lumbar vertebrae are irregular bones consisting of various named parts (Fig. 1.2). The anterior part of each vertebra is a large block of bone called the **vertebral body**. The vertebral body is more or less box-shaped, with essentially flat top and bottom surfaces, and slightly concave anterior and lateral surfaces. Viewed from above or below the vertebral body has a curved perimeter that is more or less kidney-shaped. The posterior surface of the body is essentially flat, but is obscured from thorough inspection by the posterior elements of the vertebra.

The greater part of the top and bottom surfaces of each vertebral body is smooth and perforated by tiny holes. However, the perimeter of each surface is marked by a narrow rim of smoother, less perforated bone that may even be slightly raised from the surface. This rim represents the fused **ring apophysis**, which is a secondary ossification centre of the vertebral body (see Ch. 11).

The posterior surface of the vertebral body is marked by one or more large holes known as the **nutrient foramina**. These foramina transmit the nutrient arteries of the vertebral body and the basivertebral veins (see Ch. 10). The anterolateral surfaces of the vertebral body are marked by similar, but smaller, foramina that transmit additional intra-osseous arteries.

Projecting from the back of the vertebral body are two stout pillars of bone. Each of these is

1

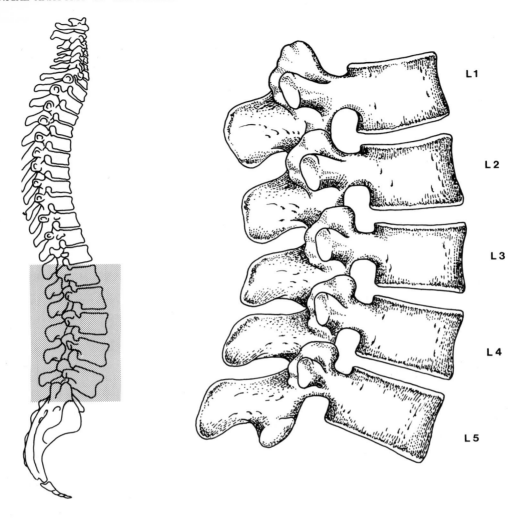

Fig. 1.1   The lumbar vertebrae and how they appear in the entire vertebral column.

called a **pedicle**. The pedicles attach to the upper part of the back of the vertebral body, and this is one feature that allows the superior and inferior aspects of the vertebral body to be identified. To correctly orientate a vertebra, view it from the side. That end of the posterior surface of the body to which the pedicles are more closely attached will be the upper (Fig. 1.2A and B).

The word 'pedicle' is derived from the Latin *pediculus*, meaning little foot, and the reason for this nomenclature is apparent when the vertebra is viewed from above (Fig. 1.2E). It can be seen that attached to the back of the vertebral body is

an arch of bone, called the **neural arch**, so-called because it surrounds the neural elements that pass through the vertebral column. The neural arch has several parts and several projections, but the pedicles are those parts that look like short legs with which it appears to 'stand' on the back of the vertebral body (Fig. 1.2E). Hence the derivation from the Latin for foot.

Projecting from each pedicle towards the midline is a sheet of bone called the **lamina** (plural: laminae). The name is derived from the Latin *lamina*, meaning leaf, or plate. The two laminae meet and fuse with one another in the midline,

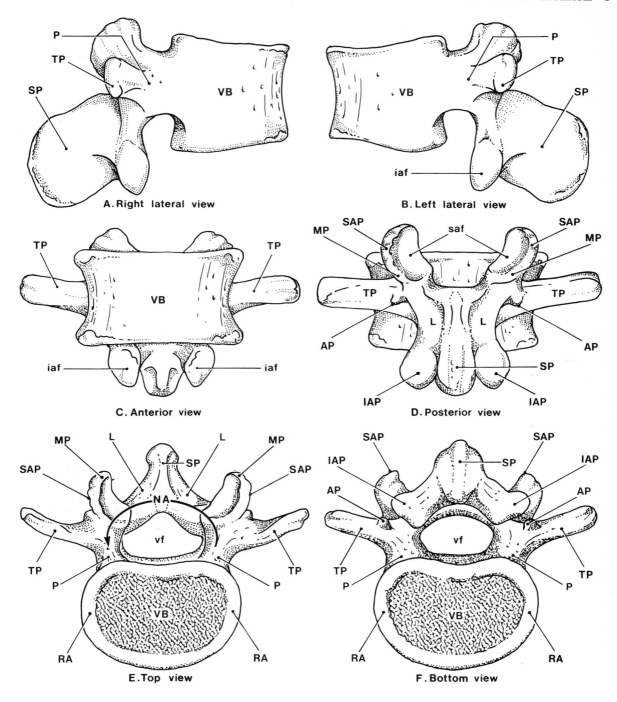

Fig. 1.2 The parts of a typical lumbar vertebra: VB — vertebral body. P — pedicle. TP — transverse process. SP — spinous process. L — lamina. SAP — superior articular process. IAP — inferior articular process. saf — superior articular facet. iaf — inferior articular facet. MP — mamillary process. AP — accessory process. vf — vertebral foramen. RA — ring apophysis. NA — neural arch.

and in a top view, the laminae look like the roof of a tent, and indeed, form the so-called 'roof' of the neural arch*.

The full extent of the laminae is seen in a posterior view of the vertebra (Fig. 1.2D). Each lamina has slightly irregular, and perhaps sharp, superior edges, but its lateral edge is rounded and smooth. There is no medial edge of each lamina because the two lamina blend in the midline. Similarly, there is no superior lateral corner of the laminae because in this direction, the lamina blends with the pedicle on that side. The inferolateral corner and inferior border of each lamina is developed into a specialised mass of bone — the **inferior articular process**.

Each vertebra presents four articular processes. Extending upwards from the junction of the lamina and pedicle on each side is a **superior articular process**, and from the lower lateral corner of the lamina projects the **inferior articular process**. The four processes are distinguished as the right and left superior articular processes and the right and left inferior articular processes. On the medial surface of each superior articular process and on the lateral surface of each inferior articular process is a smooth area of bone which in the intact spine is covered by articular cartilage. This area is known as the articular **facet** of each articular process.

Projecting posteriorly from the junction of the two laminae is a narrow blade of bone (readily gripped between the thumb and index finger), that in a side-view resembles the blade of an axe. This is the **spinous process**, so named because in other regions of the vertebral column these processes form projections under the skin that are reminiscent of the dorsal spines of fish and other animals. The base of the spinous process blends imperceptibly with the two laminae, but otherwise it presents free superior and inferior edges, and a broader posterior edge.

---

* Strictly speaking, there are two laminae in each vertebra, one on the left and one on the right, and the two meet posteriorly in the midline, but in some circles, the term 'lamina' is used incorrectly to refer to both laminae collectively. When this is the usage, the term 'hemilamina' is used to refer to what has been described above as a true lamina.

Extending laterally from the junction of the pedicle and the lamina, on each side, is a flat, rectangular bar of bone called the **transverse process**, so named because of its transverse orientation. Near its attachment to the pedicle, each transverse process bears on its posterior surface a small, irregular bony prominence called the **accessory process**. Accessory processes vary in form and size from a simple bump on the back of the transverse process, to a morepronounced mass of bone, or a definitive pointed projection of variable length.[324,341] Regardless of its actual form, the accessory process is identifiable as the only bony projection from the back of the proximal end of the transverse process. It is most evident if the vertebra is viewed from behind and from below (Fig. 1.2D and F).

Close inspection of the posterior edge of each of the superior articular processes reveals another small bump, distinguishable from its surroundings by its smoothness. Apparently because this structure reminded early anatomists of the shape of breasts it was called the **mamillary process**, derived from the Latin *mamilla*, meaning little breast. It lies just above and slightly medial to the accessory process, and the two processes are separated by a notch, of variable depth, that may be referred to as the mamillo-accessory notch.

Reviewing the structure of the neural arch, it can be seen that each arch consists of two laminae, meeting in the midline, and anchored to the back of the vertebral body by the two pedicles. Projecting posteriorly from the junction of the laminae is the spinous processes, and projecting from the junction of the lamina and pedicle, on each side, are the transverse processes. From the corners of the laminae project the superior and inferior articular processes.

The further named features of the lumbar vertebrae are not bony parts but spaces and notches. Viewing a vertebra from above, it can be seen that the neural arch and the back of the vertebral body surround a space that is large enough to perhaps just admit an examining finger. This space is the **vertebral canal**, which amongst other things transmits the nervous structures that the vertebral column protects.

In a side-view, two notches can be recognised above and below each pedicle. The superior notch is small, and is bounded inferiorly by the top of the pedicle, posteriorly by the superior articular process, and anteriorly by the uppermost posterior edge of the vertebral body. The inferior notch is deeper and more pronounced. It lies behind the lower part of the vertebral body, below the lower edge of the pedicle, and in front of the lamina and the inferior articular process. The difference in size of these notches can be used to correctly identify the upper and lower ends of a lumbar vertebra. The deeper, more obvious notch will always be the inferior.

Apart from providing this aid in orientating a lumbar vertebra, these notches have no intrinsic significance and have not been accorded a formal name. However, when consecutive lumbar vertebrae are articulated (see Fig. 1.6), the superior and inferior notches face one another and form most of what is known as the **intervertebral foramen**, whose anatomy is described in further detail in Chapter 5.

Particular features

Conceptually, a lumbar vertebra may be divided into three functional components (Fig. 1.3).

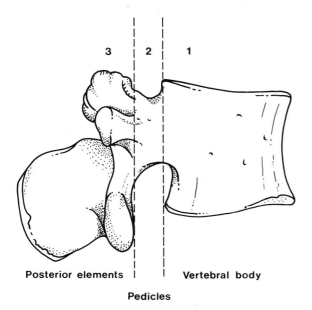

Fig. 1.3 The division of a lumbar vertebra into its three functional components.

These are the vertebral body, the pedicles, and the posterior elements consisting of the laminae and their processes. Each of these components subserves a unique function, but each contributes to the integrated function of the whole vertebra.

Vertebral body

The vertebral body subserves the weight-bearing function of the vertebra, and is perfectly designed for this purpose. Its flat superior and inferior surfaces are dedicated to supporting longitudinally applied loads.

Take two lumbar vertebrae and fit them together so that the inferior surface of one body rests on the superior surface of the other. Now squeeze them together, as strongly as you can. Feel how well they resist the applied longitudinal compression. The experiment can be repeated by placing the pair of vertebrae upright on a table (near the edge, so that the inferior articular processes can hang down over the edge). Now press down on the upper vertebra, and feel how the pair of vertebrae sustains the pressure, even up to taking your whole body weight. These experiments illustrate how the flatness of the vertebral bodies confers stability to an intervertebral joint, in the longitudinal direction. Even without intervening and other supporting structures, two articulated vertebrae can stably sustain immense longitudinal loads.

The load-bearing design of the vertebral bodies is also reflected in its internal structure. The vertebral body is not a solid block of bone, but simply a shell of cortical bone surrounding a cancellous cavity. The advantages of this design are several. First, consider the problems of a solid block of bone. Although strong, a solid block of bone is heavy. (Compare the weight of five lumbar vertebrae with that of five similarly sized stones.) More significantly, while solid blocks are suitable for maintaining static loads, solid structures are not ideal for dynamic load-bearing. Their crystalline structure tends to fracture along cleavage planes when sudden forces are applied. The reason for this is that crystalline structures cannot absorb and dissipate loads suddenly applied to them. They lack resilience, and the energy goes into breaking the bonds between the

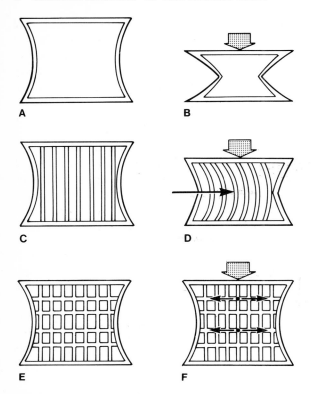

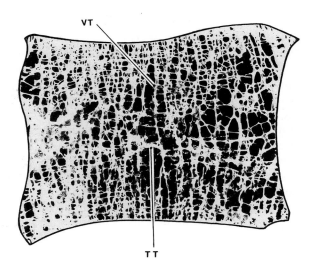

Fig. 1.5 A sagittal section of a lumbar vertebral body showing its vertical (VT) and transverse (TT) trabeculae.

Fig. 1.4 Reconstruction of the internal architecture of the vertebral body. **A**: With just a shell of cortical bone, a vertebral body is like a box, and collapses when a load is applied (**B**). **C**: Internal vertical struts brace the box (**D**). **E**: Transverse connections prevent the vertical struts from bowing, and increase the load-bearing capacity of the box. Loads are resisted by tension in the transverse connections (**F**).

constituent crystals. The manner in which vertebral bodies overcome these physical problems can be appreciated if the internal structure of the vertebral body is reconstructed.

With just an outer layer of cortical bone, a vertebral body would be merely a shell (Fig. 1.4A). This shell is not strong enough to sustain longitudinal compression, and collapses like a cardboard box (Fig. 1.4B). It needs to be reinforced. This can be achieved by introducing some vertical struts between the superior and inferior surfaces (Fig. 1.4C). A strut acts like a solid, but narrow, block of bone, and provided it is kept straight, it can sustain immense longitudinal loads. The problem with a strut, however, is that it tends to bend, or bow, when subjected to a longitudinal force. Nevertheless, a box with ver-

tical struts, even if they bend, is still somewhat stronger than an empty box (Fig. 1.4D). The load-bearing capacity of a vertical strut can be preserved, however, if it is prevented from bowing. By introducing a series of cross-beams, connecting the struts, the strength of a box can be further enhanced (Fig. 1.4E). Now, when a load is applied, the cross-beams hold the struts in place, preventing them from deforming and preventing the box from collapsing (Fig. 1.4F).

The internal architecture of the vertebral body follows this same design. The struts and cross-beams are formed by thin rods of bone called respectively vertical and transverse **trabeculae** (Fig. 1.5). The trabeculae endow the vertebral body with weight-bearing strength and resilience. Any applied load is first borne by the vertical trabeculae, and when these attempt to bow they are restrained from doing so by the horizontal trabeculae. Consequently, the load is sustained by a combination of vertical pressure and transverse tension in the trabeculae. It is the transfer of load from vertical pressure to transverse tension that endows the vertebra with resilience. The advantage of this design is that a strong, but lightweight load-bearing structure is constructed with the minimum use of material (bone).

A further benefit is that the space between

the trabeculae can be profitably used as convenient channels for the blood supply and venous drainage of the vertebral body, and under certain con- ditions as an accessory site for haemopoiesis (making blood cells). Indeed, the presence of blood in the intertrabecular spaces acts as a further useful element for transmitting the loads of weight-bearing and absorbing force.[558] When filled with blood the trabeculated cavity of the vertebral body appears like a sponge, and for this reason is sometimes referred to as the vertebral **spongiosa**.

The vertebral body is thus ideally designed, externally and internally, to sustain longitudinally applied loads. However, it is virtually exclusively dedicated to this function, and there are no features of the vertebral body that confer stability to the intervertebral joint in any other direction.

Taking two vertebral bodies, attempt to slide one over the other; backwards, forwards, sideways. Twist one vertebral body in relation to the other. Feel how easily the vertebrae move. There are no hooks, bumps or ridges on the vertebral bodies that prevent gliding or twisting movements between them. Lacking such features, the vertebral bodies are totally dependent on other structures for stability in the horizontal plane, and foremost amongst these are the posterior elements of the vertebrae.

Posterior elements

The posterior elements of a vertebra are the laminae, the articular processes, and the spinous processes (see Fig. 1.3). The transverse processes are not customarily regarded as part of the posterior elements because they have a slightly different embryological origin (see Ch. 11), but for present purposes they can be considered together with them.

Collectively, the posterior elements form a very irregular mass of bone, with various bars of bone projecting in all directions. This is because the various posterior elements are specially adapted to receive the different forces that act on a vertebra.

The inferior articular processes form obvious hooks that project downwards. In the intact lumbar vertebral column, these processes will

lock into the superior articular processes of the vertebra below, forming synovial joints whose principal function is to provide a locking mechanism that resists forward sliding and twisting of the vertebral bodies. This action can be illustrated by the following experiment.

Place two consecutive vertebrae together so that their bodies rest on one another and the inferior articular processes of the upper vertebra lock behind the superior articular processes of the lower vertebra. Slide the upper vertebra forwards and feel how the locked articular processes resist this movement. Next, holding the vertebral bodies slightly pressed together, attempt to twist them. Note how one of the inferior articular processes rams into its apposed superior articular process, and realise that further twisting can occur only if the vertebral bodies slide off one another.

The spinous, transverse, accessory and mamillary processes provide areas for muscle attachments. Moreover, the longer processes (the transverse and spinous processes) form substantial levers that enhance the action of the muscles which attach to them. The details of the attachments of muscles are described in Chapter 8, but it is worth noting at this stage that every muscle that acts on the lumbar vertebral column is attached somewhere on the posterior elements. Only the crura of the diaphragm and parts of the psoas muscles attach to the vertebral bodies. Every other muscle attaches to the transverse, spinous, accessory and mamillary processes or laminae. This emphasises how all the muscular forces acting on a vertebra are delivered first to the posterior elements.

Traditionally, the function of the laminae has been dismissed simply as a protective one. The laminae are described as forming a bony protective covering over the neural contents of the vertebral canal. While this is a worthwhile function, it is not an essential function, as demonstrated by patients who suffer no ill-effects to their nervous system when laminae have been removed at operation. In such patients, it is only under unusual circumstances that the neural contents of the vertebral canal can be injured.

The laminae serve a more significant, but subtle and therefore overlooked, function. Amongst the posterior elements they are centrally placed, and the various forces that act on the spinous and articular processes are ultimately transmitted to the laminae. By inspecting a vertebra, note how any force acting on the spinous process or the inferior articular processes must next be transmitted to the laminae. This concept is most important for the appreciation of how the stability of the lumbar spine can be compromised when a lamina is destroyed or weakened by disease, injury or surgery. Without a lamina to transmit the forces from the spinous and inferior articular processes, a vertebral body would be denied the benefit of these forces that either execute movement or provide stability.

That part of the lamina which intervenes between the superior and inferior articular process on each side is accorded a special name: the pars interarticularis, meaning 'inter-articular part'. The pars interarticularis runs obliquely from the lateral border of the lamina to its upper border. The biomechanical significance of the pars interarticularis is that it lies at the junction of the vertically orientated lamina and the horizontally projecting pedicle. It is therefore subjected to considerable bending forces as the forces transmitted by the lamina undergo a change of direction into the pedicle. To withstand these forces, the cortical bone in the pars interarticularis is generally thicker than anywhere else in the lamina.[313] However, in some individuals the cortical bone is insufficiently thick to withstand excessive or sudden forces applied to the pars interarticularis,[112] and such individuals are susceptible to fatigue fractures, or stress fractures to the pars interarticularis.[112,266,526]

Pedicles

Customarily, the pedicles are parts of the lumbar vertebrae that are simply named, and no particular function is ascribed to them. However, as with the laminae, their function is so subtle (or obvious) that is is overlooked or neglected.

The pedicles are the only connection between the posterior elements and the vertebral bodies. As described above, the bodies are designed for weight-bearing but cannot resist sliding or twisting movements, while the posterior elements are adapted to receive various forces: the articular processes locking against rotations and forward slides, and the other processes receiving the action of muscles. All forces sustained by any of the posterior elements are ultimately chanelled towards the pedicles, which then transmit the benefit of these forces to the vertebral bodies.

The pedicles transmit both tension and bending forces. If a vertebral body slides forwards, the inferior articular processes of that vertebra will lock against the superior articular processes of the next lower vertebra and resist the slide. This resistance is transmitted to the vertebral body as tension along the pedicles. Bending forces are exerted by the muscles attaching to the posterior elements. Conspicuously (see Ch. 8) all the muscles that act on a lumbar vertebra pull downwards. Therefore, muscular action is transmitted to the vertebral body through the pedicles which act as levers, and thereby are subjected to a certain amount of bending.

The pedicles are superbly designed to sustain these forces. Externally, they are stout pillars of bone. In cross-section they are found to be cylinders with thick walls. This structure enables them to resist bending in any direction. When a pedicle is bent downwards its upper wall is tensed while its lower wall is compressed. Similarly, if it is bent medially its outer wall is tensed while its inner wall is compressed. Through such combinations of tension and compression along opposite walls the pedicle can resist bending forces applied to it. In accordance with engineering principles, a beam when bent resists deformation with its peripheral surfaces; towards its centre forces reduce to zero. Consequently there is no need for bone in the centre of a pedicle, which explains why the pedicle is hollow but surrounded by thick walls of bone.

THE INTERVERTEBRAL JOINTS

When any two consecutive lumbar vertebrae are articulated they form three joints. One is formed between the two vertebral bodies. The other two are formed by the articulation of the superior ar-

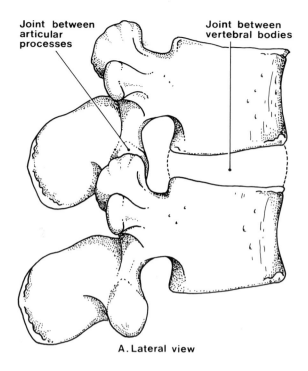

Joint between articular processes

Joint between vertebral bodies

A. Lateral view

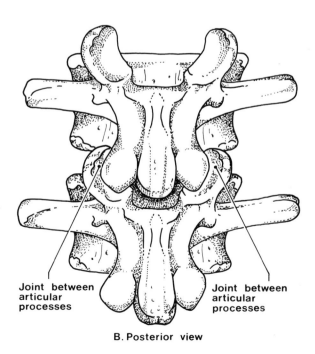

Joint between articular processes

Joint between articular processes

B. Posterior view

Fig. 1.6 The joints between two lumbar vertebrae.

ticular process of one vertebra with the inferior articular processes of the vertebra above (Fig. 1.6). The nomenclature of these joints is varied, irregular and confusing.

The joints between the articular processes have an 'official' name. Each is known as a **zygapophysial joint**.[408] Individual zygapophysial joints can be specified by using the adjectives 'left' or 'right', and the numbers of the vertebrae involved in the formation of the joint. For example, the 'left L3–4 zygapophysial joint' refers to the joint on the left, formed between the third and fourth lumbar vertebrae.

The term 'zygapophysial' is derived from the Greek words *apophysis*, meaning out-growth, and *zygos*, meaning yoke, or bridge. The term 'zygapophysis', therefore, means 'a bridging outgrowth', and refers to any articular process. The derivation relates to how, when two articulated vertebrae are viewed from the side, the articular processes appear to arch towards one another to form a bridge between the two vertebrae.

Other names that are used for the zygapophysial joints are 'apophysial joints' and 'facet' joints. 'Apophysial' predominates in the British literature and is simply a contraction of 'zygapophysial' which is the correct term. 'Facet' joint is a lazy and deplorable term. It is popularised in the American literature, probably because it is conveniently short, but it carries no formal endorsement and is essentially ambiguous. The term stems from the fact that the joints are formed by the articular facets of the articular processes; but the term 'facet' applies to any such structure in the skeleton. Every small joint has a facet. For example, in the thoracic spine, there are facets not only for the zygapohysial joints, but also for the costovertebral joints and the costotransverse joints. Facets are not restricted to zygapophysial articular processes, and strictly, the term 'facet' joint does not imply only zygapophysial joints.

Because the zygapophysial joints are located posteriorly, they are also known as the posterior intervertebral joints. This nomenclature implies that the joint between the vertebral bodies is known as the anterior intervertebral joint (Table 1.1), but this latter term is rarely, if ever, used. In fact, there is no formal name for the joint be-

Table 1.1 Systematic nomenclature of the intervertebral joints

Joints between articular processes	Joints between vertebral bodies
zygapophysial joints	(no equivalent term)
(no equivalent term)	interbody joints
posterior intervertebral joints	anterior intervertebral joints
intervertebral diarthroses	intervertebral amphiarthroses
	or intervertebral symphyses

tween the vertebral bodies, and difficulties arise if one seeks to refer to this joint. The term 'interbody joint' is descriptive and usable, but carries no formal endorsement, and is not conventional. The term 'anterior intervertebral joint' is equally descriptive, but is too unwieldy for convenient usage.

The only formal technical term for the joints between the vertebral bodies is the classification to which the joints belong. These joints are symphyses, and so, can be called **intervertebral symphyses**[408] or **intervertebral amphiarthroses** but again, these are unwieldy terms. Moreover, if this system of nomenclature were adopted, to maintain consistency the zygapophysial joints would have to be known as the intervertebral diarthroses (Table 1.1), which would compound the complexity of nomenclature of the intervertebral joints.

In this text, the terms 'zygapophysial joint' and 'interbody joint' will be used, and the details of the structure of these joints is described in the following chapters.

2. The inter-body joints and the intervertebral discs

A joint could be formed simply by resting two consecutive vertebral bodies on top of one another (Fig. 2.1A). Such a joint could adequately bear weight, and would allow gliding movements between the two bodies. However, because of the flatness of the vertebal surfaces, the joint would not allow the rocking movements that are necessary if flexion and extension or lateral bending are to occur at the joint. Rocking movements could occur only if either of two modifications were made. The first could be to introduce a curvature to the surfaces of the vertebral bodies. For example, the lower surface of a vertebral body could be curved (like the condyles of a femur). The upper vertebral body in an inter-body joint could then roll forwards on the flat upper surface of the body below (Fig. 2.1B). However, this adaptation would compromise the weight-bearing capacity and stability of the inter-body joint. The bony surface in contact with the lower vertebra would be less, and there would be a strong tendency for the upper vertebra to roll backwards or forwards whenever a weight was applied to it. This adaptation, therefore, would be inappropriate if the weight-bearing capacity and stability of the inter-body joint is to be preserved. It is noteworthy, however, that in some species where weight-bearing is not important, for example in fish, a form of ball and socket joint is formed between vertebral bodies to provide mobility of the vertebral column.[296]

The second modification, and the one that occurs in humans and most mammals, is to interpose a layer of strong, but deformable, soft tissue between the vertebral bodies. This soft tissue is provided in the form of the **intervertebral disc**. The foremost effect of an intervertebral disc is to separate two vertebral bodies. The space between the vertebral bodies allows the upper vertebra to tilt forwards without its lower edge coming into contact with the lower vertebral body (Fig. 2.1C).

The consequent biomechanical requirements of an intervertebral disc are threefold. In the first instance, it must be strong enough to sustain weight, i.e. transfer the load from one vertebra to the next, without collapsing (being squashed). Secondly, without unduly compromising its strength, the disc must be deformable to accommodate the rocking movements of the vertebrae. Thirdly, it must be sufficiently strong in order that it not be injured during movement. The structure of the intervertebral discs, therefore, should be studied with these requirements in mind.

STRUCTURE OF THE INTERVERTEBRAL DISC

Each intervertebral disc consists of two basic components: a central **nucleus pulposus**, surrounded by a peripheral **anulus fibrosus**. Although the nucleus pulposus is quite distinct in the centre of the disc, and the anulus fibrosus is distinct at its periphery, there is no clear boundary between the nucleus and the anulus within the disc. Rather, the peripheral parts of the nucleus pulposus merge with the deeper parts of the anulus fibrosus.

A third component of the intervertebral disc are two layers of cartilage which cover the top and bottom aspects of each disc. Each is called a **vertebral end-plate** (Fig. 2.2). The vertebral end-plates separate the disc from the adjacent

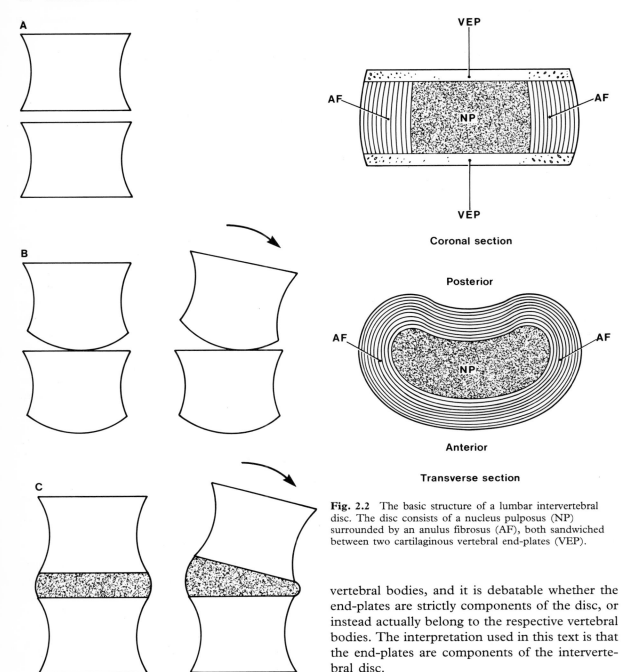

Fig. 2.1 Possible designs of an inter-body joint. **A**: The vertebral bodies rest directly on one another. **B**: Adding a curvature to the bottom of a vertebra allows rocking movements to occur. **C**: Interposing soft tissue between the vertebral bodies separates them and allows rocking movements to occur.

Fig. 2.2 The basic structure of a lumbar intervertebral disc. The disc consists of a nucleus pulposus (NP) surrounded by an anulus fibrosus (AF), both sandwiched between two cartilaginous vertebral end-plates (VEP).

vertebral bodies, and it is debatable whether the end-plates are strictly components of the disc, or instead actually belong to the respective vertebral bodies. The interpretation used in this text is that the end-plates are components of the intervertebral disc.

Nucleus pulposus

In typical, healthy, intervertebral discs of young adults, the nucleus pulposus is a semi-fluid mass of mucoid material (with the consistency, more or less, of toothpaste). Embryologically, the nucleus pulposus is a remnant of the notochord (Ch. 11). Histologically, it consists of a few cartilage cells, and some irregularly arranged collagen fibres, dispersed in a medium of semifluid ground substance (see below). Biomechanically, the fluid nature of the nucleus pulposus allows it to be deformed under pressure, but as a fluid, its volume cannot be compressed. If subjected to pressure from any direction, the nucleus will attempt to deform and will thereby transmit the applied pressure in all directions. A suitable analogy is a balloon filled with water. Compression of the balloon deforms it; pressure in the balloon rises, and stretches the walls of the balloon in all directions.

Anulus fibrosus

The anulus fibrosus consists of collagen fibres arranged in a highly ordered pattern. Foremost, the collagen fibres are arranged in between 10 and 20 sheets[29,509] called **lamellae** (from the Latin *lamella*, meaning little leaf). The lamellae are arranged in concentric rings that surround the nucleus pulposus (Figs 2.2 and 2.3). The lamellae are thick in the anterior and lateral portions of the anulus, but posteriorly they are finer and more tightly packed. Consequently the posterior portion of the anulus fibrosus is thinner than the rest of the anulus.[29,275,429]

Within each lamella, the collagen fibres lie parallel to one another passing from the vertebra above to the vertebra below. The orientation of all the fibres in any given lamellae is, therefore, the same, and measures about 65–70° from the vertical.[239,240] However, while the angle is the same, the direction of this inclination alternates with each lamellae. Viewed from the front, the fibres in one lamella may be orientated 65° to the right, but those in the next deeper lamella will be orientated 65° to the left. The fibres in the next lamella will again lie 65° to the right, and so on (Fig. 2.3). Every second lamella, therefore, has exactly the same orientation.

Vertebral end-plates

Each vertebral end-plate is a layer of cartilage about 0.6–1 mm thick[158,469,477] that covers the area on the vertebral body encircled by the ring apophysis. The two end-plates of each disc, therefore, cover the nucleus pulposus in its entirety, but peripherally, they fail to cover the entire extent of the anulus fibrosus (Fig. 2.4). Histologically, and end-plate consists of both hyaline cartilage and fibrocartilage. Hyaline cartilage occurs towards the vertebral body, and is best evident in neonatal and young discs (see

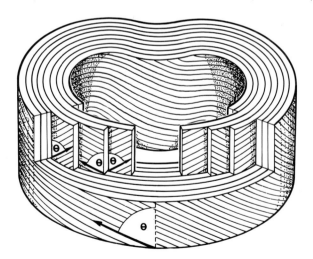

Fig. 2.3 The detailed structure of the anulus fibrosus. Collagen fibres are arranged in 10–12 concentric, circumferential lamellae. The orientation of fibres alternates in successive lamellae, but their orientation with respect to the vertical (θ) is always the same, and measures about 65°.

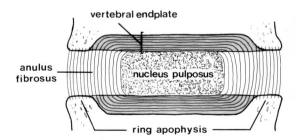

Fig. 2.4 Detailed structure of the vertebral end-plate. The collagen fibres of the inner two-thirds of the anulus fibrosus sweep around into the vertebral end-plate, forming its fibrocartilaginous component. The peripheral fibres of the anulus are anchored into the bone of the ring apophysis.

Ch. 11). Fibrocartilage occurs towards the nucleus pulposus, and in older discs the end-plates are virtually entirely fibrocartilage (Ch. 11). The fibrocartilage is formed by the insertion into the end-plate of collagen fibres of the anulus fibrosus.[429]

The collagen fibres of the inner lamellae of the anulus enter the end-plate and swing centrally within it.[102,270,509] By tracing these fibres along their entire length, it can be seen that the nucleus pulposus is enclosed around all aspects by a sphere of collagen fibres, more or less like a capsule. Anteriorly, posteriorly and laterally, this capsule is apparent as the innermost lamellae of the anulus fibrosus, but superiorly and inferiorly, the 'capsule' is absorbed into the vertebral end-plates (Fig. 2.4).

Where the end-plate is deficient, over the ring apophysis, the collagen fibres of the most superficial lamellae of the anulus insert directly into the bone of the vertebral body[270] (Fig. 2.4). In their original form, in younger discs, these fibres attach to the vertebral end-plate which fully covers the vertebral bodies in the developing lumbar spine, but they are absorbed secondarily into bone when the ring apophysis ossifies (see Ch. 11).

Because of the attachment of the anulus fibrosus to the vertebral end-plates, the end-plates are strongly bound to the intervertebral disc. In contrast, the end-plates are only weakly attached to the vertebral bodies,[102,270] and can be wholly torn from the vertebral bodies in certain forms of spinal trauma.[351] It is for this, and other morphological reasons that the end-plates are regarded as constituents of the intervertebral disc rather than as parts of the vertebral bodies.[101,102,158,477,478,508]

Over some of the surface area of the vertebral end-plate (about 10%), the subchondral bone of the vertebral body is deficient, and pockets of the marrow cavity abut against the surface of the end-plate or penetrate a short distance into it.[360,469] These pockets facilitate the diffusion of nutrients from blood vessels in the marrow space, and are important for the nutrition of the end-plate and intervertebral disc (see Ch. 10).

DETAILED STRUCTURE OF THE INTERVERTEBRAL DISC

Constituents

Glycosaminoglycans

As a class of chemicals, **glycosaminoglycans (GAGs)** are present in most forms of connective tissue. They are found in skin, bone, cartilage, tendon, heart valves, arterial walls, synovial fluid, and the aqueous humour of the eye. Chemically, they are long chains of polysaccharides, each chain consisting of a repeated sequence of two molecules called the **repeating unit**[97,560] (Fig. 2.5). These repeating units consist of a sugar molecule and a sugar molecule with an amine attached, and the nomenclature 'glycosaminoglycan' is designed to reflect the sequence of 'sugar-amine — sugar — sugar-amine — sugar. . .' in their structure.

The length of individual GAGs varies, but is characteristically about 20 repeating units.[560] Each different GAG is characterised by the particular molecules that make up its repeating unit. The GAGs found in human intervertebral discs are chrondoitin-6-sulphate, chondroitin-4-sulphate, keratan sulphate and hyaluronic acid.[79,368] The structures of the repeating units of these molecules are shown in Figure 2.6.

Proteoglycans

Proteoglycans are very large molecules consisting of many glycosaminoglycans linked to proteins. They occur in two basic forms: proteoglycan

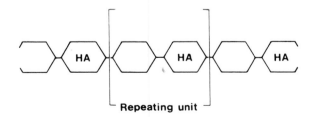

Fig. 2.5 The molecular structure of a mucopolysaccharide. The molecule consists of a chain of sugar molecules, each being a six-carbon ring (hexose). Every second sugar is a hexose-amine (HA). The chain is a repetition of identical pairs of hexose, hexose-amine units called the repeating unit.

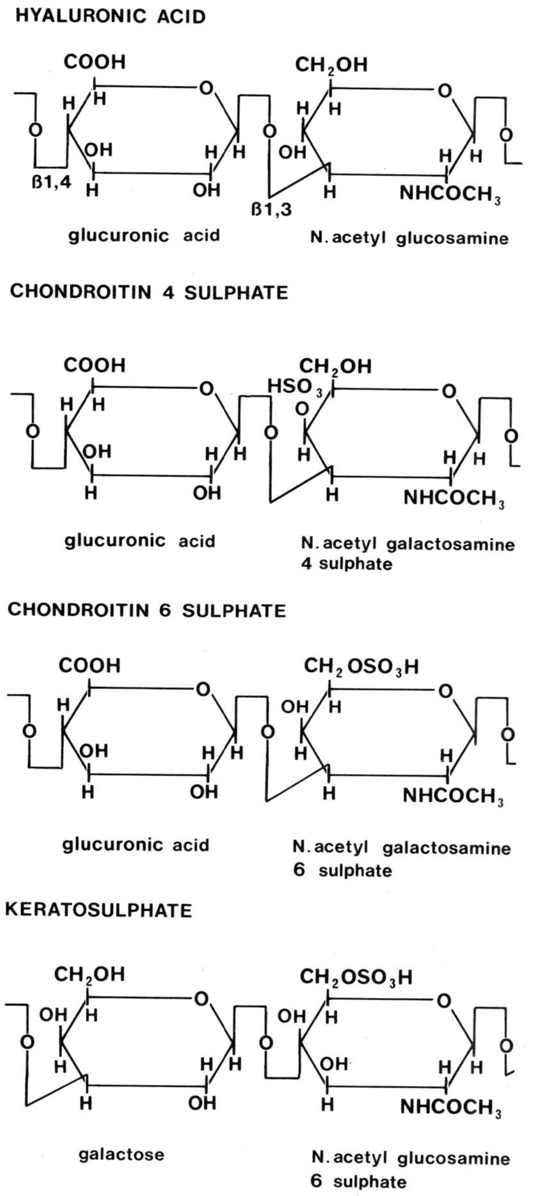

HYALURONIC ACID

glucuronic acid   N. acetyl glucosamine

CHONDROITIN 4 SULPHATE

glucuronic acid   N. acetyl galactosamine
4 sulphate

CHONDROITIN 6 SULPHATE

glucuronic acid   N. acetyl galactosamine
6 sulphate

KERATOSULPHATE

galactose   N. acetyl glucosamine
6 sulphate

Fig. 2.6 The chemical structure of the repeating units of the glycosaminoglycans.

units, and proteoglycan **aggregates**. Proteoglycan units are formed when several glycosaminoglycans are linked to a polypeptide chain known as a core protein[79,539] (Fig. 2.7). A single core protein may carry as few as six, or as many as 60 polysaccharide chains.[560] The glycosaminoglycans are joined to the core protein by covalent bonds involving special sugar molecules.[79,368] Keratan sulphate chains are bound principally towards the 'head' end of the core protein, while the longer, chondroitin sulphate chains are dispersed along the rest of the core protein[78,79,368,539] (Fig. 2.7).

Proteoglycan aggregates are formed when several proteoglycan units are linked to a chain of hyaluronic acid. A single hyaluronic chain may bind 20 to 100 proteoglycan units.[79] The linkage between the proteoglycan units and the hyaluronic acid is stabilised by a relatively small mass of protein known as the **link protein**[79] (Fig. 2.7).

Large proteoglycans that aggregate with hyaluronic acid are characteristic of hyaline cartilage and they occur in immature intervertebral discs.[368] They are rich in chondroitin sulphate, carrying about 100 of these chains each with an average molecular weight of about 20 000. They carry 30 to 60 keratan sulphate chains each with a molecular weight of 4000 to 8000.[368]

Moderately sized and small proteoglycans that aggregate with hyaluronic acid occur in older articular cartilage and are relatively richer in keratan sulphate.[368]

Large and moderately sized proteoglycans that do not aggregate with hyaluronic acid are the major proteoglycans that occur in the mature nulceus pulposus.[368]

In vivo, proteoglycan units and aggregates are convoluted to form complex, three-dimensional molecules, like large and small tangles of cotton wool (Fig. 2.8). Physico-chemically, these molecules have the property of attracting and retaining water (compare this with the water-absorbing properties of a ball of cotton wool). The volume enclosed by a proteoglycan molecule, and into which it can attract water is known as its **domain**.[560]

The water-binding capacity of a proteoglycan molecule is partially a property of its size and physical shape, but the main force that holds water to the molecule stems from the ionic, carboxyl (COOH) and sulphate (SO_4) radicals of the glycosaminoglycan chains (Fig. 2.6). These radicals attract water electrically, and the water-binding capacity of a proteoglycan can be shown

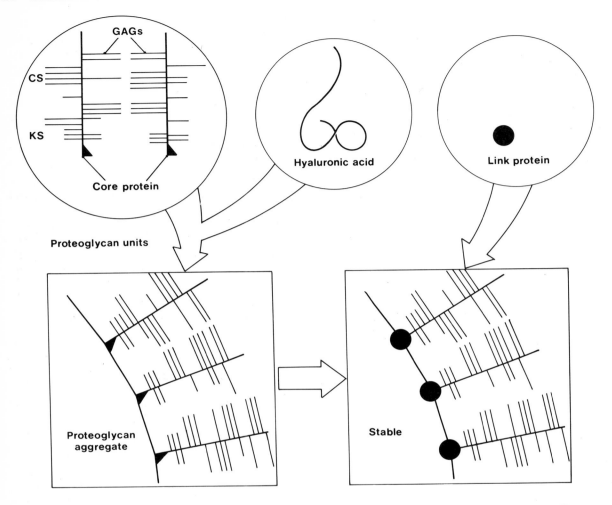

Fig. 2.7 The structure of proteoglycans. Proteoglycan units are formed by many GAGs linked to a core protein. Keratan sulphate chains (KS) tend to occur closer to the head of the core protein. Longer chains of chondroitin sulphate (CS) are attached along the entire length of the core protein. Proteoglycan aggregates are formed when several protein units are linked to a chain of hyaluronic acid. Their linkage is stabilised by a link protein.

to be proportional to the density of these ionic radicals in its structure. In this respect, sulphated glycosaminoglycans attract water more strongly than other mucopolysaccharides of similar size that lack sulphate radicals. Furthermore, it is readily apparent that because the chondroitin sulphates have both sulphate and carboxyl radicals in their repeating units (Fig. 2.6), they will have twice the water-binding capacity of keratan sulphate which, although carrying a sulphate radical, lacks a carboxyl radical. The water-binding capacity of any proteoglycan, therefore, will be largely dependent on the concentration of chondroitin sulphate within its structure.[539]

Collagen

Fundamentally, collagen consists of strands of protein molecules. The fundamental unit of collagen is the **tropocollagen** molecule, which itself consists of three polypeptide chains wound around one another in a helical fashion and held together end to end by hydrogen bonds (Fig. 2.9). Collagen is formed when many tropocolla-

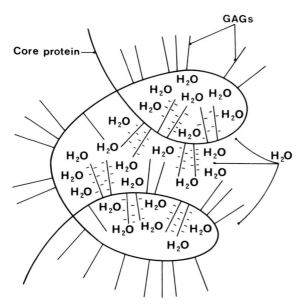

Fig. 2.8 A sketch of a coiled proteoglycan unit illustrating how the ionic radicals on its glycosaminoglycans (GAGs) attract water into its 'domain'.

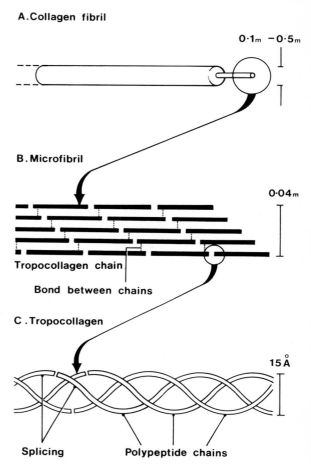

Fig. 2.9 The structure of collagen. A collagen fibril (**A**) is made up of several microfibrils (**B**). Each microfibril consists of several chains of tropocollagen (**C**) held together side-to-side by covalent bonds involving hydroxylysine molecules (⦂). Tropocollagen consists of three polypeptide chains wound around one another in a helical fashion. Tropocollagen chains are formed by the peptide chains in consecutive molecules splicing and being held together by electrostatic bonds between their ends.

gen molecules are arrayed end-on and side by side. When only a few tropocollagen chains are arrayed side by side, the structure formed is known as a small collagen **fibril**. When the structure is made thicker, by the addition of further layers of tropocollagen chains, it becomes a **large fibril**. The aggregation of several large fibrils forms a collagen **fibre**. The tropocollagen chains within a collagen fibre are held together, side by side, by covalent bonds involving a molecule of hydroxylysine[40,237,400] (Fig. 2.9).

There are 11 types of collagen found in connective tissue.[155] Each type is genetically determined and differs in the chemical nature of the polypeptide chains that form the tropocollagen molecules found in the collagen fibre, and in the microstructure of the fibre. The different types of collagen are named by Roman numerals as types I, II, III through to type XI.

Types I, II, III, V and XI exhibit the typical triple helical structure described above. Types IV and VII are long-chain molecules that bear a globular extension at one end and whose triple helix is interrupted periodically by non-helical segments. Types VI, VIII, IX and X are much

shorter molecules with interrupted or uniform helical segments that bear globular extensions at one or both ends.[155]

Type I, II and III molecules form most of the collagen fibres of the body. Types I and II are typical of musculoskeletal tissues. Their distribution is shown in Table 2.1. Type I collagen is essentially tensile in nature and is found in tissues that are typically subjected to tension and com-

Table 2.1 Genetic types of collagen and their distribution on connective tissues

Type	distribution
I	skin, bone, tendon, meniscus, dentine, anulus fibrosus
II	cartilage, vitreous humour, nucleus pulposus
III	dermis, heart, blood vessels, synovium
IV	basement membrane
V	co-distributed with type I
VI	vessels, viscera, muscle
VII	ectodermal basement membranes
VIII	Descemet's membrane
IX	cartilage, vitreous humour
X	epiphysial plates
XI	co-distributed with type II

pression. Type II collagen is more elastic in nature and is typically found in tissues habitually exposed to pressure.

Type III collagen is typical of the dermis, blood vessels and synovium. Type IV collagen occurs only in basement membranes; type VII is found in basement membranes of ectodermal origin; and type VIII is found in Descemet's membrane of the cornea; type X has been found only in epiphysial plates; type VI is characteristically found in blood vessels, viscera and muscles while type IX occurs in cartilage.[155]

The principal types of collagen found in the intervertebral disc are types I and II. Other types of collagen occur in much lesser amounts. Type V collagen is regularly associated with type I collagen and is co-distributed with it, but its concentration is only about 3% of that of type I collagen. Similarly, type XI co-exists with type II but at only about 3% of its concentration.[155] Type IX collagen occurs in discs at about 2% of the concentration of type II collagen; its function appears to be to link proteoglycans to collagen fibres.[155] Small amounts of type VI collagen occur in both the nucleus pulposus and anulus fibrosus, and traces of type III collagen occur within the nucleus pulposus and inner anulus fibrosus, but the functions of these latter two types are still unknown.[155]

Both type I and type II collagen are present in

the anulus fibrosus, but type I is the predominant form.[13,40,73,156,157,197,237] Type II collagen predominates in the nucleus pulposus. Type I collagen is absent from the central portions of the nucleus, or is present only in small amounts. This difference in distribution within the intervertebral disc correlates with the different biomechanical roles of the anulus fibrosus and the nucleus pulposus. From a knowledge of the biochemistry of the collagen in the intervertebral disc, it can be anticipated that the nucleus pulposus, with only type II collagen, will be involved more in processes involving pressure, while the anulus fibrosus, containing both types I and type II collagen, will be involved in both tension-related and pressure-related processes.

An important property of collagen and proteoglycans is that they can bind together. The binding involves both electrostatic and covalent bonds,[45,97,197,373,435,495] and these bonds contribute to the strength of structures whose principal constituents are proteoglycans and collagen. Bonds are formed directly between proteoglycans and type I and type II collagen, or indirectly through type IX collagen.

Microstructure

Nucleus pulposus

The nucleus pulposus is approximately 70–90% water,[45,209,399,400,453,478] although the exact fraction varies with age (see Ch. 12). Proteoglycans are the next major component, and they constitute about 65% of the dry weight of the nucleus.[45,209] The water of the nucleus is contained within the domains of these proteoglycans. Only about 25% of the proteoglycans occur in an aggregated form.[539] The majority are in the form of freely dispersed proteoglycan units that lack a functional binding site that would enable them to aggregate with hyaluronic acid.[368]

About two-thirds of the proteoglycan aggregates in the nucleus pulposus are smaller than those typically found in articular cartilage.[78] Each consists of about 8–18 proteoglycan units closely spaced on a short chain of hyaluronic acid.[78]

Interspersed through the proteoglycan medium are thin fibrils of type II collagen, that serve to hold proteoglycan aggregates together.[269,502] The mixture of proteoglycan units, aggregates and collagen fibres within the nucleus pulposus is referred to collectively as the **matrix** of the nucleus.

Collagen constitutes 15–20% of the dry weight of the nucleus,[45,79] and the remainder of the nucleus consists of some elastic fibres and small quantities of various other proteins known as non-collagenous proteins.[45,126,375,399,400,517] These include the link proteins of the proteoglycans[197,375] and other proteins involved in stabilising the structure of large collagen fibrils[197] and other components of the nuclear matrix;[375] but the function of many of these non-collagenous proteins remains unknown.[375]

Embedded in the proteoglycan medium of the nucleus are cartilage cells, and in the newborn there are also some remnant cells of the notochord[373] (see Ch. 11). The cartilage cells are located predominantly in the regions of the vertebral end-plates, and are responsible for the synthesis of the proteoglycans and collagen of the nucleus pulposus.[360,539] The type III collagen that occurs in the intervertebral disc is characteristically located around the cells of the nucleus pulposus and the inner anulus fibrosus.[155]

It is the presence of water, in large volumes, that endows the nucleus pulposus with its fluid properties, and the proteoglycans and collagen fibrils account for its 'thickness' and viscosity, or 'stickiness'.

Anulus fibrosus

Water is also the principal structural component of the anulus fibrosus, amounting to 60–70% of its weight.[45,209,399,400,453,478] Collagen makes up 50–60% of the dry weight of the anulus,[13,45,126,400] and the tight spaces between collagen fibres and between separate lamellae are filled with a proteoglycan gel, which binds the collagen fibres and lamellae together,[539] to prevent them from buckling or fraying. Proteoglycans make up about 20% of the dry weight of the anulus,[45] and it is this gel that binds the water of the anulus. About 50–60% of the proteoglycans of the anulus fibrosus are aggregated, principally in the form of large aggregates.[78]

Interspersed among the collagen fibres and lamellae are chondrocytes and fibroblasts that are responsible for synthesising the collagen and the proteoglycan gel of the anulus fibrosus. The fibroblasts are located predominantly towards the periphery of the anulus, while the chondrocytes occur in the deeper anulus, towards the nucleus.[360,539]

From a biochemical standpoint, it can be seen that the nucleus pulposus and anulus fibrosus are similar. Both consist of water, collagen and proteoglycans. The differences lie only in the relative concentrations of these components, and in the particular type of collagen that predominates in each part. The nucleus pulposus consists predominantly of proteoglycans and water, with some type II collagen. The anulus fibrosus also consists of proteoglycans and a large amount of water, but is essentially 'thickened' by a high concentration of (principally type I) collagen.

The anulus fibrosus also contains a notable quantity of elastic fibres.[77,241,242,277] Elastic fibres constitute about 10% of the anulus fibrosus, and are arranged circularly, obliquely and vertically within the lamellae of the anulus.[277] They appear to be concentrated towards the attachment sites of the anulus with the vertebral end-plate.[278]

Vertebral end-plates

The chemical structure of the vertebral end-plate resembles and parallels that of the rest of the disc. It consists of proteoglycans and collagen fibres with cartilage cells aligned along the collagen fibres.[469] It resembles the rest of the disc by having a higher concentration of water and proteoglycans and a lower collagen content towards its central region that covers the nucleus pulposus, with a reciprocal pattern over the anulus fibrosus. Across the thickness of the end-plate, the tissue nearer bone contains more collagen while that nearer the nucleus pulposus contains more proteoglycans and water.[469] This resemblance to the rest of the disc means that at a chemical level the end-plate does not constitute an additional barrier to diffusion. Small molecules pass through an essentially uniform, chemical environment to get from the vertebral body to the centre of the disc.

Metabolism

The intervertebral disc is metabolically active, although at a relatively low rate, and its constituents regularly undergo turnover. Thus, in addition to the structural proteins described above, the disc is endowed with enzymes that synthesise its matrix and enzymes that break it down such as collagenase, elastase and other proteinases.[375,480] The activity of these degradative enzymes, and therefore the balance between degradation and synthesis, is controlled by other enzymes known as proteinase inhibitors.[375]

FUNCTIONS OF THE DISC

The principal functions of the disc are to allow movement between vertebral bodies and to transmit loads from one vertebral body to the next. Having reviewed the detailed structure of the intervertebral disc, it is possible to appreciate how this structure accommodates these functions.

Weight-bearing

Both the nucleus pulposus and the anulus fibrosus are involved in weight-bearing. The anulus participates in two ways: independently; and in concert with the nucleus pulposus. Its independent role will be considered first.

Although the anulus is 60–70% water, its densely packed collagen lamellae make it a turgid, relatively stiff body. In a sense, the collagen lamellae endow the anulus with 'bulk'. As long as the lamellae remain healthy and intact and are held together by their proteoglycan gel, the anulus will resist buckling and will be capable of sustaining weight in a passive way, simply on the basis of its bulk.

A suitable analogy for this phenomenon is a thick book like a telephone directory. If the book is wrapped into a semi-cylindrical form and stood on its end, its weight-bearing capacity can be tested and appreciated. So long as the pages of the book do not buckle, the book standing on end can sustain large weights.

It has been shown experimentally that, under briefly applied loads, a disc with its nucleus removed maintains virtually the same axial load-bearing capacity as an intact disc.[358] These observations demonstrate that the anulus fibrosus is able to act as a passive space-filler, and to act alone in transmitting weights from one vertebra to the next. The disc does not necessarily need a nucleus pulposus to do this. The anulus alone can be enough.

The liability of an isolated anulus fibrosus, however, is that if subjected to prolonged weight-bearing it will tend to deform, i.e. it will be slowly squashed by any sustained weight. Sustained pressure will buckle the collagen lamellae and water will be squeezed out of the anulus. Both processes will lessen the height of the anulus. The binding of the collagen by proteoglycan gel will not be enough to prevent this prolonged deformation. Some form of additional bracing mechanism is required. This is provided by the nucleus pulposus.

As a ball of fluid, the nucleus pulposus may be deformed, but its volume cannot be compressed. Thus, when a weight is applied to a nucleus from above, it tends to reduce the height of the nucleus, and the nucleus tries to expand radially, i.e. outwards towards the anulus fibrosus. This radial expansion exerts a pressure on the anulus that tends tends to stretch its collagen lamellae outwards; but the tensile properties of the collagen resist this stretch, and the collagen lamellae of the anulus oppose the outward pressure exerted on them by the nucleus (Fig. 2.10A).

For any given load applied to the disc, an equilibrium will eventually be attained in which the radial pressure exerted by the nucleus will be exactly balanced by the tension developed in the anulus. In a healthy disc with intact collagen lamellae, this equilibrium is attained with minimum radial expansion of the nucleus. The anulus fibrosus is normally so thick and strong that during weight-bearing it resists any tendency for the disc to bulge radially. Application of a 40 kg load to an intervertebral disc causes only 1 mm of vertical compression and only 0.5 mm of radial expansion of the disc.[249]

The other direction in which the nucleus exerts its pressure is towards the vertebral end-plates

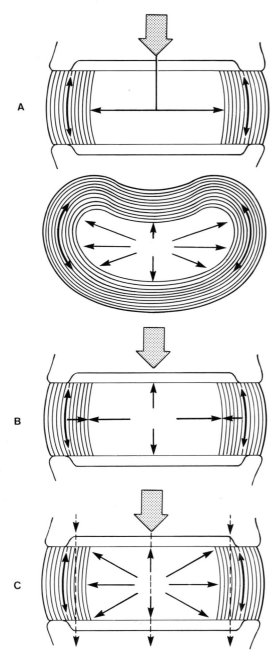

Fig. 2.10 The mechanism of weight transmission in an intervertebral disc. **A:** Compression raises the pressure in the nucleus pulposus. This is exerted radially onto the anulus fibrosus and the tension in the anulus rises. **B:** The tension in the anulus is exerted on the nucleus preventing it from expanding radially. Nuclear pressure is then exerted on the vertebral end-plates. **C:** Weight is borne, in part, by the anulus fibrosus, and by the nucleus pulposus. The radial pressure in the nucleus braces the anulus, and the pressure on the end-plates transmits the load from one vertebra to the next.

(Fig. 2.10B), but because the end-plates are applied to the vertebral bodies, they too will resist deformation. The situation that arises, therefore, is that when subjected to a load, the nucleus attempts to deform, but it is prevented from doing so. Radially it is constrained by the anulus fibrosus, and upwards and downwards it is constrained by the vertebral end-plates and vertebral bodies. All that the nucleus can do is exert its raised pressure against the anulus and the end-plates.

This achieves two things. The pressure exerted on the end-plates serves to transmit part of the applied load from one vertebra to the next, thereby lessening the load borne by the anulus fibrosus. Secondly, the radial pressure on the anulus fibrosus braces it and prevents the anulus from buckling. This aids the anulus in its own capacity to transmit weight.

The advantage of the co-operative action of the nucleus and the anulus is that the disc can sustain loads that otherwise might tend to buckle an anulus fibrosus acting alone.[468] The essence of the combined mechanism is the fluid property of the nucleus pulposus. The water content of the nucleus makes the disc a turgid body that resists compression, and the water content of the nucleus is, therefore, of criticial importance to the disc. Because the water content of the nucleus is, in turn, a function of its proteoglycan content, the normal mechanics of the disc will ultimately depend on a normal proteoglycan content of the nucleus pulposus. Any change in the proteoglycan and water content of the nucleus will inevitably alter the mechanical properties of the disc (see Ch. 12).

A further property of the disc is its capacity to absorb and store energy. As the nucleus tries to expand radially, energy is used to stretch the collagen of the anulus fibrosus. The collagen fibres are elastic and stretch like springs, and as such they store the energy that went into stretching them. If the load applied to the disc is released, the elastic recoil of the collagen fibres causes the energy stored in them to be exerted back onto the nucleus pulposus, where it is used to restore any deformation that the nucleus may have undergone. This combined action of the nucleus and anulus endows the disc with a resilience or 'springiness'.

In essence, the fluid nature of the nucleus enables it to translate vertically applied pressure into circumferential tension in the anulus. In a static situation, this tension balances the pressure in the nucleus; but if the applied load is released, the tension is used to restore any deformation of the disc that may have occurred. Biochemically, this mechanical property of the disc is due to the presence of proteoglycans and water in the nucleus, and the tensile properties of the type I collagen in the anulus fibrosus.

In a more global sense, the resilience of the intervertebral disc enables it to act as a 'shock absorber'. If a force is rapidly applied to a disc, it will be diverted momentarily into stretching the anulus fibrosus. This brief diversion attenuates the speed at which a force is transmitted from one vertebra to the next. The size of the force is not lessened. Ultimately, it is fully transmitted to the next vertebra. However, by temporarily diverting the force into the anulus fibrosus, a disc can protect its underlying vertebra by slowing the rate at which the applied force is transmitted to that vertebra.

Movements

It is somewhat artificial to consider the movements of an inter-body joint, as in vivo movement of any lumbar vertebra always involves movement not only at the inter-body joint but at the zygapophysial joints as well. However, in order to establish principles relevant to the appreciation of the role played by inter-body joints in the movements of the intact lumbar spine, it is worthwhile to consider the inter-body separately, as if they were capable of independent movement.

If unrestricted by any of the posterior elements of the vertebrae, two vertebral bodies united by an intervertebral disc can move in virtually any direction. In weight-bearing they can press together. Conversely, if distracted, they can separate. They can slide forwards, backwards or sideways; they can rock forwards, backwards and sideways, or in any direction in between these; and they can twist. Deformation of the disc accommodates all of these movements, but at the same time, the disc confers varying degrees of stability to the inter-body joint during these

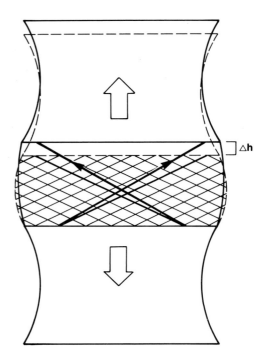

Fig. 2.11 Distraction of the inter-body joint. Separation of the vertebral bodies increases the height of the intervertebral disc (Δ h), and all the collagen fibres in the anulus fibrosus are lengthened and tensed, regardless of their orientation.

movements. The mechanics of the disc during compression (weight-bearing) has already been described, but a study of each of the other movements of the inter-body joint illustrates how well the disc is designed to also accommodate and stabilise these movements.

During *distraction* all points on one vertebral body move an equal distance perpendicularly from the upper surface of the other vertebral body (Fig. 2.11). Consequently, the attachments of every collagen fibre in the anulus fibrosus are separated an equal distance. Every fibre is, therefore, strained, and every fibre in the anulus resists distraction. Because of the density of collagen fibres in the anulus fibrosus, distraction is strongly resisted by the anulus. The capacity of the discs in this regard is illustrated by how well they sustain the load of the trunk and lower limbs in activities like hanging by the hands. Hanging by the arms, however, is not a common activity of

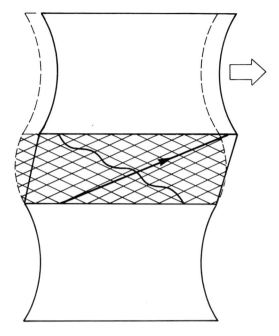

Fig. 2.12 Sliding movements of an inter-body joint. Those fibres of the anulus that are orientated in the direction of movement have their points of attachment separated, and therefore, they are stretched. Fibres in every second lamella of the anulus have their points of attachment approximated, and these fibres are relaxed.

daily living, and vertebral distraction is not a particularly common event. On the other hand, distraction is induced clinically, in the form of traction. Therefore, the mechanics of distraction are of relevance to physiotherapists. A further description of the mechanics of traction, however, is deferred until Chapter 7, when it is considered in the context of the whole lumbar spine.

In pure *sliding* movements of the inter-body joint, all points on one vertebra move an equal distance parallel to the upper surface of the next vertebra (Fig. 2.12). This movement is resisted by the anulus fibrosus, but the fibres of the anulus act differently according to their location within the anulus and in relation to the direction of movement. In forward sliding, the fibres at the sides of the disc lie in a plane more or less parallel to the direction of movement and run obliquely between the vertebral bodies, but in opposite directions in each successive lamella. Con-

sequently, during forward sliding, only half of the fibres in the lateral anulus will be strained, for only half of the fibres have their points of attachment separated by the movement. The other half have their points approximated (Fig. 2.12). Therefore, only half the fibres in the lateral anulus contribute to resisting forward sliding.

Fibres in the anterior and posterior anulus also contribute resistance, but not as greatly as the lateral fibres. Although the movement separates the points of attachment of all the fibres in the anterior and posterior anulus, the separation is not in the principal direction of orientation of the fibres. These fibres run either to the left or to the right, whereas the movement is forwards. The effect of forward sliding is simply to incline the planes of the lamellae in the anterior and posterior anulus anteriorly. Under these circumstances, the degree of stretch imparted to the anterior and posterior anulus is less than that imparted to the lateral anulus whose fibres are stretched principally longitudinally.

Bending or *rocking* movements involve the lowering of one end of the vertebral body and the raising of the opposite end. This necessarily causes distortion of the anulus fibrosus and the nucleus pulposus, and it is the fluid content of the nucleus and anulus that permits this deformation. In forward bending, the anterior end of the vertebral body lowers, while the posterior end rises. Consequently, the anterior anulus will be compressed and will tend to buckle[76,481,483,558] (Fig. 2.13). The nucleus pulposus will also be compressed but predominantly anteriorly. The elevation of the posterior end of the vertebral body relieves pressure on the nucleus pulposus posteriorly, but at the same time, stretches the posterior anulus.

The anterior anulus buckles because it is directly and selectively compressed by the tilting vertebral body, and because it is not braced internally by the nucleus pulposus. Although the nucleus is compressed anteriorly, it is relieved posteriorly, and is able to deform posteriorly.

Mathematical analyses indicate that if the disc is not otherwise loaded (e.g. also bearing weight), there should be no rise in nuclear pressure during bending of an inter-body joint, as the volume of the nucleus pulposus remains unchanged.[240] Ex-

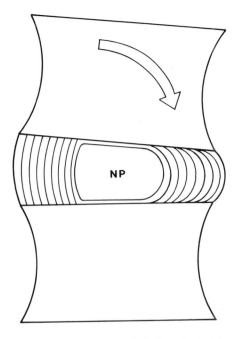

Fig. 2.13 Rocking movement of the inter-body joint. Rocking causes compression of the anulus fibrosus in the direction of movement, and stretching of the anulus on the opposite side.

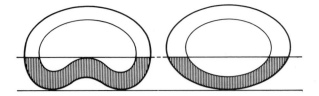

Fig. 2.14 Discs that are concave posteriorly have a greater portion of anulus fibrosus located posteriorly. Therefore, concave discs have more anulus available to resist the posterior stretch that occurs in flexion.

perimental studies, however, show that in cadaveric discs, 5° of bending is associated with a rise in nuclear pressure of about 0.7 kpcm^{-2}.[387]. This rise is the same regardless of the load carried by the disc, and therefore, the relative increase in disc pressure caused by bending decreases as greater external loads are applied. The increase in disc pressure amounts to about 22% of the total disc pressure for loads of 2 kpcm^{-2}, but is only 5% for loads of 10 kpcm^{-2}.[387]

The large increases in disc pressure seen in vivo during bending of the lumbar spine are not intrinsically due to the bending, but are the result of the additional compressive loads applied to the discs by the action of the back muscles that control the bending (see Ch. 8).

When an inter-body joint bends, the anterior compression deforms the nucleus pulposus which tries to 'escape' the anterior compression by moving backwards. If at the same time a load is applied to the disc, nuclear pressure will rise, and this will be exerted on the posterior anulus which is already stretched by the separation of the ver-

tebral bodies posteriorly. A normal anulus will adequately resist this combination of tension and pressure, but because the posterior anulus is the thinnest portion of the entire anulus, its capacity to resist is readily compromised.

Previous injury, or erosion as a result of disc disease, may weaken some of the lamellae of the posterior anulus, and the remaining lamellae may be insufficient to resist the tension and posterior pressure that occurs in loaded forward bending. Consequently, the pressure of the nucleus may rupture the remaining lamellae, and extrusion, or herniation, of the nucleus pulposus may result (see Ch. 14). The resistance to this type of injury is proportional to the density of collagen fibres in the posterior anulus. Thicker anuli afford more protection than thinner ones, but the shape of the posterior anulus also plays a role.

Discs that are concave posteriorly have a greater cross-sectional area of anulus posteriorly than do discs with an elliptical shape, even if the anulus is the same thickness (Fig. 2.14). Thus, concave discs are better designed than posteriorly convex discs to withstand forward bending and injury during this movement,[240] and this difference has a bearing on the pattern of injuries seen in intervertebral discs (see Ch. 14).

During *twisting* movements of the inter-body joint, all points on the lower surface of one vertebra will move circumferentially in the direction of the twist, and this has a unique effect on the anulus fibrosus. Because of the alternating direction of orientation of the collagen fibres in the anulus, only those fibres inclined in the direction of movement will have their points of attachment separated. Those inclined in the opposite direction will have their points of attachment

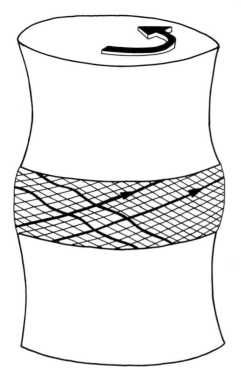

Fig. 2.15 Twisting movements of the inter-body joint. Those fibres of the anulus that are orientated in the direction of the twist have their points of attachment separated, and are therefore, stretched. Fibres in every second lamella of the anulus have their points of attachment approximated, and these fibres are relaxed.

approximated (Fig. 2.15). Thus, at any time, the anulus resists twisting movements with only half of its complement of collagen fibres. Half of the number of lamellae in the anulus will be stretched, while the other half will be relaxed. This is one of the reasons why twisting movements of an inter-body joint are the most likely to injure the anulus (see Ch. 14).

REVIEW

From the preceding accounts it is evident that the different components of an intervertebral disc act in different ways, both independently and co-operatively, during the various functions of the disc. The nucleus pulposus is designed to sustain and transmit pressure. It is principally involved in weight-bearing, when it transmits loads and braces the anulus fibrosus. During bending it deforms in a passive manner, unless the joint is additionally loaded, in which case its weight-bearing functions is superimposed on the mechanics of bending. The nucleus pulposus does not participate in the other movements of the inter-body joint. These are resisted by the anulus fibrosus.

In all movements, the anulus fibrosus acts like a ligament to restrain movements and stabilise the joint to some degree. Whenever the attachments of individual collagen fibres are separated, these fibres will be stretched and will resist the movement. All fibres resist distraction, and all are involved in weight-bearing. In other movements, the participation of individual collagen fibres will depend on their orientation with respect to the movement. In this way, the alternating oblique orientation of the collagen fibres of the anulus fibrosus optimises the capacity of the anulus to restrain various movements in various directions.

If the fibres of the anulus were arranged perpendicular to the vertebral bodies, they would be optimally orientated to resist distraction. However, they would afford virtually no resistance to sliding movements of the joint. The advantage of the oblique orientation is that each fibre can offer a component of resistance both vertically and horizontally, and therefore, the anulus fibrosus can participate in resisting movements in all directions. The degree of obliquity governs the extent to which a fibre resists horizontal movement, versus vertical movement, and it can be shown mathematically that the orientation of 65° is optimal for the various strains that an anulus is called upon to sustain.[240] A steeper orientation would enhance resistance to distraction, but would compromise resistance to sliding and twisting. Reciprocally, a flatter orientation would enhance resistance to twisting, but would compromise resistance to distraction and bending. The alternation of the direction of fibres in alternate lamellae of the anulus fibrosus is integral to the capacity of the disc to resist twisting. Half of the lamellae are dedicated to resisting twisting to the right; the other half resist twisting to the left. For a more detailed analysis of the mechanics of the anulus fibrosus, the reader is referred to the papers of Hickey and Hukins,[240] Hukins,[262] Broberg,[75] and Farfan and Gracovetsky.[167]

3. The zygapophysial joints

The lumbar zygapophysial joints are formed by the articulation of the inferior articular processes of one lumbar vertebra with the superior articular processes of the next vertebra. The joints exhibit the features typical of synovial joints. The articular facets are covered by articular cartilage, and a synovial membrane bridges the margins of the articular cartilages of the two facets in each joint. Surrounding the synovial membrane is a joint capsule that attaches to the articular processes a short distance beyond the margin of the articular cartilage (Fig. 3.1).

DETAILED STRUCTURE

Articular facets

Viewed from behind (Fig. 3.1), the articular facets of the lumbar zygapophysial joints appear as straight surfaces, suggesting that the joints are planar. However, viewed from above (Fig. 3.2), the articular facets vary both in the shape of their articular surfaces and in the general direction they face. Both of these features have significant ramifications in the biomechanics of these joints and consequently of the lumbar spine, and should be understood and appreciated.

In the transverse plane, the articular facets may be flat or planar, or may be curved to varying extents[258] (Fig. 3.3). The curvature may be little different from a flat plane (Fig. 3.3D), or may be more pronounced, with the superior articular facets depicting a 'C' shape (Fig. 3.3E), or a 'J' shape (Fig. 3.3F). The relative incidence of flat and curved facets at various vertebral levels is shown in Table 3.1.

The orientation of a lumbar zygapophysial joint

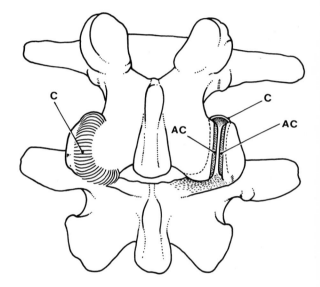

Fig. 3.1 A posterior view of the L3–4 zygapophysial joints. On the left, the capsule of the joint (C) is intact. On the right, the posterior capsule has been resected to reveal the joint cavity, the articular cartilages (AC), and the line of attachment of the joint capsule (broken lines). The upper joint capsule (C) attaches further from the articular margin than the posterior capsule.

is, by convention, defined by the angle made by the average plane of the joint with respect to the sagittal plane (Fig. 3.3). In the case of joints with flat articular facets the plane of the joint is readily depicted as a line parallel to the facets. The average plane of joints with curved facets is usually depicted as a line passing through the anteromedial and posterolateral ends of the joint cavity (Fig. 3.3). The incidence of various orientations at different levels is shown in Figure 3.4.

The variations in the shape and orientation of

27

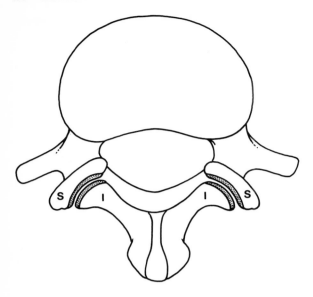

Fig. 3.2 A top view of an L3–4 zygapophysial joint showing how the joint space and articular facets are curved in the transverse plane. I — inferior articular process L3. S — superior articular process L4.

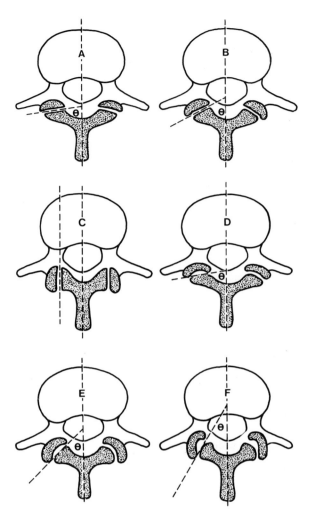

Fig. 3.3 The varieties of orientation and curvature of the lumbar zygapophysial joints. **A**: Flat joints orientated close to 90° to the sagittal plane. **B**: Flat joints orientated at 60° to the sagittal plane. **C**: Flat joints orientated parallel (0°) to the sagittal plane. **D**: Slightly curved joints with an average orientation close to 90° to the sagittal plane. **E**: 'C' shaped joints orientated at 45° to the sagittal plane. **F**: 'J' shaped joints orientated at 30° to the sagittal plane.

the lumbar zygapophysial joints govern the role of these joints in preventing forward displacement and rotatory dislocation of the intervertebral joint. The extent to which a given joint can resist forward displacement depends on the extent to which its superior articular facets face backwards. Reciprocally, the extent to which the joint can resist rotation is related to the extent to which its superior articular facets face medially.

In the case of planar zygapophysial joints the analysis is straightforward. In a joint with an oblique orientation, the superior articular facets face backwards and medially (Fig. 3.5A). Because

of their backward orientation these facets can resist forward displacement. If the upper vertebra in a joint attempts to move forwards, its inferior articular processes will impact against the superior articular facets of the lower vertebra, and this impaction will prevent further forward movement (Fig. 3.5A).

Similarly, the medial orientation of the superior

Table 3.1 The incidence of flat and curved lumbar zygapophysial joints at different segmental levels (Based on Horwitz and Smith[258])

	Joint level and % incidence of feature				
	L1–2	L2–3	L3–4	L4–5	L5–S1
Flat	44	21	19	51	86
Curved	56	76	81	49	14
Number of specimens	11	40	73	80	80

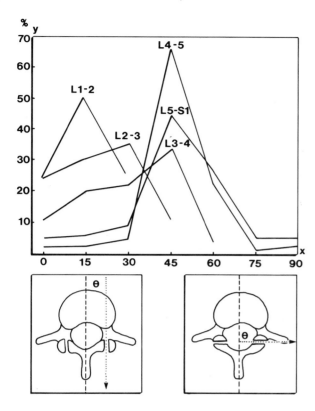

Fig. 3.4 The orientation of lumbar zygapophysial joints with respect to the sagittal plane: incidence by level. (Based on Horwitz and Smith[258]). y axis: proportion of specimens showing particular orientation — x axis: orientation (degrees from sagittal plane).

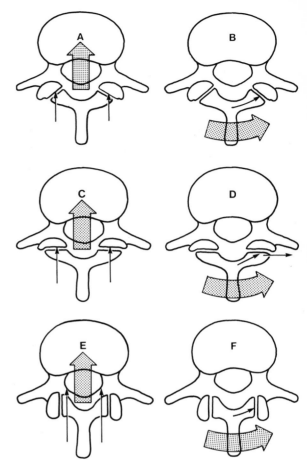

Fig. 3.5 The mechanics of flat lumbar zygapophysial joints. A flat joint at 60° to the sagittal plane affords resistance to both forward displacement (**A**) and rotation (**B**). A flat joint at 90° to the sagittal plane strongly resists forward displacement (**C**), but during rotation (**D**), the inferior articular facet can glance off the superior articular facet. A flat joint parallel to the sagittal plane offers no resistance to forward displacement (**E**), but strongly resists rotation (**F**).

articular facets allows them to resist rotation. As the upper vertebra attempts to rotate, say, anti-clockwise as viewed from above, its right inferior articular facet will impact against the right superior articular facet of the vertebra below, and further rotation will be arrested (Fig. 3.5B).

Maximum resistance to forward displacement will be exerted by the superior articular facets that are orientated at 90° to the sagittal plane, for then the facets face fully backwards and the entire articular surface directly opposes the movement (Fig. 3.5C). Such facets, however, are less capable of resisting rotation, for during rotation the inferior articular facet impacts the superior articular facet at an angle and is able to glance off the superior articular facet (Fig. 3.5D).

Joints orientated parallel to the sagittal plane

afford no resistance to forward displacement. The inferior articular facets are able simply to slide past the superior articular facets (Fig. 3.5E). However, such joints provide substantial resistance to rotation (Fig. 3.5F).

In essence, therefore, the closer a joint is orientated towards the sagittal plane the less it is able to resist forward displacement. Resistance is greater the closer a joint is orientated at 90° to the sagittal plane.

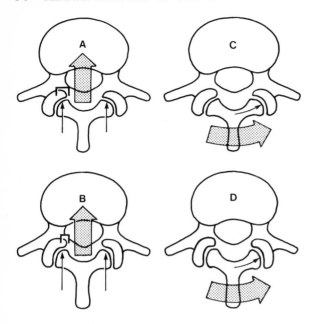

Fig. 3.6 The mechanics of curved lumbar zygapophysial joints. **A**: 'C' shaped joints have a wide anteromedial portion which faces backwards (indicated by the bracket), and this portion resists forward displacement. **B**: 'J' shaped joints have a narrower anteromedial portion (bracket) that nonetheless resists forward displacement. **C** and **D**: Both 'C' shaped and 'J' shaped joints resist rotation as their entire articular surface impacts.

In the case of joints with curved articular surfaces the situation is modified to the extent that particular portions of the articular surface are involved in resisting different movements. In curved joints, the anteromedial end of the superior articular facet faces backwards, and it is this portion of the facet that will resist forward displacement. As the upper vertebra attempts to move forwards, its inferior articular facets will impact against the anteromedial portion of the superior articular facets of the vertebra below (Fig. 3.6A). The degree of resistance will be proportional to the surface area of the backward-facing, anteromedial portion of the superior articular facet. Thus, 'C' shaped facets (Fig. 3.6A) have a larger surface area facing backwards and afford greater resistance than 'J' shaped facets (Fig. 3.6B) which have only a small portion of their articular surface facing backwards.

Rotation is well resisted by both 'C' shaped and 'J' shaped facets, for virtually the entire articular surface is brought into contact by this movement (see Fig. 3.6C and D).

The further significance of variations in orientation of zygapophysial joints in relation to the biomechanical requirements of joints at different levels, the age changes they suffer, and their liability to injury is explored in Chapters 5, 12 and 14.

Articular cartilage

There are no particular, or unique, features of the cartilage of normal lumbar zygapophysial joints. However, it is appropriate to revise the histology of articular cartilage as it relates to the zygapophysial joints, to provide a foundation for later chapters on age-related changes in these joints.

Articular cartilage covers the facets of the superior and inferior articular processes, and as a whole, assumes the same concave or convex curvature as the underlying facet. In a normal joint the cartilage is thickest over the centre of each facet, rising to a height of about 2 mm.[122,328] Histologically, four zones may be recognised in the cartilage[328] (Fig. 3.7). The superficial, or tangential zone consists of 3–4 layers of ovoid cells whose long axes are orientated parallel to the cartilage surface. Deep to this zone is a transitional zone in which cartilage cells are arranged in small clusters of 3–4 cells. Next deeper is a radial zone which constitutes most of the cartilage thickness. It consists of clusters of 6–8 large cells whose long axes lie perpendicular to the cartilage surface. The deepest zone is the calcified zone which uniformly covers the subchondral bone plate, and constitutes about 1/6 th of the total cartilage thickness. Conspicuously, the radial zone of cartilage is identifiable only in the central regions of the cartilage. Towards the periphery, the calcified zone is covered only by the transitional and tangential zones. As is typical of all articular cartilage, the cartilage cells of the zygapophysial joints are embedded in a matrix of glycosaminoglycans and type II collagen; but the most superficial layers of the tangential zone, forming the surface of the cartilage, lack glycosaminoglycans, and consist only of collagen fibres running parallel to the cartilage surface.

The articular cartilage rests on a thickened

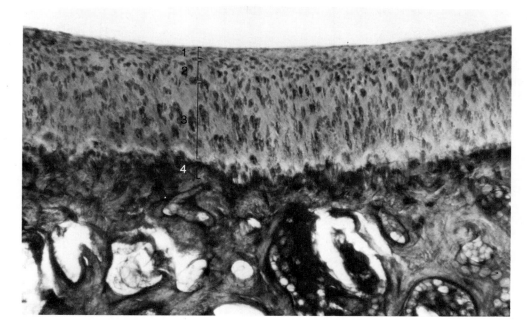

Fig. 3.7 A histological section of the cartilage of a lumbar zygapophysial joint showing the 4 zones of cartilage: 1 — superficial zone. 2 — transitional zone. 3 — radial zone. 4 — calcified zone.

layer or bone known as the **subchondral bone** (Fig. 3.7). In normal joints there are no particular features of the subchondral bone. However, the age and degenerative changes that affect the articular cartilage also affect the subchondral bone, and these changes are described in Chapter 12.

Capsule

Around its dorsal, superior and inferior margins each lumbar zygapophysial joint is enclosed by a fibrous capsule, formed by collagen fibres passing more or less transversely from one articular process to the other (Figs 3.1 and 3.8). Along the dorsal aspect of the joint the outermost fibres of the capsule are attached about 2 mm from the edge of the articular cartilage, but some of the deepest fibres attach into the margin of the articular cartilage[515,533] (Figs 3.8 and 3.9). At the superior and inferior poles of the joint, the capsule attaches further from the osteochondral junctions, creating subcapsular pockets over the superior and inferior edges of both the superior and inferior articular processes, which in the intact joint are filled with fat[329] (Fig. 3.8). Anteri-

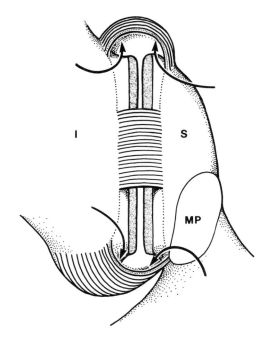

Fig. 3.8 A posterior view of a right lumbar zygapophysial joint in which the posterior capsule has been partially removed to reveal the joint cavity and the subcapsular pockets (arrows). I — inferior articular process. S — superior articular process. MP — mamillary process.

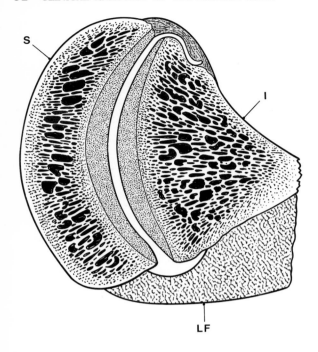

Fig. 3.9 A transverse (horizontal) section through a lumbar zygapophysial joint. Note how the posterior capsule is fibrous and attaches to the inferior articular process (I) well beyond the articular margin, but at its other end it attaches to the superior articular process (S) and the margin of the articular cartilage. The anterior capsule is formed by the ligamentum flavum (LF).

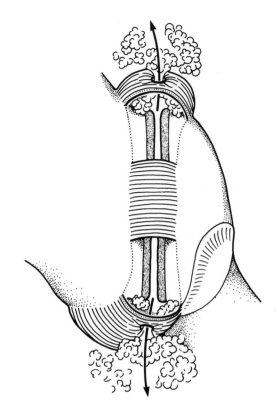

Fig. 3.10 A right lumbar zygapophysial joint viewed from behind. Portions of the capsule have been removed to show how the fat in the subcapsular pockets communicates to the extra-capsular fat through foramina in the superior and inferior capsules.

orly, the fibrous capsule of the joint is replaced entirely by the ligament flavum (see Ch. 4), which attaches close to the articular margin[329,456,573] (Fig. 3.9).

The joint capsule is thick dorsally, and it is reinforced by some of the deep fibres of the multifidus muscle[218,328,515] (see Ch. 8). At the superior and inferior poles of the joint, the capsule is abundant and loose.[329] Superiorly, it balloons upwards towards the base of the next transverse process. Inferiorly, it balloons over the back of the lamina (Fig. 3.8). In both the superior and inferior parts of the capsule there is a tiny hole, or foramen, that permits the passage of fat from within the capsule to the extra-capsular space[329] (see Fig. 3.10).

Synovium

There are no particular features of the synovium of the lumbar zygapophysial joints that distinguish it from the synovium of any typical synovial joint. It attaches along the entire peripheral margin of the articular cartilage on one facet and extends across the joint to attach to the margin of the opposite articular cartilage. Basically it lines the deep surface of the fibrous capsule and the ligamentum flavum, but it is also reflected in parts to cover the various intra-articular structures of the lumbar zygapophysial joints.

Intra-articular structures

There are two principal types of intra-articular structures in the lumbar zygapohysial joints. They are fat, and what may be referred to as 'meniscoid' structures. The fat basically fills any left-over space underneath the capsule. It is located principally in the subcapsular pockets at the

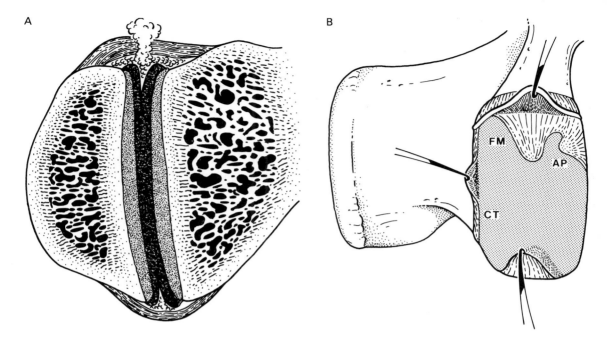

Fig. 3.11 Intra-articular structures of the lumbar zygapohysial joints. **A**: A coronal section of a left zygapophysial joint showing fibro-adipose meniscoids projecting into the joint cavity from the capsule over the superior and inferior poles of the joint. **B**: A lateral view of a right zygapophysial joint, in which the superior articular process has been removed to show intra-articular structures projecting into the joint cavity across the surface of the inferior articular facet.

The superior capsule is retracted to reveal the base of a fibro-adipose meniscoid (FM) and an adipose tissue pad (AP). Another fibro-adipose meniscoid at the lower pole of the joint is lifted from the surface of the articular cartilage. A connective tissue rim (CT) has been retracted along the posterior margin of the joint.

superior and inferior poles of the joint (Fig. 3.10). Externally it is covered by the capsule, while internally it is covered by the synovium. It communicates with the fat outside the joint through the foramina in the superior and inferior capsules. Superiorly, this extra-capsular fat lies lateral to the lamina and dorsal to the intervertebral foramen.[328,329] Inferiorly, it lies dorsal to the upper end of the lamina of the vertebra, and separates the bone from the overlying multifidus muscle.

There have been many studies and differing interpretations of the meniscoid stuctures of the lumbar zygapophysial joints,[49,132,133,145,202,222, 223,307–309,329,356,503,570,576] but the most recent and most comprehensive study of these structures identifies three types.[62,146]

The simplest and smallest structure is the **connective tissue rim**. This is simply a wedge-shaped thickening of the internal surface of the capsule that, along the dorsal and ventral margins of the joint, fills the space left by the curved margins of the articular cartilages (Fig. 3.11). The second type of structure is an **adipose tissue pad**. These are found principally at the supero-ventral and infero-dorsal poles of the joint. Each consists of a fold of synovium enclosing some fat and blood vessels (Fig. 3.11). At the base of the structure, the synovium is reflected onto the joint capsule to become continuous with the synovium of the rest of the joint, and the fat within the structure is continuous with other fat within the joint. These adipose tissue pads project into the joint cavity for a short distance (about 2 mm).

The largest of the meniscoid structures is the **fibro-adipose meniscoid**. These project from the inner surface of the superior and inferior capsules. They consist of a leaf-like fold of synovium that encloses fat, collagen and some blood vessels

(Fig. 3.11). The fat is located principally in the base of the structure, where it is continuous with the rest of the fat within the joint, and where it communicates with the extra-capsular fat through the superior and inferior capsular foramina. The collagen is densely packed and is located towards the apex of the structure. Fibro-adipose menioscoids are long, and project up to 5 mm into the joint cavity.

Differing and conflicting interpretations have marked the literature on zygapophysial intra-articular structures, and there is no conventional, universal nomenclature that can be ascribed to them. However, it is clear from their histology that none is really a meniscus which resembles the menisci of the knee joint or the temperomandibular joint. They do, nonetheless, resemble the intra-articular structures found in the small joints of the hand.[475,476] The connective tissue rims described above are most easily interpreted as a thickening of the joint capsule that simply acts as a space filler, although it may be that they also serve to increase the surface area of contact when articular facets are impacted, and thereby transmit some load.[202,329]

The adipose tissue pads and the fibro-adipose meniscoids have been interpreted as serving a protective function.[62] During flexion of an intervertebral joint, the inferior articular facet slides upwards some 5–8 mm along the superior articular facet.[248,329] This movement results in cartilages of the upper portion of the inferior facet and the lower portion of the superior facet to become exposed. The adipose tissue pads and the fibro-adipose meniscoids are suitably located to cover these exposed articular surfaces, and afford them some degree of protection during this movement.

There is also another form of intra-articular structure derived from the articular cartilage, but it is apparently formed artificially by traction on the cartilage. This structure is described in Chapter 12, and the clinical relevance of all intra-articular structures is considered in Chapter 14.

4. The ligaments of the lumbar spine

Topographically, the ligaments of the lumbar spine may be classified into four groups:

1. Those ligaments that interconnect the vertebral bodies.
2. Those ligaments that interconnect the posterior elements.
3. The ilio-lumbar ligament.
4. False ligaments.

LIGAMENTS OF THE VERTEBRAL BODIES

The two named ligaments that interconnect the vertebral bodies are the anterior and posterior longitudinal ligaments. Intimately associated with these ligaments are the anuli fibrosi of the intervertebral discs, and it must be emphasised that although described as part of the intervertebral disc, each anulus fibrosus is both structurally and functionally like a ligament. In fact, on the basis of size and strength, the anuli fibrosi can be construed as the principal ligaments of the vertebral bodies, and for this reason their structure bears reiteration in the context of the ligaments of the lumbar spine.

Anuli fibrosi

As described in Chapter 2, each anulus fibrosus consists of collagen fibres running from one vertebral body to the next and arranged in concentric lamellae. Furthermore, the deeper lamellae of collagen are continuous with the collagen fibres in the fibrocartilaginous vertebral end-plates (Ch. 2). By surrounding the nucleus pulposus these inner layers of the anulus fibrosus

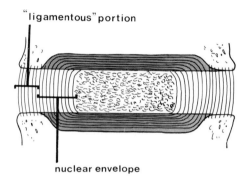

"ligamentous" portion

nuclear envelope

Fig. 4.1 The anulus fibrosus as a ligament. The inner fibres of the anulus which attach to the vertebral end-plate form an internal capsule that envelopes the nucleus pulposus. The outer fibres of the anulus which attach to the ring apophysis constitute the 'ligamentous' portion of the anulus fibrosus.

constitute a capsule or envelope around the nucleus, whereupon it could be inferred that their principal function is to retain the nucleus pulposus (Fig. 4.1).

In contrast, the outer fibres of the anulus fibrosus are attached to the ring apophysis (Ch. 2). For various reasons it is these fibres that could be inferred to be the principal 'ligamentous' portion of the anulus fibrosus. Foremost, like other ligaments, they are attached to separate bones and consist largely of type I collagen which is designed to resist tension (Ch. 2). Such tension arises during rocking or twisting movements of the vertebral bodies. During these movements the peripheral edges of the vertebral bodies undergo more separation than their more central parts, and the tensile stresses applied to the peripheral anulus are greater than those applied to the inner anulus. In resisting these movements the peripheral fibres of the anulus fibrosus are subject to the same demands as conventional ligaments, and function accordingly.

As outlined in Chapter 2 and considered further in Chapter 7, the anulus fibrosus functions as a ligament in resisting distraction, bending, sliding and twisting movements of the intervertebral joint. Thus, the anulus fibrosus is called upon to function as a ligament whenever the lumbar spine moves. It is only during weight-bearing that it functions in concert with the nucleus pulposus.

Anterior longitudinal ligament

Conventional descriptions maintain that the anterior longitudinal ligament is a long band which covers the anterior aspects of the the lumbar vertebral bodies and intervertebral discs[556] (Fig. 4.2). Although well developed in the lumbar region, this ligament is not restricted to that region. Inferiorly it extends onto the sacrum, and superiorly it continues into the thoracic and cervical regions to cover the anterior surface of the entire vertebral column.

Structurally, the anterior longitudinal ligament is said to consist of several sets of collagen fibres.[556] There are short fibres that span each interbody joint, covering the intervertebral disc and attaching to the margins of the vertebral bodies (Figs 4.2 and 4.3). These fibres are inserted into the bone of the anterior surface of the vertebral bodies or into the overlying periosteum.[182,542] Some early authors interpreted these fibres as being part of the anulus fibrosus,[102] and there is a tendency in some contemporary circles to interpret these fibres as constituting a 'disc capsule'. However, embryologically, their attachments are always associated with cortical bone, as are ligaments in general, whereas the anulus fibrosus proper is attached to the vertebral end-plate.[182] Even those fibres of the adult anulus that attach to bone do so by being secondarily incorporated into the ring apophysis (Ch. 2), which is not cortical bone. Because of these developmental differences the deep, short fibres of the anterior longitudinal lig-

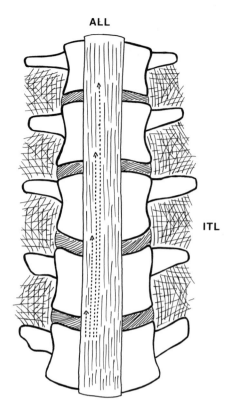

Fig. 4.2 Classical descriptions of the anterior longitudinal ligament (ALL) and the intertransverse ligaments (ITL). The arrows indicate the span of various fibres in the anterior longitudinal ligament stemming from the L5 vertebra.

ament should not be interpreted as part of the anulus fibrosus.

Covering the deep, unisegmental fibres of the anterior longitudinal ligament are several layers of increasingly longer fibres. There are fibres that span two, three and even four or five interbody joints. The attachments of these fibres, like those of the deep fibres, are into the upper and lower ends of the vertebral bodies.

Although the ligament is primarily attached to the anterior margins of the lumbar vertebral bodies, it is also secondarily attached to their concave anterior surfaces. The main body of the ligament bridges this concavity, but some collagen fibres from its deep surface blend with the periosteum covering the concavity. Otherwise, the space be-

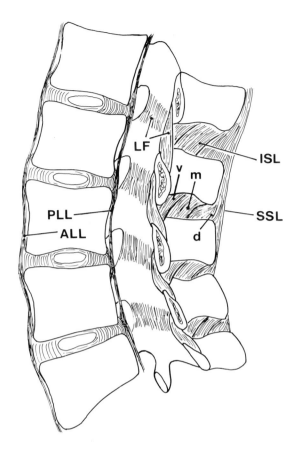

Fig. 4.3 A median sagittal section of the lumbar spine to show its various ligaments. ALL — anterior longitudinal ligament. PLL — posterior longitudinal ligament. SSL — supraspinous ligament. ISL — interspinous ligament: v — ventral part; m — middle part; d — dorsal part. LF — ligamentum flavum, viewed from within the vertebral canal, and in sagittal section at the midline.

Comment

It is only in the thoracic spine that the anterior longitudinal ligament has an unambiguous structure for there it stands in isolation from any prevertebral muscles. In the lumbar region the structure of the anterior longitudinal ligament is rendered ambiguous by the attachment of the crura of the diaphragm to the first three lumbar vertebrae. Although formal studies have not been completed, detailed examination of the crura and their attachments suggests that many of the tendinous fibres of the crura are prolonged caudally beyond the upper three lumbar vertebrae such that these tendons appear to constitute much of what has otherwise been interpreted as the lumbar anterior longitudinal ligament. Thus, it may be that the lumbar anterior longitudinal ligament is to a greater or lesser extent not strictly a ligament but more a prolonged tendon attachment.

Posterior longitudinal ligament

Like the anterior longitudinal ligament, the posterior longitudinal ligament is represented throughout the vertebral column. In the lumbar region, it forms a narrow band over the backs of the vertebral bodies, but expands laterally over the backs of the intervertebral discs to give it a serrated, or saw-toothed, appearance (Fig. 4.4). Its fibres mesh with those of the anuli fibrosi, but penetrate through the anuli to attach to the posterior margins of the vertebral bodies.[542] The deepest and shortest fibres of the posterior longitudinal ligament span two intervertebral discs. Starting at the superior margin of one veretebra, they attach to the inferior margin of the vertebra two levels above, describing a curve concave laterally as they do so. Longer, more superficial fibres span three, four and even five vertebrae (Figs 4.3 and 4.4).

The posterior longitudinal ligament serves to resist separation of the posterior ends of the vertebral bodies, but because of its polysegmental disposition, its action is exerted over several interbody joints, not just one.

tween the ligament and bone is filled with loose areolar tissue, blood vessels and nerves. Over the intervertebral discs, the anterior longitudinal ligament is only loosely attached to the front of the anuli fibrosi by loose areolar tissue.

Because of its strictly longitudinal disposition, the anterior longitudinal ligament serves principally to resist vertical separation of the anterior ends of the vertebral bodies. In doing so, it functions during extension movements of the intervertebral joints, and resists anterior bowing of the lumbar spine (see Ch. 5).

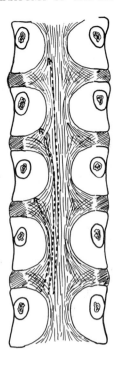

Fig. 4.4 The posterior longitudinal ligament. The dotted lines indicate the span of some of the constituent fibres of the ligament arising from the L5 vertebra.

LIGAMENTS OF THE POSTERIOR ELEMENTS

The named ligaments of the posterior elements are the ligamentum flavum, the interspinous ligaments, and the supraspinous ligaments. In some respects, the capsules of the zygapophysial joints act like ligaments to prevent certain movements, and in a functional sense they can be considered to be one of the ligaments of the posterior elements. Indeed, their biomechanical role in this regard is quite substantial (see Ch. 7). However, their identity as capsules of the zygapophysial joints is so clear that they have been described formally in that context.

Ligamentum flavum

The ligamentum flavum is a short, but thick, ligament that joins the laminae of consecutive vertebrae. At each intersegmental level, the ligamentum flavum is a paired structure, being represented symmetrically on both left and right sides. On each side, the upper attachment of the ligament is to the lower half of the anterior surface of the lamina and the inferior aspect of the pedicle (Figs 4.3 and 4.5). Its smooth surface blends perfectly with the smooth surface of the upper half of the lamina. Traced inferiorly, on each side, the ligament divides into a medial and a lateral portion.[397,456,573] The medial portion passes to the back of the next lower lamina and attaches to the rough area located on the upper quarter, or so, of the dorsal surface of that lamina (Fig. 4.5). The lateral portion passes in front of the zygapophysial joint formed by the two vertebrae that the ligament connects. It attaches to the anterior aspects of the inferior and superior articular processes of that joint, and forms its anterior capsule. The most lateral fibres extend along the root of the superior articular process as far as the next lower pedicle to which they are attached.[573]

Histologically, the ligamentum flavum consists of 80% elastin and 20% collagen.[573] It is, therefore, essentially an elastic ligament, and as such differs from all the other ligaments of the lumbar spine. This difference has prompted speculation as to its implied unique function. Its elastic nature has been said to aid in restoring the flexed lumbar spine to its extended position, while its lateral division is said to serve to prevent the anterior capsule of the zygapophysial joint being nipped within the joint cavity during movement. While all of these suggestions are consistent with the elastic nature of the ligament, the importance of these functions for the mechanics of the lumbar spine is unknown. It is questionable whether the ligamentum flavum contributes significantly to producing extension,[532] and no disabilities have been reported in patients in whom the ligamentum flavum has been excised, at single or even multiple levels. Biomechanical studies have revealed that the ligamentum flavum serves to pre-stress the intervertebral disc, exerting a disc pressure of about 0.70 kg/cm^{2,393} but the biological significance of this effect remains obscure.

A plausible explanation for the unique nature of the ligamentum flavum relates more to its location than to its possible biomechanical functions. The ligamentum flavum lies immedi-

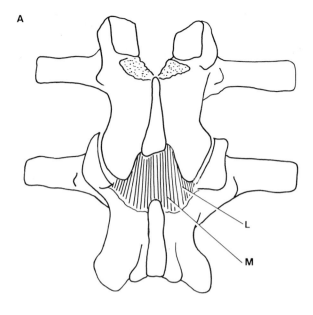

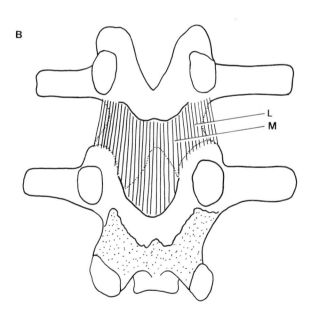

Fig. 4.5 The ligamentum flavum at the L2–3 level.
A: posterior view. **B**: anterior view (from within the vertebral canal). The medial (M) and lateral (L) divisions of the ligament are labelled. The shaded areas depict the sites of attachment of the ligamentum flavum at the levels above and below L2–3. In Fig. 4.4B the silhouettes of the lamina and inferior, articular processes behind the ligament are indicated by the dotted lines.

ately behind the vertebral canal, and therefore, immediately adjacent to the nervous structures within the canal. As a ligament it serves to resist excess separation of the vertebral lamina. A collagenous ligamentum in the same location would not function as well. A collagenous ligament could resist separation of the laminae, but when the laminae were approximated a collagenous ligament would buckle. Were the ligament to buckle into the vertebral canal it would encroach upon the spinal cord or spinal nerve roots, and possibly damage them. On the other hand, by replacing such a collagenous ligament with an elastic one, this buckling would be prevented. From a resting position, an elastic ligament stretches and thins. When relaxed again, the ligament simply assumes it original thickness. Buckling does not occur or is minimal. Therefore, by endowing the ligamentum flavum with elastic tissue, the risk of nerve root compromise is reduced.

Interspinous ligaments

The interspinous ligaments connect adjacent spinous processes. The collagen fibres of these ligaments are arranged in a particular manner, with three parts being identified[238] (see Fig. 4.3). The ventral part consists of fibres passing posterocranially from the dorsal aspect of the ligamentum flavum to the anterior half of the lower border of the spinous process above. The middle part forms the main component of the ligament, and consists of fibres that run from the anterior half of the upper border of one spinous process to the posterior half of the lower border of the spinous process above. The dorsal part consists of fibres from the posterior half of the upper border of the lower spinous process that pass behind the posterior border of the upper spinous process, to form the supraspinous ligament. Anteriorly, the interspinous ligament is a paired structure, the ligaments on each side being separated by slit-like midline cavity filled with fat. This cavity is not present more posteriorly.

The fibres of the interspinous ligament are disposed to resist separation of the spinous processes, and hence would be involved in limiting forward bending movements of the intervertebral joint.

Comment

Only the ventral and middle parts of the inter-spinous ligament constitute true ligaments for only they exhibit connections to separate adjacent bones. The dorsal part of the ligament appears to pass from the upper border of one spinous process to the dorsal edge of the next above, but here the ligament does not assume a bony attachment; it blends with the supraspinous ligament whose actual identity as a ligament can be questioned (see below).

Supraspinous ligament

The supraspinous ligament lies in the midline. It runs posterior to the posterior edges of the lumbar spinous processes, to which it is attached, and bridges the interspinous spaces (Fig. 4.3). The ligament is well-developed only in the upper lumbar region. Its lower limit varies. It terminates at the L3 spinous process in about 22% of individuals, and at L4 in 73%; it bridges the L4–5 interspace in only 5% of indivduals, and is regularly lacking at L5–S1.[238,466]

Upon close inspection, the nature of the supraspinous ligament as a ligament can be questioned. It consists of three parts: a superficial, middle and a deep.[466] The superficial layer is subcutaneous and consists of longitudinally running collagen fibres that span three to four successive spinous processes. It varies considerably in size from a few extremely thin fibrous bundles to a robust band, 5–6 mm wide and 3–4 mm thick, with most individuals exhibiting intermediate forms.[466]

The middle layer is about 1 mm thick and consists of intertwining tendinous fibres of the dorsal layer of thoracolumbar fascia (see Ch. 8) and the aponeurosis of longissimus thoracis (see Ch. 8).

The deep layer consists of very strong, tendinous fibres derived from the aponeurosis of longissimus thoracis. As these tendons pass to their insertions on the lumbar spinous processes they are aggregated in a parallel fashion creating a semblance of a supraspinous ligament, but they are clearly identifiable as tendons. The deepest of these tendons arch ventrally and caudally to reach the upper border of a spinous process,

thereby constituting the dorsal part of the inter-spinous ligament at that level. The deep layer of the supraspinous ligament is reinforced by tendinous fibres of the multifidus muscle (see Ch. 8).

It is thus evident that the supraspinous ligament consists largely of tendinous fibres derived from the back muscles, and is therefore not truly a ligament. Only the superficial layer lacks any continuity with muscle, and this layer is not present at lower lumbar levels. Lying in the subcutaneous plane, dorsal to the other two layers and therefore displaced from the spinous processes, the superficial layer may be rejected as a true ligament and is more readily interpreted as a very variable condensation of the deep or membranous layer of superficial fascia that anchors the midline skin to the thoracolumbar fascia.

At the L4 and L5 levels where the superficial layer is lacking, there is no semblance of a longitudinally orientated, midline supraspinous ligament and the true nature of the 'ligament' is revealed. Here, the obliquely orientated tendinous fibres of the thoracolumbar fascia decussate dorsal to the spinous processes and are fused deeply with the fibres of the aponeurosis of longissimus thoracis that attach to the spinous processes.

ILIO-LUMBAR LIGAMENT

The ilio-lumbar ligaments are present bilaterally, and on each side they connect the transverse process of the fifth lumbar vertebra to the ilium. In brief, each ligament extends from the tip of its transverse process to an area on the anteromedial surface of the ilium and the inner lip of the iliac crest. In greater detail, the ligament can be found to consist of five parts[484] (Fig. 4.6).

The **anterior ilio-lumbar ligament** is a well-developed ligamentous band whose fibres arise from the entire length of the antero-inferior border of the L5 transverse process, from as far medially as the body of the L5 vertebra to the tip of the transverse process. The fibres from the medial end of the transverse process cover those from the lateral end, and collectively they all pass posterolaterally, in line with the long axis of the transverse process, to attach to the ilium. Addi-

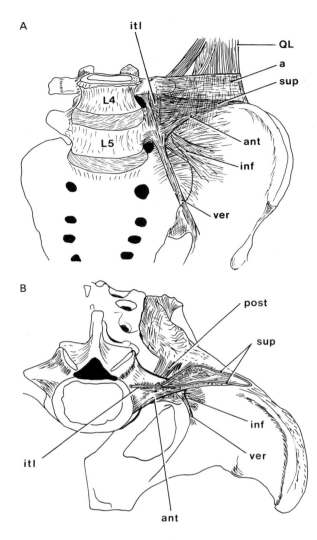

Fig. 4.6 The left ilio-lumbar ligament. (Based on
Shellshear and Macintosh[484]). **A**: front view. **B**: top view.
sup — superior ilio-lumbar ligament. ant — anterior
ilio-lumbar ligament. inf — inferior ilio-lumbar ligament.
ver — vertical ilio-lumbar ligament. post — posterior
ilio-lumbar ligament. itl — intertransverse ligament. a —
anterior layer of thoracolumbar fascia. QL — quadratus
lumborum.

tional fibres of the anterior ilio-lumbar ligament
arise from the very tip of the transverse process,
so that beyond the tip of the transverse process
the ligament forms a very thick bundle. The
upper surface of this bundle forms the site of attachment for the fibres of the lower end of the
quadratus lumborum muscle.

The **superior ilio-lumbar ligament** is
formed by anterior and posterior thickenings of
the fascia that surrounds the base of the
quadratus lumborum muscle. These thickenings
are attached in common to the antero-superior
border of the L5 transverse process near its tip.
Lateral to this, they separate to pass respectively
in front of and behind the quadratus lumborum
muscle to attach eventually to the ilium. Inferiorly, they blend with the anterior ilio-lumbar
ligament to form a trough from which the
quadratus lumborum arises.

The **posterior ilio-lumbar ligament** arises
from the tip and posterior border of the L5 transverse process and inserts into the ligamentous
area of the ilium behind the origin of the
quadratus lumborum. The deepest fibres of the
longissimus lumborum arise from the ligament in
this area.

The **inferior ilio-lumbar ligament** arises
from the lower border of the L5 transverse process and from the body of L5. Its fibres pass
downwards and laterally across the surface of the
anterior sacro-iliac ligament to attach to the
upper and posterior part of the iliac fossa. These
fibres are distinguished from the anterior sacro-
iliac ligament by their oblique orientation.

The **vertical ilio-lumbar ligament** arises
from the antero-inferior border of the L5 transverse process and descends almost vertically to
attach to the posterior end of the ilio-pectineal
line of the pelvis. Its significance lies in that it
forms the lateral margin of the channel through
which the L5 ventral ramus enters the pelvis.

Through its various parts, the ilio-lumbar ligament forms a strong bond between the L5
vertebra and the ilium with different parts sub-
serving different functions. As a whole, the
ligament is disposed to prevent forward sliding
of the L5 vertebra on the sacrum, and the relevance of this function is explored in Chapter 5.
It also resists twisting of the L5 vertebra.[92] Forward bending is resisted by the posterior band of
the ligament, while lateral bending is resisted by
its anterior band.[326]

It is noteworthy that the ilio-lumbar ligament
is present only in adults. In neonates and children
it is represented by a bundle of muscle.[342] This
muscle is gradually replaced by ligamentous tis-

sue. Replacement starts near the transverse process and spreads towards the ilium. The structure is substantially ligamentous by the third decade of age, although some muscle fibres persist. From the fifth decade the ligament contains no muscle, but exhibits hyaline degeneration. From the sixth decade, the ligament exhibits fatty infiltration, hyalinisation, myxoid degeneration and calcification. The identity of the muscles that form the ilio-lumbar ligament is discussed in Chapter 8.

FALSE LIGAMENTS

There are several structures in the lumbar spine that carry the name 'ligament', but for various reasons this is not a legitimate term. These structures are the intertransverse ligaments, the transforaminal ligaments and the mamillo-accessory ligament.

Intertransverse ligaments

The so-called intertransverse ligaments (see Fig. 4.2) have a complicated structure that can be interpreted in various ways. They consist of sheets of connective tissue extending from the upper border of one transverse process to the lower border of the transverse process above. Unlike other ligaments they lack a distinct border medially or laterally, and their collagen fibres are not as densely packed, nor are they as regularly orientated as are the fibres of true ligaments. Rather, their appearance is more like that of a membrane.[542] The medial and lateral continuations of these membranes suggest that rather than being true ligaments, these structures form part of a complex fascial system that serves to separate or demarcate certain paravertebral compartments. Indeed, the only 'true' ligament recognised in this area is the ligament of Bourgery which connects the base of a transverse process to the mammillary process below.[542]

In the intertransverse spaces, the intertransverse ligaments form a septum that divides the anterior musculature of the lumbar spine from the posterior musculature, and embryologically the ligaments arise from the tissue that separates the epaxial and hypaxial musculature (Ch. 11). Laterally, the intertransverse ligaments can be interpreted as dividing into two layers: an anterior layer, otherwise known as the anterior layer of thoracolumbar fascia, that covers the front of the quadratus lumborum muscle; and a posterior layer that blends with the aponeurosis of the transversus abdominis to form the middle layer of thoracolumbar fascia (see Ch. 8).

Towards the medial end of each intertransverse space, the intertransverse ligament splits into two leaves[329] (Fig. 4.7). The dorsal leaf continues medially to attach to the lateral margin of the lamina of the vertebra that lies opposite the intertransverse space. Inferiorly, it blends with the capsule of the adjacent zygapophysial joint. The ventral leaf curves forwards and extends forward over the lateral surface of the vertebral bodies until it eventually blends with the lateral margins of the anterior longitudinal ligament. In covering the lateral aspect of the vertebral column it forms a membranous sheet that closes the outer end of the intervertebral foramen. This part of the leaf is marked by two perforations which transmit structures into and out of the intervertebral foramen. The superior opening transmits the nerve

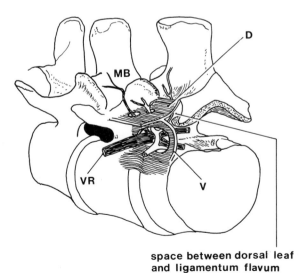

**space between dorsal leaf
and ligamentum flavum**

Fig. 4.7 The ventral and dorsal leaves of the intertransverse ligament. (Based on Lewin et al.[329]) D — dorsal leaf. V — ventral leaf. VR — ventral ramus of spinal nerve. MB — medial branch of dorsal ramus.

branches to the psoas muscle. The inferior opening transmits the ventral ramus of the spinal nerve and the spinal branches of the lumbar arteries and veins.

Enclosed between the ventral and dorsal leaves of the intertransverse ligament is a wedge-shaped space, called the superior articular recess. This recess serves to accommodate movements of the sub-adjacent zygapophysial joint. It is filled with fat that is continuous with the intra-articular fat in the joint below, through the foramen in its superior capsule. The superior articular process of this joint projects into the bottom end of the recess, and during extension movements of the joint, its inferior articular process moves inferiorly pulling the superior articular recess, like a sleeve, over the medial end of the superior articular process. During this process the fat in the recess acts as a displaceable space-filler. At rest, it maintains the space in the recess, but is easily moved out to accommodate the superior articular process. A reciprocal mechanism operates at the inferior pole of the joint where a pad of fat over the vertebral lamina maintains a space between the lamina and the multifidus muscle, into which the inferior articular process can move.

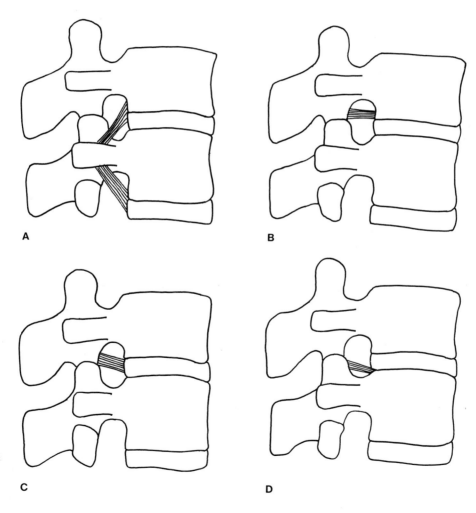

Fig. 4.8 The transforaminal ligaments. (Based on Golub and Silverman.[207]) **A**: Superior and inferior corporotransverse ligaments. **B**: Superior transforaminal ligament. **C**: Middle transforaminal ligament. **D**: Inferior transforaminal ligament.

Transforaminal ligament

The transforaminal ligaments are narrow bands of collagen fibres that traverse the outer end of the intervertebral foramen. Five types of such bands have been described, according to their specific attachments[207] (Fig. 4.8). These are the superior corporotransverse ligament which connects the lower posterolateral corner of a vertebral body with the accessory process of the transverse process of the same vertebra. The inferior corporotransverse ligaments connect the lower posterolateral corner of a vertebral body with the transverse process below. Superior transforaminal ligaments bridge the inferior vertebral notches, and inferior transforaminal ligaments bridge superior vertebral notches. Mid-transforaminal ligaments run from the posterolateral corner of an anulus fibrosus to the zygapophysial joint capsule and ligamentum flavum behind.

Transforaminal ligaments are not always present. The overall incidence of all types is around 47%, with the superior corporotransverse being the most common type (27%).[207] For two reasons, they are not strictly ligaments. First, their structure more resembles bands of fascia than ligaments proper. Secondly, except for the inferior corporotransverse ligament, they do not connect two separate bones; and the mid-transforaminal variety is not connected to any bones. Accordingly, they are more correctly interpreted as bands of fascia, and in view of their location it is most likely that they represent thickenings in the ventral leaf of the intertransverse ligament.

Mamillo-accessory ligament

A tight bundle of collagen fibres, of variable thickness, bridges the tips of the ipsilateral mamillary and accessory processes of each lumbar vertebra (Fig. 4.9). This structure has been called the mamillo-accessory ligament,[58] but it is not a true ligament because it connects two points on the same bone. Moreover, its cord-like structure resembles more a tendon than a ligament and, indeed, it has been interpreted as representing a tendon of the semispinalis musculature in the lumbar region.[58] The ligament may be ossified, converting the mamillo-accessory

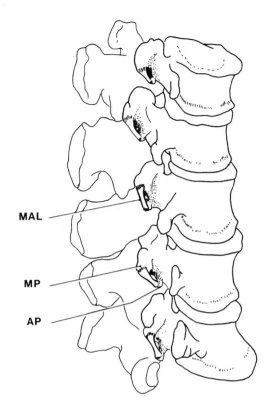

Fig. 4.9 The mamillo-accessory ligaments (MAL). MP — mamillary process. AP — accessory process. Note the foramina under the ligaments, through which pass the medial branches of the lumbar dorsal rami.

notch into a bony foramen. The prevalence of this change was found in one study to be 10% at the L5 level,[58] while in another study it was 28% at L5, 10% at L4 and 3% at L3.[406]

The ligament has no biomechanical significance, but its significance lies in the fact that it covers the medial branch of the dorsal ramus of the spinal nerve as it runs through the mamillo-accessory notch. Furthermore, when the ligament is ossified, the foramen it forms can be an apparent anomaly evident on computed tomographic (CT) scans.[47] Ossification of the ligament, however, is a normal phenomenon without any pathological significance. It has been suggested that the ligament may be a site of entrapment of the nerve beneath it[70] but this has not been verified clinically.

5. The lumbar lordosis and the vertebral canal

THE LUMBAR LORDOSIS

The intact lumbar spine is formed when the five lumbar vertebrae are articulated to one another (Fig. 5.1). Anteriorly the vertebral bodies are separated by the intervertebral discs and are held together by the anterior and posterior longitudinal ligaments. Posteriorly the articular processes form the zygapophysial joints, and consecutive vertebrae are held together by the supraspinous, interspinous and intertransverse ligaments and the ligamenta flava.

Although the lumbar vertebrae can be articulated to form a straight column of vertebrae, this is not the shape assumed by the intact lumbar spine in the upright posture. The reason for this is that the sacrum, on which the lumbar spine rests, is tilted forwards, so that its upper surface is inclined downwards and forwards. From radiographs taken in the supine position, the size of this angle with respect to the horizontal plane of the body has a mean value of about 42° to 45°,[233,493,554] and is said to increase by about 8° upon standing.[233]

If a straight lumbar spine articulated with the sacrum it would consequently be inclined forwards. To restore an upward orientation and to compensate for the inclination of the sacrum, the intact lumbar spine must assume a curve (Fig. 5.1). This curve is known as the lumbar **lordosis**.

The junction between the lumbar spine and the sacrum is achieved through joints like those between the lumbar vertebrae. Anteriorly, the body of the L5 vertebra forms an inter-body joint with the first sacral vertebra, and the intervertebral disc of this joint is known as the lumbosacral disc. Posteriorly, the inferior articular processes

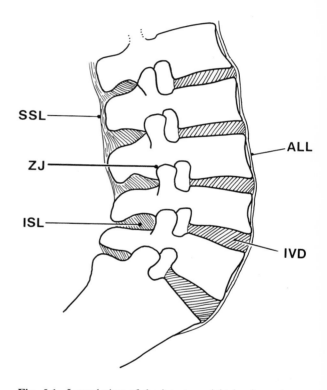

Fig. 5.1 Lateral view of the intact, upright lumbar spine, showing its curved shape. ALL — anterior longitudinal ligament. IVD — intervertebral disc. ZJ — zygapophysial joint. SSL — supraspinous ligament. ISL — interspinous ligament.

of L5 and the superior articular processes of the sacrum form synovial joints known either as the L5–S1 zygapophysial joints or as the lumbosacral zygapophysial joints. A ligamentum flavum is present between the laminae of L5 and the sacrum, and an interspinous ligament connects the

45

L5 and S1 spinous processes. However, there is no supraspinous ligament at the L5–S1 level, [238] nor are there intertransverse ligaments, the latter having been replaced by the ilio-lumbar ligament.

The shape of the lumbar lordosis is achieved as result of several factors. The first of these is the shape of the lumbosacral intervertebral disc. This disc is unlike any of the other lumbar intervertebral discs in that it is wedge-shaped. Its posterior height is about 6–7 mm less than its anterior height.[478] Consequently, when the L5 vertebra is articulated to the sacrum its lower surface does not lie parallel to the upper surface of the sacrum. It is still inclined forwards and downwards but less steeply than the top of the sacrum. The angle formed between the bottom of the L5 vertebra and the top of the sacrum varies from individual to individual over the range 6–29°, and has an average size of about 16°[478] (Fig. 5.2).

The second factor that generates the lumbar lordosis is the shape of the L5 vertebra. Like the lumbosacral disc, the L5 vertebral body is also wedge-shaped. The height of its posterior surface is some 3 mm less than the height of its anterior surface.[199] As a consequence of the wedge shape of both the L5 body and the lumbosacral disc the upper surface of L5 lies much closer to a horizontal plane than does the upper surface of the sacrum.

The remainder of the lumbar lordosis is completed simply by inclination of the vertebrae above L5. Each vertebra is inclined slightly backwards in relation to the vertebra below. As a result of this inclination, the anterior parts of the anuli fibrosi and the anterior longitudinal ligament are stretched. Posteriorly, the intervertebral discs are compressed slightly, and the inferior articular processes slide downwards in relation to the superior articular processes of the vertebra below, and may impact either the superior articular process or the pedicle below. The latter phenomemon has particular bearing on the weight-bearing capacity of the zygapophysial joints and is described further in Chapter 7.

The form of the curve thus achieved is such that in the upright posture the L1 vertebra is brought to lie vertically above the sacrum. The exact shape of the lumbar lordosis at rest varies from individual to individual, and it is difficult

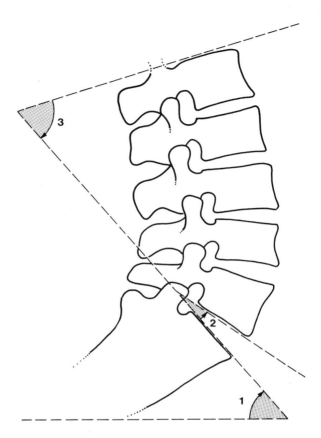

Fig. 5.2 Some of the angles used to describe the lumbar spine. 1: Angle formed by the top of the sacrum and the horizontal plane. Mean value about 50°. 2: Angle between the bottom of L5 and the top of the sacrum. Mean value 16°. 3: Angle between the top of L1 and the sacrum, used to measure the lumbar lordosis. Mean value about 70°.

to define what might be called the 'normal' lumbar lordosis.

Various parameters have been used by different investigators to quantify the curvature of the lumbar lordosis, although they all involve measuring one or other of the angles formed by the lumbar vertebral bodies (Fig. 5.2). Some have used the angle formed by the planes through the top surface of L1 and the top surface of the sacrum,[228,439] and this could be called the 'L1–S1 lordosis angle'. Fernand and Fox[176] measured the angles between the top of L2 and the top of the sacrum, and between the top of L2 and the bottom of L5, which they respectively called the 'lumbosacral lordotic angle' and the 'lumbolumbar lordotic angle'. Others have measured the angle between the top of L3 and the sacrum,[521] or the angle formed between planes that bisect the L1–L2 disc and the L5–S1 disc.[172,446] Consequently the measures obtained in these various studies differ somewhat from one another. Nevertheless they all show substantial ranges of variation.

In radiographs taken in the supine position, the angle between the top of L1 and the top of the sacrum varies from 20° to more than 60°, but has an average value of about 50°.[228] In the standing position, this same angle has been measured as 67° (±3° standard deviation) in children, and 74° (±7° standard deviation) in young males.[433] The angle between the top of L2 and the sacrum has a range of 16° to 80° and mean value of 45°.[176] A value greater than 68° is considered to indicate a hyperlordotic curve.[176] However, despite a common belief that excessive lordosis is a risk factor for low-back pain, comparison studies reveal that there is no correlation between the shape of the lumbar lordosis and the presence or absence of back pain symptoms.[228,446,521]

The foremost structural liability of the lumbar spine stems from the inclination of the sacrum. Because of the downward slope of the superior surface of the sacrum, there is a constant tendency for the L5 vertebra, and hence the entire lumbar spine, to slide forwards down this slope under the influence of the weight of the trunk; more so whenever additional weights are borne by the lumbar spine. In turn, there is a similar, though lesser, tendency for the L4 vertebra to slide down the upper surface of the L5 vertebra. However, the lumbar spine is adapted to offset these tendencies, and these adaptations are seen in the structure of the articular processes and ligaments of the L5 and other lumbar vertebrae.

As described in Chapter 3, the lumbar zygapophysial joints provide a bony locking mechanism that resists forward displacement, and the degree to which a joint affords such resistance is determined by its orientation. The more a superior articular process faces backwards, the greater the resistance it offers to forward displacement.

To resist the tendency for the L5 vertebra to slip forwards, the superior articular processes of the sacrum face considerably backwards. The average orientation of the L5–S1 zygapophysial joints with respect to the sagittal plane is about 45°, with most lumbosacral zygapophysial joints assuming this orientation (see Ch. 3, Fig. 3.4). Only a minority of joints assume a greater or lesser angle. Joints with a greater angle, i.e. facing backwards even more, provide greater resistance to forward displacement of L5, but they provide less resistance to axial rotation, or twisting movements, of L5. Joints with an angle less than 45° provide greater protection against rotation but less against forward displacement. An angle of 45° is, therefore, a satisfactory compromise, allowing the lumbosacral zygapophysial joints to resist both rotation and forward displacement.

The L4–5 zygapophysial joints are also orientated at about 45° (Ch. 3, Fig. 3.4), and thereby resist forward displacement of the L4 vertebra. Above L4 the slopes of the upper surfaces of the vertebral bodies are horizontal or inclined backwards, and there is no tendency, at rest, for the upper lumbar vertebrae to slide forwards. Consequently, there is less need for the upper lumbar zygapophysial joints to face backwards, and their angle of orientation is progressively less than 45° (Ch. 3, Fig. 3.4). Such resistance as may be required to resist forward displacement of these joints during flexion of the lumbar spine is nevertheless afforded by the curved shape of their articular surfaces. Although their general orientation is closer to the sagittal plane, the anteromedial ends of the articular surfaces of the upper lumbar joints face backwards and can resist forward displacement, if required (Ch. 3).

The second mechanism that stabilises the lumbar lordosis is provided by the ligaments of the lumbar spine. At all levels, any tendency for a vertebra to slide forwards will be resisted by the anulus fibrosus of the underlying intervertebral disc. However, the anuli fibrosi are spared undue strain in this regard by the bony locking mechanism of the zygapophysial joints. Bony impaction will occur before the intervertebral discs are strained. However, should the mechanism of the zygapophysial joints be compromised by unsuitable orientation or by disease or injury, then the resistance of the anuli fibrosi will be invoked to a greater extent.

By connecting the L5 transverse processes to the ilium, the ilio-lumbar ligaments, through their sheer size, provide a strong additional mechanism that prevents the L5 vertebra from sliding forwards. The tension sustained through the ilio-lumbar ligament is evident in the size of the L5 transverse processes. These are unlike the transverse processes of any other lumbar vertebra. Instead of thin flat bars, they are thick and pyramidal in shape. Moreover, instead of stemming just from the posterior end of the pedicle, they have an enlarged base that extends forwards along the pedicle as far as the vertebral body. This modification of structure can be interpreted as due to the modelling of the bone in response to the massive forces transmitted through the L5 transverse processes and the ilio-lumbar ligaments.

The anterior longitudinal ligament, and in a similar way, the anterior fibres of the anuli fibrosi, play a further role in stabilising the lumbar lordosis. If the lumbar spine bows forwards, the anterior ends of the vertebral bodies will attempt to separate, but this separation will be resisted by the anterior longitudinal ligament and the anterior fibres of the anuli fibrosi. Eventually, an equilibrium will be established in which any force tending to separate the vertebral bodies will be balanced exactly by the tension in the anterior ligaments. Any increase in force will be met by increased tension in the ligaments. In this way, the anterior ligaments endow the curved lumbar spine with a resilience. This mechanism is analogous to the 'springiness' that can be felt in a long wooden rod, or a plastic ruler that is stood on its end and deformed into an arc.

One of the advantages of a curved lumbar spine lies in this resilience. By being curved, the lumbar spine is protected to an appreciable extent from compressive forces and shocks. In a straight lumbar spine, an axial, compressive force would be transmitted through the vertebral bodies and intervertebral discs, and the only mechanism to protect the lumbar vertebrae would be the shock-absorbing capacity of the intervertebral discs (Ch. 2). In contrast, in a curved lumbar spine, compressive forces are transmitted through the posterior ends of the intervertebral discs while the anterior ends of the vertebral bodies tend to separate. In other words, compression tends to accentuate the lumbar lordosis. This tendency will tense the anterior ligaments which, in turn, will resist the accentuation. In this way, some of the energy of the compressive force is diverted into stretching the anterior ligaments instead of being transmitted directly into the next vertebral body. This mechanism and other advantages of the lumbar lordosis are explored in further detail in Chapter 7.

THE VERTEBRAL CANAL

In the intact lumbar spine, the vertebral foramina of the five lumbar vertebrae are aligned to form a continuous channel called the **vertebral canal** (Fig. 5.3). The anterior wall of this canal is formed by the posterior surfaces of the lumbar vertebrae, the intervening discs and the posterior longitudinal ligament. The posterior wall is formed by the lamina of the vertebrae and the intervening ligamenta flava. Because operations on the lumbar spine are most frequently performed with the patient in the prone position, the anterior and posterior walls of the vertebral canal are by convention alternatively referred to as the **floor** and **roof** of the vertebral canal, respectively.

The floor of the vertebral canal is not absolutely flat because the posterior surfaces of the lumbar vertebral bodies exhibit slight curves, both transversely and longitudinally. The posterior surfaces of the L1 to L3 vertebrae regularly exhibit a slight transverse concavity. In contrast, L5 is slightly convex, while L4 exhibits and intermediate curvature.[319] Along the sagittal plane, the lumbar vertebra present a slightly concave posterior surface, so that in profile the floor of the vertebral canal presents a scalloped appearance.[318] This scalloping is believed to be produced by the pulsatile, hydrostatic pressure of the cerebrospinal fluid in the dural sac which occupies the vertebral canal.[318]

The lateral walls of the vertebral canal are formed by the pedicles of the lumbar vertebrae. Between the pedicles the lateral wall is deficient where the superior and inferior vertebral notches

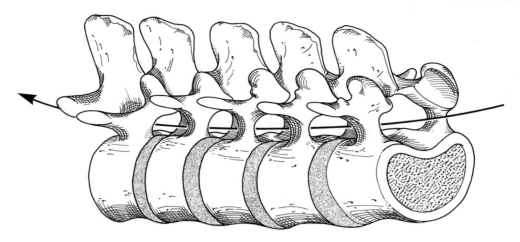

Fig. 5.3 Lateral view of a prone lumbar spine with an arrow depicting the vertebral canal.

appose one another to form the intervertebral foramina. Each intervertebral foramen is bounded
anteriorly by an intervertebral disc, the adjacent
lower third of the vertebral body above, and the
uppermost portion of the vertebral body below
(Fig. 5.4). Above and below, each intervertebral
foramen is bounded by a pedicle, while posteriorly it is bounded by a vertebral lamina and a
zygapophysial joint. More accurately, the posterior boundary of each intervertebral foramen is
the lateral portion of the ligamentum flavum that
covers the anterior aspect of the lamina and
zygapophysial joint (Ch. 4).

Subdivisions of the vertebral canal, recognised
by surgeons because of their relationship to the
spinal nerve roots,[67,104,128,553] are the so-called
radicular canals. These are not true canals because they do not have boundaries around all
their aspects. More accurately, they are only subdivisions of the space of the vertebral canal and
intervertebral foramina, through which the spinal
nerve roots run (see Ch. 9), but in so far as they
form a series of bony relations to the course of
the nerve roots they may be regarded as canals.

Each radicular canal is a curved channel running around the medial aspect of each pedicle in
the lumbar spine, and each can be divided into
three segments.[553] The uppermost, or retrodiscal
segment, lies above the level of the pedicle. Its
anterior wall is formed by the intervertebral disc
in this region, while its posterior wall is formed

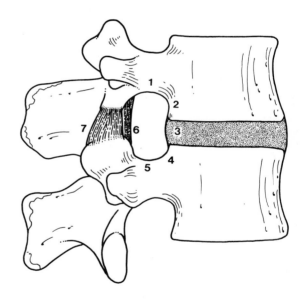

Fig. 5.4 Lateral view of the boundaries of an
intervertebral foramen. 1 — Pedicle. 2 — Back of
vertebral body. 3 — Intervertebral disc. 4 — Back of
vertebral body. 5 — Pedicle. 6 — Ligamentum flavum. 7
— Zygapophysial joint.

by the uppermost end of a superior articular process (Fig. 5.5). This segment lacks a lateral wall
because it lies opposite the level of an intervertebral foramen. Similarly, it has no medial wall,
for in this direction it is simply continuous with
the rest of the vertebral canal.

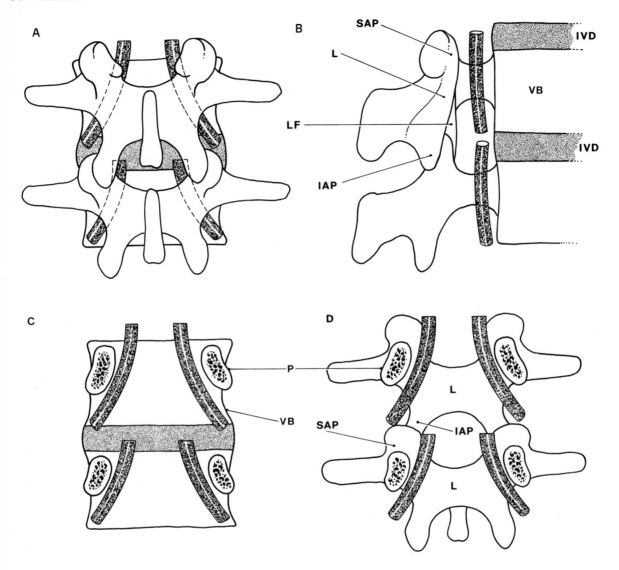

Fig. 5.5 The radicular canals. **A**: The location of the radicular canals (shaded), in a dorsal view of the lumbar spine. **B**: A view of the radicular canals from within the vertebral canal, showing their lateral, anterior and posterior boundaries. **C**: The anterior and lateral boundaries of the radicular canals, viewed from behind. **D**: The posterior and lateral boundaries of the radicular canals, as seen from within the vertebral canal, looking at its roof. The ligamentum flavum has not been included (see Fig. 4.5B). IVD — intervertebral disc. VB — vertebral body. SAP — superior articular process. IAP — inferior articular process. LF — ligamentum flavum. P — pedicle. L — lamina.

The parapedicular segment lies immediately medial to the pedicle, which therefore forms its lateral wall. Anteriorly, this segment is related to the back of the vertebral body, while posteriorly it is covered by the vertebral lamina and the an-teromedial edge of the superior articular process that projects from this lamina (Fig. 5.5). Technically, this segment of the radicular canal is simply the lateral portion of the vertebral canal opposite the level of a pedicle, and for this reason

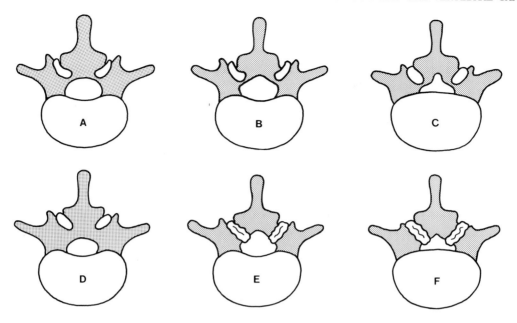

Fig. 5.6 The shape of the vertebral canal in transverse section. **A**: Oval outline of upper lumbar vertebrae. **B**: Triangular shape of lower lumbar vertebrae. **C**: Trefoil shape found at lower lumbar levels. **D**: Congenital spinal stenosis. **E**. Acquired spinal stenosis of a triangular vertebral canal, due to arthrosis of the zygapophysial joints. **F**: Acquired spinal stenosis of a trefoil vertebral canal, due to arthrosis of the zygapophysial joints.

this segment is also known as the **lateral recess** (of the vertebral canal). A lateral recess is therefore present on both sides of the vertebral canal opposite each of the lumbar pedicles.

The third segment of the radicular canal is formed by the upper part of the intervertebral foramen: that part behind the vertebral body and below the upper pedicle (Fig. 5.5).

The anatomical relevance of the radicular canals is that the lumbar nerve roots run along them, and the anatomy of these nerves is described in Chapter 9. The clinical relevance lies in the propensity for the nerve roots to be compressed by structural alterations in one or other of the structures that form boundaries to the canals.

Another concept of relevance to nerve root compression concerns narrowing of the vertebral canal. The shape and size of the lumbar vertebral canal governs the amount of space available for the nerves that the canal transmits, and if this space is in any way lessened by encroachment of the boundaries of the canal, the condition is re-ferred to as **canal stenosis** or **spinal stenosis**.[30,138,148,300,546–548]

In transverse section, the lumbar vertebral canal varies in shape. It is oval at upper lumbar levels, becoming triangular more caudally, sometimes assuming a trefoil shape at lower lumbar levels[426] (Fig. 5.6). The term 'trefoil' refers to a triangular shape in which the angles are stretched or accentuated.[140] The basal angles of the triangular, or trefoil, outline are formed by the lateral recesses of the vertebral canal.

The shape and size of the vertebral canal can be abnormally small as a result of aberrations in the development of the neural arch. In relation to the size of the vertebral canal, the pedicles may be too thick or the articular process may be too large. In effect, the space left in the vertebral canal becomes relatively too small for the volume of nerves that it has to transmit. This condition is called congenital or developmental spinal stenosis,[30] but by itself, developmental stenosis does not not cause compression of nerves. It only renders the patient more likely to compression in the face of the slightest aberration of the boundaries of the vertebral canal.[30,300]

Acquired spinal stenosis occurs whenever any of the structures surrounding the vertebral canal is affected by disease or degeneration that results in enlargement of the structure into the space of the vertebral canal. Examples of such processes include buckling of the ligamentum flavum, osteophytes from the zygapophysial joints or intervertebral discs, and intervertebral disc herniations or bulges.[30,104,300,547] Such changes may occur at single levels in the vertebral canal or at multiple levels, and symptoms may arise either from the disease process that caused the changes or as a result of compression of one or more nerves by the encroaching structure. The pathogenesis of symptoms in spinal stenosis is described further in Chapter 13.

6. Basic biomechanics

Because of its jargon and mathematical flavour, biomechanics is a subject that is often daunting and overwhelming to students of anatomy. However, certain biomechanical concepts are indispensible for the description and interpretation of the movements and age changes of the lumbar spine. It is, therefore, appropriate to review and summarise these concepts as a prelude to the chapters discussing these topics.

MOVEMENTS

There are two types of motion that a bone may undergo: **translation** and **rotation**. The essence of translation is that every point on the bone moves in the same direction and to the same extent (Fig. 6.1). Translation occurs whenever a single force or a nett single force acts on a bone, and any force that tends to cause translation is called a **shear** force.

Rotation is characterised by all the points on a bone moving in parallel around a curved path centred on some fixed point. The points move in a similar direction but to different extents depending on their radial distance from the fixed point which is known as the centre of rotation (Fig. 6.2). Rotation occurs when two unaligned forces act in opposing directions on different parts of the bone, forming what is known as a force couple (Fig. 6.2), and the nett force tending to cause rotation is referred to as the **torque**. Depending on circumstances torque may be the result of two opposed forces which may both be muscular actions, or they may be a muscular action and a ligamentous resistance, or they may be gravity opposed by either muscular action or ligamentous resistance.

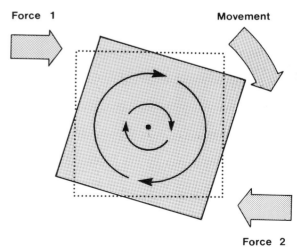

Fig. 6.2 Rotation. Two unaligned, opposite forces (*a force couple*) cause the points in a body to move around a stationary centre.

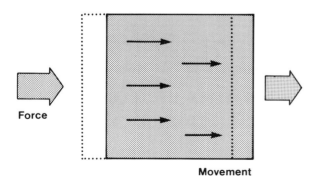

Fig. 6.1 Translation. A single nett force causes all points in a body to move in parallel, in the same direction to the same extent.

53

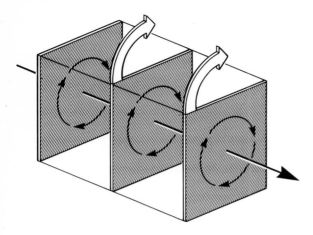

Fig. 6.3 During rotation, the points in any plane of a body move around a centre located in that plane. A line formed by these centres is the axis of rotation of the body.

When a rotating bone is considered in three dimensions, it can be seen that all the points throughout the bone can be grouped into individual planes that all lie parallel to the direction of motion (Fig. 6.3). In each plane, the points move about a centre located in that plane, and when all the centres of all the planes are lined up they depict a straight line 'that forms what is known as the **axis of rotation** of the bone'.

There is nothing special about an axis of rotation in a biological sense. The points along an axis of rotation do not have any unique biological properties. An axis of rotation is only a mathematical phenomenon created by the nett effect of forces acting on a bone. For any rotation, it can be shown that there is a region where all opposing forces cancel out and no nett force acts, and this will be the axis of rotation. The axis remains stationary because no nett force acts on it. Meanwhile, all the points surrounding the axis are subjected to a nett force, and motion will occur around the stationary axis. Thus, a formal definition of an axis of rotation can be 'that region that does not move when two or more opposing, unaligned forces act on a bone'.

The location of any axis of rotation is not an intrinsic property of the bone which moves around it. It is a property of the forces that may happen to act on the bone, and different forces will create a different axis of rotation. So-called

'normal' axes of rotation occur only when, during repetitions of a movement, the same forces are consistently applied. With each repetition the axis of rotation occurs consistently in the same place. However, if at any time one of the applied forces is altered, a new axis will occur.

PLANES OF MOVEMENT

Both translation and rotation can occur in either of two opposite senses which can be variously defined according to circumstances or convention. For example, the motion can be upwards or downwards, forwards or backwards, clockwise or anticlockwise, and in some conventions positive (+) or negative (−). Furthermore, in three-dimensional space, translation or rotation can occur in any of three fundamental planes. In anatomical terms, these planes are the sagittal, coronal and horizontal planes (Fig. 6.4). Backward or forward rotations are movements in the sagittal plane as are translations in the backward or forward direction. Side-bending is rotation in the coronal plane, and twisting is rotation in the horizontal plane. A sideways gliding movement across the horizontal plane would be horizontal translation, while movements up or down are described as coronal translations.

Biomechanists prefer to define movements in relation to three imaginary axes drawn through the body, which are labelled X,Y and Z.[558,559] The X axis passes sideways through the body; the Y axis passes through it vertically; and the Z axis passes through it from back to front (Fig. 6.5). Movements can then be described as along or around any particular axis. Thus, sagittal translation is translation along the Z axis; sideways gliding movements are translations along the X axis; and up and down movements are along the Y axis. Forward bending is rotation around the X axis; side-bending is rotation about the Z axis; and twisting movements are rotations around the Y axis.

The advantage of the biomechanists' convention is that the dimensions of movements are accurately and unambiguously defined. However, the terms 'X', 'Y' and 'Z' are unfamiliar and anonymous to all except to those who use them regularly. The terms 'sagittal', 'coronal' and

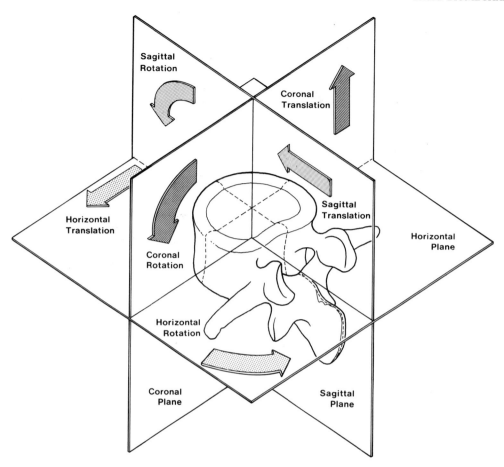

Fig. 6.4 Planes and directions of motion: anatomical system.

'horizontal' are somewhat more meaningful because of their use in other areas of anatomy, and are the terms used in this text. For reference, the equivalence of various terms derived from the anatomical system, the biomechanists' convention and colloquial vocabulary is shown in Table 6.1.

Because of difficulties in appreciating the distinctions between translations and rotations in the horizontal and coronal planes, the term 'axial' has been introduced in Table 6.1. Thus, the term 'axial rotation' replaces 'horizontal rotation' to refer to rotation in the horizontal plane, i.e. around the long axis of the body. The term 'axial translation' replaces 'coronal translation' to refer to movement up or down, or along the long axis of the body, and to distinguish this movement

from sideways translations in the horizontal plane, which are described as horizontal or lateral translations.

To specifiy the direction of axial translations the terms 'cephalad', meaning towards the head, and 'caudad', meaning towards the tail, are used in Table 6.1. Although perhaps cumbersome and unfamiliar, these terms are accurate and applicable in all situations. The more familiar terms 'upward' and 'downward' are applicable for axial translations in the upright position, but they are not strictly applicable to describe motions of vertebra in patients who might be lying down. To overcome this difficulty, the more colloquial terms of 'distraction' and 'compression' are more usually used instead of 'cephalad' and 'caudad

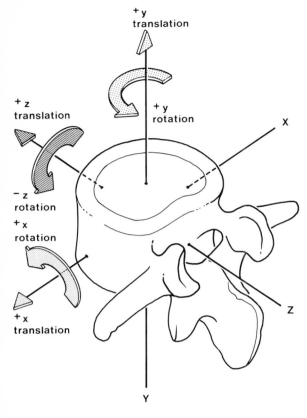

Fig. 6.5 Axes and directions of motion: biomechanical system.

axial translation'. Similarly, the term 'lateral bending' is more convenient and is preferred to 'coronal rotation'.

In this text, the term 'sagittal' rotation is strictly used, to refer to forward and backward rotatory movements. Although the terms 'flexion' and 'extension' are commonly used to describe this motion, these terms are insufficiently accurate when applied to movements of individual lumbar vertebrae. Flexion and extension are not pure movements of the lumbar vertebrae, for as will be shown in Chapter 7, these movements involve a combination of both sagittal translation and sagittal rotation. The terms 'flexion' and 'extension' may be used to describe forward bending and backward bending of the lumbar spine in a general sense, but in relation to movements of individual vertebrae it should be understood that the terms refer to a combination of both sagittal rotation and sagittal translation.

The relevance of these explicit definitions of motion is extensive. In the first instance, the motion of individual vertebrae is often complex, and no single term can described the motion. Nevertheless, it can always be describe as some combination of the fundamental movements listed in Table 6.1. Furthermore, each component of motion of the lumbar spine is exerted and resisted by different mechanisms, and to ap-

Table 6.1 Descriptive terms of motion

Anatomical system	Biomechanical system	Colloquial description
anterior sagittal translation	+ Z translation	forward slide or glide
posterior sagittal translation	– Z translation	backward slide
cephalad coronal translation	+ Y translation	longitudinal or axial distraction
caudad coronal translation	– Y translation	longitudinal or axialc ompression
left horizontal translation	+ X translation	left lateral slide
right horizontal translation	– X translation	right lateral slide
anterior sagittal rotation	+ X rotation	forward bend, 'flexion'
posterior sagittal rotation	– X rotation	backward bend, 'extension'
left coronal rotation	– Z rotation	left lateral bend
right coronal rotation	+ Z rotation	right lateral bend
left horizontal rotation*	+ Y rotation	left (axial) rotation
right horizontal rotation*	– Y rotation	right (axial) rotation

* The direction of rotation is defined according to the direction of movement of the most anterior point on the bone.

preciate how these mechanisms act, each needs to be analysed in relation to the particular component of motion that it controls. This type of analysis is undertaken in Chapter 7.

STRESS-STRAIN

To stretch a collagen fibre, a force must be aplied to it. Once it starts to stretch, the fibre resists elongation by generating a resisting force generated by the chemical bonds between collagen fibrils, between tropocollagen molecules, between collagen fibres, and between collagen fibres and proteoglycans (see Ch. 2). By convention the applied or elongating force is known as the applied **stress** and the extent to which a fibre is elongated is known as the **strain**. Stress is measured in units of force (newtons) and strain is measured as the fractional or percentage increase in length relative to initial length. Thus a fibre of length L_0 when stretched to a new length L_1 undergoes a strain of L_1/L_0 or $L_1/L_0 \times 100\%$.

Particular terms are used to specify different types of stress and strain according to the direction in which a structure is deformed. When a structure is stretched longitudinally the deforming force is known as **tension** and the structure undergoes tension strain. If a structure is squashed the deforming stress is **compression** and it undergoes compression strain. The latter is measured as the fractional or percentage decrease in height of the structure. Forces that cause two vertebrae to slide with respect to one another are referred to as **shear** forces and the strain that occurs in the intervening intervertebral disc is referred to as shear strain. The distinction between shear and tension is that tension conventionally applies to forces exerted along the long axis of a structure whereas shear forces are applied across this axis. When an object twists, it is said to undergo **torsion**. A force that causes torsion is a torque and the resultant strain is referred to as torsion strain.

At rest, single collagen fibres are usually buckled, and the wavy shape they assume is referred to as **crimp**.[125,299,481,482] When stress is applied to a collagen fibre the first effect is to straighten this crimp. Little energy is required to do this as there are no major chemical bonds that maintain

the crimp. Thus, a crimped collagen fibre will elongate in response to little applied force. However, once crimp has been removed, the collagen fibres start to resist strongly any further elongation. The stress attempts to break the bonds between the collagen fibrils and tropocollagen molecules. Energy is required to oppose, strain and perhaps eventually break these bonds. Consequently, more force is required to produce further elongation of the collagen fibre. If sufficient force is applied, the bonds may break, and when this occurs in a substantial number of bonds, the collagen fibre ceases to resist elongation and is said to 'fail'. Once the collagen fibre has failed, only small forces are required to tear apart its, now unbonded, component fibrils and molecules.

The mechanical behaviour of collagen fibres subject to stress can be depicted graphically,[1] as in Figure 6.6. Such graphs are known as stress-strain curves. The curve exhibits three main regions. The first region, known as the 'toe' phase, reflects the phase when crimp is being removed from the collagen fibre. The second, or linear, region is the steep slope along the middle of the curve. Mathematical calculations reveal

STRESS

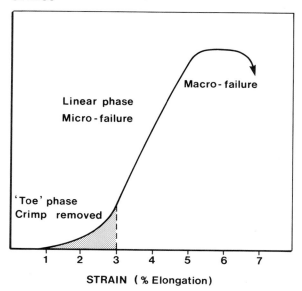

Fig. 6.6 Stress-strain curve of collagen. (Based on Abraham[1], and Shah et al.[482]).

that the junction of the toe phase and the linear region represents the point where crimp has been maximally removed from the fibre, and the stress starts to stretch the collagen fibre longitudinally.[1,482] The linear region represents the phase when bonds within and between collagen fibrils are being strained and some are being broken. The peak of the curve represents the phase of failure of the collagen fibre, when substantial numbers of bonds are irreversibly broken. As depicted by the last part of the curve, once failure has occurred, elongation can continue with ever decreasing amounts of stress being required.

A key feature of the mechanical properties of collagen is that bonds within and between collagen fibrils start to be strained and broken somewhere after 3% and 4% elongation of the fibre has occurred. Consequently, about 4% elongation is the maximum a fibre can sustain without risking microscopic damage.

Collagenous tissues, like ligaments and joint capsules, behave in a similar manner to isolated collagen fibres, and exhibit similar stress-strain curves[409,411,481,482] but certain additional mechanical events are involved (Fig. 6.7). In addition to

the removal of crimp, the 'toe' phase may represent the removal of any macroscopic slack in the ligament. During the second phase, collagen fibres are being re-arranged in the stressed structure. Fibres that, at rest, are curved or run obliquely in the three-dimensional lattice of the ligament or capsule, are straightened to line up with the applied force. Thus, when the three-dimensional lattice is stressed, any bonds between separate collagen fibres and between collagen fibres and their surrounding proteoglycan matrix are strained. Furthermore, to make way for the re-arrangement of collagen fibres, water and proteoglycans may need to be displaced from between the collagen fibres.

All of these processes require energy: energy to strain the bonds, to move the collagen fibres and proteoglycans, and to squeeze out water. Thus, to achieve continued elongation more force must be applied, and this creates the steep slope of the second phase (Fig. 6.7). Eventually, after the collagen fibres, proteglycans and water have been re-arranged, the bonds within individual collagen fibres are strained. In the face of increasing stress, these bonds and those between collagen fibres will fail and the entire structure fails.

What proportion of collagen fibres need to fail before macroscopic failure of a ligament or capsule occurs is not known, and it is not possible to predict the stress-strain curves for different structures on the basis of the number or nature of their constituent collagen fibres. Therefore, the mechanical behaviour of different structures has to be derived empirically by subjecting several samples of the same structure to known stresses and obtaining average stress-strain curves representative of the particular structure.

The value of stress-strain curves is that they graphically depict the mechanical properties of collagenous (and other) structures, notably their strength and the way in which they resist elongation. In turn, the mechanical behaviour reflects the biochemical properties of the structure, for alterations in the proteoglycan content and the bonding within and between collagen fibres will affect the way a ligament or a capsule can resist applied forces.

To a certain extent, physical examination involves obtaining a stress-strain curve for a joint,

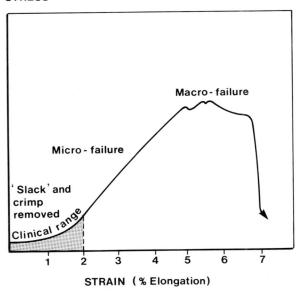

Fig. 6.7 Stress-strain curve for a ligament. (Based on Nordin and Frankel,[409] and Noyes.[411])

and its capsule or ligaments. When passive movement is induced, a stress is applied, and strain is reflected both in terms of the range of movement observed and in the form of the palpated resistance to movement. It is important to realise, however, that clinical examination studies only the early part of the stress-strain curve, no further than just beyond the toe phase.[409] The limit is well within the 4% elongation at which microscopic injury occurs. Physical examination rarely (and shouldn't) enter into the second phase for then it is actually inducing micro-failure of the structure, and risks macro-failure. Physical examination, therefore, gains access to only a part of the total stress-strain curve possible. Nevertheless, it does detect some of the physical properties of the structure examined, which can be interpreted in the light of knowledge of the microstructure and biochemistry of the structure examined, and knowledge of its total mechanical behaviour as determined in cadaveric and postmortem material.

STIFFNESS

The stiffness of a given structure is its resistance to deformation, and can be measured by the force required to produce a unit elongation or deformation.[531] In mathematical terms, it is the slope of the stress-strain curve of a structure. Stiffer structures resist deformation and the slope of their stress-strain curve will be steeper. In biochemical terms, stiffness implies a greater degree of bonding between collagen fibres, or between collagen fibres and their surrounding matrix.

INITIAL RANGE OF MOVEMENT

If a joint is moved passively or actively by a constant force, a point is reached where no further movement appears possible. The resistance in the capsule and ligaments of the joint balances exactly the force attempting to move the joint. The distance moved by the joint up to this point is known as the **initial range of movement**. If a stress-strain curve were constructed for the joint, the initial range of movement would be found to occur somewhere early in the second phase of

the curve, just after the 'toe' phase when collagen bonding is starting to resist the movement.

Application of a greater force would strain the resisting structures further and a new, greater initial range of movement would be perceived. The amount of increased range would be dependent both on the increase in force and on the stiffness of the joint and its ligaments. However, to obtain a substantially greater initial range of movement, considerably larger forces would need to be applied to most joints and ligaments. Such larger forces are not usually possible during normal clinical examination.

With the forces used in clinical examination, the initial range of movement remains early in the second phase of the stress-strain curve, and even if the applied force varies somewhat with the strength of the examiner, the resistance of the joint is such that the differences in perceived range of movement are not great. Consequently, the initial range of movement as perceived from clinical examination falls in a narrow range and can be called the normal range of movement.

CREEP

Initial ranges of movement are usually measured on the basis of a brief application of force. The force is applied until range of movement is maximal, and once the range is measured, the force is released. However, if a constant force is left applied to a collagenous structure for a more prolonged period, further movement is detectable. This movement is small in amplitude, occurs slowly, almost imperceptibly, and is consequently known as **creep**.

Graphically, creep is seen as continued displacement when a constant force is maintained at some point on a stress-strain curve (Fig. 6.8). The time over which creep can be measured is optional, and various studies have employed times varying from minutes to hours.[285,286,305,357,531]

The biochemical and structural basis of creep is not known for certain, but it appears to be due to the gradual re-arrangement of collagen fibres, proteoglycans and water in the ligament or capsule being stressed. Forces of short duration may not act long enough to squeeze water out of a

STRESS

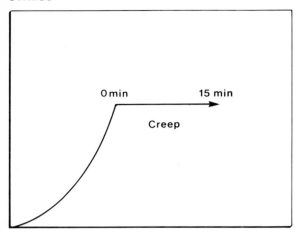

ELONGATION

Fig. 6.8 Stress-strain curve illustrating creep. Despite maintenance of a constant load, elongation occurs with the passage of time.

ligament or to allow the re-arrangement of collagen that could possibly occur. The force is removed before maximal displacement has had a chance to occur. In contrast, sustained forces allow for these displacements to occur, whereupon the ligament or capsule can elongate slightly as a result of the internal re-adjustment of its constituents.

The academic relevance of creep is that it provides an indirect, though readily obtainable, measure of the interactions of collagen, proteoglycans and water in a ligament or capsule. By studying the creep of structures one can determine how these interactions vary with age or in the face of disease processes or injury. However, creep is not just a laboratory phenomenon, for it occurs regularly in activities of daily living.

Many occupational groups, e.g. stonemasons, bricklayers, roofing carpenters and the like, regularly submit their lumbar spines to prolonged load-bearing in flexion. Once they achieve such a posture there is often little movement away from it, and their lumbar joints will creep. The possible significance of this phenomenon is discussed below in the section on 'hysteresis'.

HYSTERESIS

Most structures, and certainly all biological tissues, exhibit differences in mechanical behaviour during loading versus unloading. Loading produces a characteristic stress-strain curve, but gradual release of the load produces a different stress-strain curve. Restoration of the initial length of a ligament occurs at a lesser rate and to a lesser extent than did deformation (Fig. 6.9). This difference in behaviour is referred to as **hysteresis**, and reflects the amount of energy lost when the structure was initially stressed.

When a structure is deformed the energy applied to it goes into deforming the structure and into straining the bonds within it. For collagenous tissues, some of the energy goes into displacing proteoglycans and water, re-arranging the collagen fibres, and perhaps even into breaking some of the bonds between collagen fibres. Once used in this way, this energy is not immediately available to restore the structure to its original shape. Displaced water, for example, does not remain in the structure exerting some

STRESS

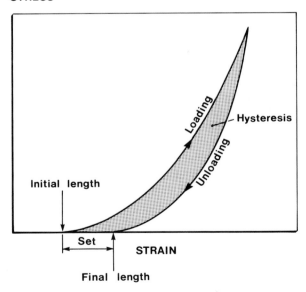

Fig. 6.9 Stress-strain curve illustrating hysteresis. When unloaded, a structure regains shape at a rate different to that at which it deformed. Any difference between the initial and final shape is the 'set'.

sort of back-pressure attempting to restore its original form. It is squeezed out of the structure, and the energy used to displace the water is no longer available to the system. If chemical bonds are broken, they cannot act to restore the form of the structure.

Thus, with less energy available to restore the structure, the rate and extent of its restoration is reduced. When all applied forces are completely removed, the final length of the ligament or capsule may remain greater than its original length (or less in the case of compressed structures). This difference between initial and final length is referred to as a 'set'.

In general, hysteresis and a residual set do not occur if a structure is stressed only in the toe phase of its stress-strain curve for bonds within and between the collagen fibres are not broken. However, the further a structure is stressed beyond its toe phase, more bonds are broken and the greater the hysteresis and set.[1]

In time, collagen fibres and proteoglycans in a structure may be re-arranged into their usual configuration, and any displaced water is eventually reabsorbed, restoring the structure to its original form. Under these circumstances any set disappears, and the structure regains its original size.

A set often occurs after creep. When the applied force is released the structure does not immediately spring back to its original shape, although it may do so in time. However, if bonds between or within collagen fibres have been broken, the set may not disappear until and unless the bonds are exactly reconstituted. If the original bonds are not reformed, or if new bonds are formed in the set position, the set may persist indefinitely.

This phenomenon has implications in the interpretation of trauma to ligaments or capsules. The energy lost in breaking the tissue may not be recoverable, and the original structure is not fully reformed. Healing may occur in a set position, and this may compromise the mechanical function of the structure. Healing in a set position effectively lengthens the ligament, and it will therefore accommodate greater than normal initial ranges of movement, which may not be desirable.

The phenomena of creep and hysteresis are also of particular relevance to the interpretation of sustained insults to ligaments and capsules. A ligament may be subjected to forces well within its load-bearing capacity, but if these forces are sustained for prolonged periods, the ligament will creep, and because of hysteresis, eventual release of the load does not result in the immediate restoration of the form and microstructure of the ligament. The ligament requires time to reform fully. In the meantime, the mechanical properties of the ligament have been altered. Its stress-strain capacity is different from normal, and until the structure is fully reformed it cannot be expected to sustain re-applied loads in the normal, or accustomed, way. Therefore, the structure may be liable to injury during this vulnerable period of restoration.

Such processes may underlie what might otherwise be called 'fatigue' in a ligament or capsule. After prolonged strain, ligaments, capsules and intervertebral discs of the lumbar spine may creep, and they may be liable to injury if sudden forces are unexpectedly applied during their vulnerable, recovery phase.

FORCES AND MOMENTS

When an object is free to move and is acted upon by a force it will accelerate in the same direction as the applied force (Fig. 6.10). The force (F) is related to the acceleration (a) by the equation

$$F = ma$$

where m is the mass of the object in kilograms. In the metre-kilogram-second system the unit of force is a newton (N) and has the dimensions of kilogram metres per second squared ($kg.m.sec^{-2}$).

For an object in the Earth's field of gravity, its weight is produced by the force of gravity trying to accelerate it towards the centre of the Earth (Fig. 6.10). The mass of the object (m) is related to its weight by the acceleration produced by the Earth's gravitational field, i.e.

$$Weight = F = mg$$

where g equals $9.8 \ m.sec^{-2}$. An object in the Earth's gravitational field therefore exerts a

A

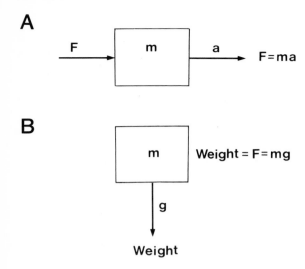

B

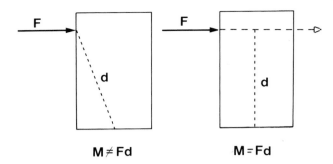

Fig. 6.12 Moments are calculated not using the distance between the fixed point and the site of application of the force but the perpendicular distance between the fixed point and the direction of the force.

Fig. 6.10 The nature of forces. **A**: A force (F) acting on a mass (m) imparts an acceleration (a) on the mass in the same direction as the force. **B**: When gravity acts downwards on an object the force it exerts is the weight of the object which is proportional to its mass (m) and the gravitational acceleration of the Earth (g).

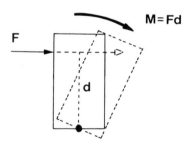

Fig. 6.11 The nature of moments. When a force acts eccentrically on an object that is fixed at some point, the force tends to bend or rotate the object. This bending effect is a moment (M) whose magnitude is proportional to the magnitude of the force (F) and the perpendicular distance (d) between the fixed point and the direction of the force.

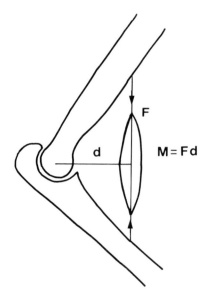

Fig. 6.13 Muscles exert moments on joints that they move. The magnitude of the moment (M) is proportional to the force (F) exerted by the muscle and the perpendicular distance (d) between the line of action of the muscle and the axis of rotation of the joint.

downward force whose magnitude in newtons is about ten times its mass measured in kilograms.

If an object is acted upon by a force but is fixed at some point, the object is not free to move in the direction of the applied force. Instead, it will tend to bend or rotate about the fixed point (Fig. 6.11). A force that causes bending is known as a **moment**, and its magnitude is proportional to both the magnitude of the force applied and the perpendicular distance between the line of force and the fixed point, i.e.

$$\text{Moment} = Fd$$

The unit of measure of a moment is newton-metres whose dimensions are $kg.m^2.sec^{-2}$.

Intuitively it should be obvious that the bending capacity of a moment will be greater either if the force aplied is greater or if the distance from the fixed point is greater. (Compare the effort required to bend a short object versus a longer object of the same material.)

It is critical to appreciate that a moment is not calculated according to the distance between the fixed point and the point on the object at which the force is applied. It is calculated according to the perpendicular distance between the fixed

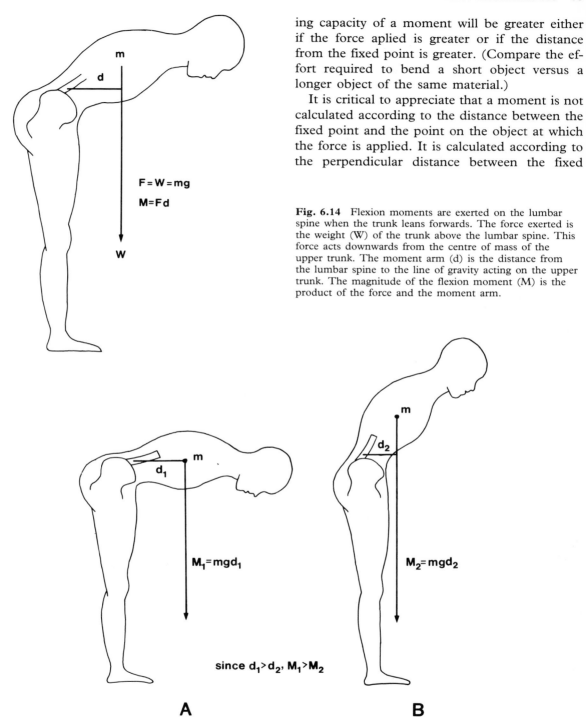

Fig. 6.14 Flexion moments are exerted on the lumbar spine when the trunk leans forwards. The force exerted is the weight (W) of the trunk above the lumbar spine. This force acts downwards from the centre of mass of the upper trunk. The moment arm (d) is the distance from the lumbar spine to the line of gravity acting on the upper trunk. The magnitude of the flexion moment (M) is the product of the force and the moment arm.

$F = W = mg$

$M = Fd$

W

m

d

$M_1 = mgd_1$

d_1

m

$M_2 = mgd_2$

d_2

m

since $d_1 > d_2$, $M_1 > M_2$

A

B

Fig. 6.15 Different angles of flexion of the trunk result in moments of different magnitude being applied to the lumbar spine. Even though the mass of the trunk (m) remains the same, different moments result from differences in the moment arms (d) that occur.

point and the **direction** of the force (Fig. 6.12). This distance is referred to as the **moment arm**.

The concept of moments applies to all situations where joints bend whether they are acted upon by muscles or by gravity. The moment generated by a muscle is the product of the force exerted by the muscle and the perpendicular distance between the axis of rotation of the joint and the line of action of the muscle (Fig. 6.13). In the case of the vertebral column, movements such as flexion are frequently exerted by gravity. The force involved is the weight of the trunk leaning forwards of the lumbar spine and is ex-

erted vertically downwards on the centre of mass of the trunk (Fig. 6.14). The magnitude of the force acting on a given joint in the lumbar spine is calculated as the mass of the trunk above that joint multiplied by **g**. The moment arm is the perpendicular distance from the joint in question to the line of action of the force (Fig. 6.14). Clearly, the further a subject leans forward the longer this moment arm and the greater the resultant moment. Conversely, the more upright a subject stands the shorter the moment arm and the smaller the flexion moment (Fig. 6.15).

7. Movements of the lumbar spine

The principal movements exhibited by the lumbar spine and its individual joints are axial compression, axial distraction, flexion, extension, axial rotation, and lateral flexion. Horizontal translation does not naturally occur as an isolated, pure movement, but is involved in axial rotation.

AXIAL COMPRESSION

Axial compression is the movement that occurs during weight-bearing in the upright posture. With respect to the inter-body joints, the weight-bearing mechanisms of the intervertebral discs have already been described in Chapter 2, where it was explained how the nucleus pulposus and anulus fibrosus co-operate to transmit weight from one vertebra to the next. It is now appropriate to add further details, relating in particular to the behaviour of other elements of the lumbar spine in weight-bearing.

During axial compression both the anulus fibrosus and nucleus pulposus bear the load and transmit it to the vertebral end-plates (Ch. 2). Biomechanical studies have shown that the load is evenly distributed over the end-plate, there being no greater load over the nucleus pulposus than over the anulus fibrosus.[257] However, other studies reveal that with the application of excessive loads to normal intervertebral discs, end-plates tend to fracture in their central region, i.e. over the nucleus pulposus, rather than over the anulus.[76,276,443,558] This suggests either that the central portion of the end-plate does bear greater loads, or that this portion is weaker than the peripheral parts of the end-plate. With the application of very great loads, the entire end-plate may fracture.[443,536,558]

In this context, it is noteworthy that the end-plates are the weakest components of the intervertebral disc in the face of axial compression. During static (slow) loading of a disc, nuclear pressure rises and acts on the anulus fibrosus and the end-plates. The anulus bulges radially while the end-plates tend to bow towards the vertebral bodies.[240,468] Provided the anulus is healthy and intact, increasing the load causes one or other of the end-plates to fail, by fracturing, sooner than the anulus fibrosus fails, by rupturing.[76,443,558] This phenomenon has particular ramifications in the pathology of compression injuries of the lumbar spine and disc degeneration (see Ch. 14), and has its basis in the relative strengths of the anulus fibrosus and the bone of the vertebral body.

The resistance of an end-plate to fracture depends on the strength of the subchondral and cancellous bone beneath it. If the underlying bone cannot sustain the pressure exerted on the end-plate the end-plate will give way and fracture. In this regard, calculations have shown that the anulus fibrosus can withstand a pressure of 3.2×10^7 Nm^{-2}, but cancellous none yields at 3.4×10^6 Nm^{-2}.[240] Consequently, end-plates would be expected to fail sooner than the anulus fibrosus when the disc is subjected to axial compression.

With respect to the vertebral bodies, experiments have shown that in adults under the age of 40, between 25–55% of the weight applied to a vertebral body is borne by the trabecular bone.[470] The rest is borne by the cortical shell.

65

In older individuals this proportion changes, for reasons explained in Chapter 12.

Another factor that increases the load-bearing capacity of the vertebral body is the blood within its marrow spaces and intra-osseous veins (see Ch. 10). Compression of the vertebral body and bulging of the end-plates causes blood to be extruded from the vertebra.[468] Because this process requires energy, it buffers the vertebral body, to some extent, from the compressive loads applied to it.[558]

During axial compression, particularly with sustained loading, water is squeezed out of the intervertebral discs[76,468,552] and various calculations and experiments have shown that the amount of water loss is between 5–11%.[240,311,539] This water loss underlies the creep characterisitcs of the intervertebral discs during axial compression.

During compression, intervertebral discs undergo an inital period of rapid creep, deforming about 1.5 mm in the first 2–10 minutes, depending on the size of the applied load.[285,286,358] Subsequently, a much slower but definite creep continues at about 1 mm per hour.[358] Depending on age, a plateau is attained by about 90 minutes, beyond which no further creep occurs.[286]

Creep underlies the variation in height changes undergone by individuals during activities of daily living. Over a 16 hour day, the pressure sustained by intervertebral discs during walking and sitting causes loss of fluid from the discs which results in a 10% loss in disc height.[539] Given that intervertebral discs account for just under a quarter of the height of the vertebral column, the 10% fluid loss results in individuals being 1–2% shorter at the end of a day.[452,538] This height is restored during sleep or reclined rest, when the vertebral column is not axially compressed and the discs are rehydrated by the osmotic pressue of the disc proteoglycans.[539] Moreover, it has been demonstrated that rest in the supine position with the lower limbs flexed and raised brings about a more rapid return to full disc height than does rest in the extended supine position.[538]

The pressure within intervertebral discs can be measured using special needles,[386,390,391] and disc pressure measurement, or discometry, provides an index of the stresses applied to a disc in various postures and movements. Several studies have addressed this issue, although for technical reasons, virtually all have studied only the L3–4 disc.

In the upright standing posture, the load on the disc is about 70 kPa.[390] Holding a weight of 5 kg in this posture raises the disc pressure to about 700 kPa.[22,390] The changes in disc pressure during other movements and manœuvres is described in Chapter 8.

Although the interbody joints are designed as the principal weight-bearing components of the lumbar spine (Ch. 2), there has been much interest in the role that the zygapophysial joints play in weight-bearing. The earliest studies in this regard provided indirect estimates of the load borne by the zygapophysial joints based on measurements of intra-discal pressure, and it was reported that the zygapophysial joints carried approximately 20% of the vertical load applied to an intervertebral joint.[386] This conclusion, however, was later retracted.[387]

Subsequent studies have variously reported that the zygapophysial joints can bear 28%[339] or 40%[224] of a vertically applied load. To the contrary, others have reported that 'compression did not load the facet joints. . .very much',[376] and that 'provided the lumbar spine is slightly flattened. . .all the intervertebral compressive force is resisted by the disc'.[9]

Reasons for these differences in conclusions relate to the experimental techniques used and to the differing appreciation of the anatomy of the zygapophysial joints and their behaviour in axial compression.

Although the articular surfaces of the lumbar zygapophysial joints are curved in the transverse plane (Ch. 3), in the sagittal and coronal planes they run straight up and down (although see Ch. 11). Thus, zygapophysial joints, in a neutral position, cannot sustain vertically applied loads. Their articular surfaces run parallel to one another and parallel to the direction of the applied load. If an intervertebral joint is axially compressed, the articular surfaces of the zygapophysial joints will simply slide past one another. For the zygapophysial joints to participate in weight-bearing in erect standing, some aberration in their orientation must occur, and either

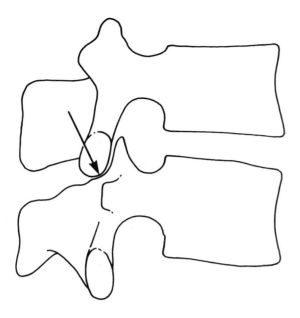

Fig. 7.1 When a vertebra rocks backwards, its inferior articular processes impact the lower face of the superior articular processes of the vertebra below.

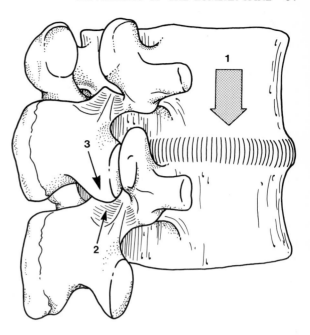

Fig. 7.2 If an intervertebral joint is compressed (1), the inferior articular processes of the upper vertebra impact the lamina below (2), allowing weight to be transmitted through the inferior articular processes (3).

of two mechanisms may operate singly or in combination to recruit the zygapophysial joints into weight-bearing.

If a vertebra is caused to rock backwards on its intervertebral disc without also being allowed to slide backwards, the tips of its inferior articular processes will be driven into the superior articular facets of the vertebra below (Fig. 7.1). Axial compression of the intervertebral joint will then result in some of the load being transmitted through the region of impaction of the zygapophysial joints. By rocking a pair of lumbar vertebrae one can readily determine by inspection that the site of impaction in the zygapophysial joints falls on the inferior medial portion of the facets. Formal experiments have shown this to be the site where maximal pressure is detected in the zygapophysial joints of vertebra loaded in extension.[136]

Another mechanism does not involve the zygapophysial joint surfaces but rather, the tips of the inferior articular processes. With severe, or sustained, axial compression intervertebral discs may be narrowed to the extent that the inferior articular processes of the upper vertebra are lowered until their tips impact the lamina of the

vertebra below (Fig. 7.2). Alternatively, this same impact may occur if an intervertebral joint is axially compressed while also tilted backwards, as is the case in a lordotic lumbar spine bearing weight.[6,136,572] Axial loads can then be transmitted through the inferior articular processes to the lamina.

It has been shown that under the conditions of erect sitting the zygapophysial joints are not impacted and bear none of the vertical load on the intervertebral joint; but in prolonged standingwith a lordotic spine, the impacted joints at each segmental level bear an average of some 16% of the axial load.[6,9] In this regard, the lower joints (L3–4, L4–5, L5–S1) bear a relatively greater proportion (19%), while the upper joints (L1–2, L2–3) bear less (11%).[6] Other studies have shown that the actual load borne by impaction of inferior articular processes varies from 3–18% of the applied load, and critically depends on the tilt of the intervertebral joint.[572] It has also been estimated that pathological disc space narrowing can result in some 70% of the axial load being borne by the inferior articular processes and laminae.[9]

It is thus evident that weight-bearing occurs through the zygapophysial joints only if the inferior articular processes impact either the superior articular facets or the lamina of the vertebra below. Variations in the degree of such impactions account for the variations in the estimates of the axial load carried by the zygapophysial joints,[572] and why the highest estimates of the load borne are reported in studies in which the intervertebral joints have been loaded in the extended position.[224,330,339,357,450]

Although the preceding account of axial compression emphasises the role of the discs and zygapophysial joints in weight-bearing, other components of the lumbar spine also participate. The shape of the lordotic lumbar spine allows the anterior longitudinal ligament and the anterior portions of the anuli fibrosi to be involved in weight-bearing. Because of the curvature of the lordosis, the posterior parts of the intervertebral discs and the zygapophysial joints are compressed, but the anterior ligaments are stretched. Axial loading of a lordotic spine tends to accentuate the lordosis and, therefore, increase the strain in the anterior ligaments. By increasing their tension, the anterior ligaments can resist this accentuation and share in the load-bearing.

In this way, the lordosis of the lumbar spine provides an axial load-bearing mechanism additional to those available in the intervertebral discs and the zygapophysial joints. Moreover, as described in Chapter 5, the tensile mechanism of the anterior ligaments imparts a resilience to the lumbar spine. The energy delivered to the ligaments is stored in them as tension, and can be used to restore the curvature of the lumbar spine to its original form, once the axial load is removed.

AXIAL DISTRACTION

Compared to axial compression and other movements of the lumbar spine, axial distraction has been studied far less. One study provided data on the stress-strain and stiffness characteristics of lumbar intervertebral discs, and revealed that the discs are not as stiff in distraction as in compres-

sion.[357] This is understandable, for the discs are designed principally for weight-bearing and would be expected to resist compression more than tension. In a biological sense, this correlates with the fact that humans spend far more time bearing compressive loads — in walking, standing and sitting — than sustaining tensile loads, as might occur in brachiating (tree-climbing) animals.

The other study that has focused on individual elements of the lumbar intervertebral joints examined the tensile properties of the zygapophysial joint capsules. In this study,[114] zygapophysial joints were subjected to longitudinal (axial) tensions and their capsules were found to be remarkably strong, to the extent that, if necessary, they could bear twice the body weight. The ramification of this study does not lie in the role of zygapophysial joints in axial distraction, but rather, in the capacity of zygapophysial joint capsules to resist anterior sagittal rotation, or flexion, of the lumbar spine. This is described in a later section below.

There has been one study[529] that has described the behaviour of the whole (cadaveric) lumbar spine during sustained axial distraction (traction). Application of a 9 kg weight to stretch the lumbar spine resulted in an initial mean lengthening of 7.5 mm. Lengthening was greater (9 mm) in lumbar spines of young subjects, and less in the middle aged (5.5 mm) and the elderly (7.5 mm). Sustained traction over 30 minutes resulted in a creep of a further 1.5 mm. Removal of the load revealed an immediate 'set' of about 2.5 mm which reduced to only 0.5 mm by 30 minutes after removal of the load. Younger spines demonstrated a more rapid creep and did not show a residual 'set'. The amount of distraction was greater in spines with healthy discs (11–12 mm) and substantially less (3–5 mm) in spines with degenerated discs.

Some 40% of the lengthening of the lumbar spine occurred as a result of flattening of the lumbar lordosis, with 60% due to actual separation of the vertebral bodies. The major implication of this observation is that the extent of distraction achieved by traction (using a 9 kg load) is not great. It amounts to 60% of 7.5 mm of actual vertebral separation, which is equivalent to about

0.9 mm per intervertebral joint. This revelation seriously compromises those theories that maintain that lumbar traction exerts a beneficial effect by 'sucking back' disc herniations, and it is suggested that other mechanisms of the therapeutic effect of traction be considered.[529]

The other implication of this study relates to the fact that the residual 'set' after sustained traction is quite small (0.5 mm), amounting to about 0.1 mm per intervertebral joint. Moreover, this is the residual 'set' in spines not subsequently reloaded by body weight. One would expect that, in living patients, a 0.1 mm 'set' would naturally be obliterated the moment the patient rose and started to bear axial compression. Thus, any effect achieved by therapeutic traction must be phasic, i.e. occurring during the application of traction; and not due to some maintained lengthening of the lumbar spine.

FLEXION

During flexion, the entire lumbar spine leans forwards (Fig. 7.3). This is achieved basically by the 'unfolding' or straightening of the lumbar lordosis. At the full range of forward flexion the lumbar spine assumes a straight alignment or is curved slightly forwards, tending to reverse the curvature of the original lordosis (Fig. 7.3). The reversal occurs principally at upper lumbar levels. Reversal may occur at the L4–5 level, but does not occur at the L5–S1 level.[430,433] Forward flexion is, therefore, achieved for the most part by each of the lumbar vertebrae rotating from their backward tilted position in the upright lordosis to a neutral position, in which the upper and lower surfaces of adjacent vertebral bodies are parallel to one another. This relieves the posterior compression of the intervertebral discs and zygapophysial joints, present in the upright lordotic lumbar spine. Some additional range of movement is achieved by the upper lumbar vertebrae rotating further forwards and compressing their intervertebral discs anteriorly.

It may appear that during flexion of the lumbar spine, the movement undergone by each vertebral body is simply anterior sagittal rotation. However, there is a concomitant component of forward translation as well.[433,532] If a vertebra

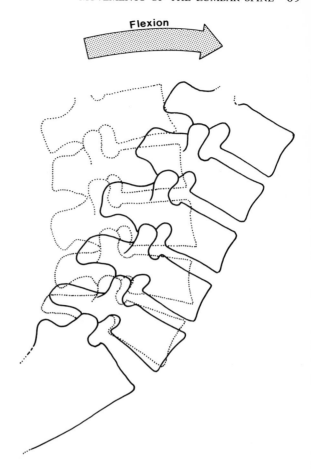

Fig. 7.3 During flexion, the lumbar lordosis unfolds and the lumbar spine straightens and leans forwards on the sacrum. The curvature of the lordosis may be reversed at upper lumbar levels, but not at L5–S1.

rocks forwards over its intervertebral disc, its inferior articular processes are raised upwards and slightly backwards (Fig. 7.4A). This opens a small gap between each inferior articular facet and the superior articular facet in the zygapophysial joint. As the lumbar spine leans forwards, gravity or muscular action causes the vertebrae to slide forwards, and this motion closes the gap between the facets in the zygapophysial joints (Fig. 7.4B). Furhter forward translation will be arrested once impaction of the zygapophysial joints is re-established, but nonetheless a small forward translation will have occurred. At each intervertebral joint, therefore,

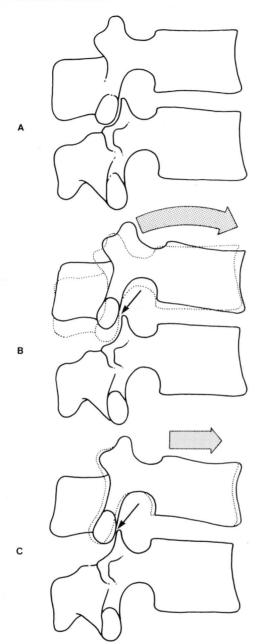

Fig. 7.4 The components of flexion of a lumbar intervertebral joint. **A**: The lateral parts of the right superior articular process have been cut away to reveal the contact between the inferior and superior articular facets in the neutral position. **B**: Sagittal rotation causes the inferior articular processes to lift upwards, leaving a gap between them and the superior articular facets. This gap allows for anterior sagittal translation. **C**: Upon translation, the inferior articular facets once again impact the superior articular facets.

flexion involves a combination of anterior sagittal rotation and a small amplitude anterior translation.

The zygapophysial joints play a major role in maintaining the stability of the spine in flexion, and much attention has been directed in recent years to the mechanisms involved. To appreciate these mechanisms, it is important to recognise that flexion involves both anterior sagittal rotation and anterior sagittal translation, for these two components are resisted and stabilised in different ways by the zygapophysial joints.

Anterior sagittal translation is resisted by the direct impaction of the inferior articular facets of a vertebra against the superior articular facets of the vertebra below, and this process has been fully described in Chapter 3. This mechanism becomes increasingly important the further the lumbar spine leans forward, for with a greater forward inclination of the lumbar spine, the upper surfaces of the lumbar vertebral bodies are inclined dowards (Fig. 7.5), and there will be a tendency for the vertebrae above to slide down this inclination. The force generating this movement is gravity, and it exerts a forward shear on the intervertebral joint. A primary role of the zygapophysial joints is to resist this forward shear, and thereby maintain stability of the lumbar spine as it leans forwards.

The cardinal ramification of the anatomy of the zygapophysial joints with respect to forward shear is that in joints with flat articular surfaces, the load will be borne evenly across the entire articular surface (Ch. 3), but in joints with curved articular surfaces, the load is concentrated on the anteromedial portions of the superior and inferior articular facets (Ch. 3). Formal experiments have shown that during flexion, the highest pressures are recorded at the medial end of the lumbar zygapophysial joints,[136] and this has further bearing on the age changes seen in these joints (Ch. 12).

The anterior sagittal rotation component of flexion is resisted by the zygapophysial joints in a different way. The mechanism involves tension in the joint capsule. Flexion involves an upward sliding movement of each inferior articular process, in relation to the superior articular process, in each zygapophysial joint, and the amplitude of this movement is about 5–7 mm.[329] This move-

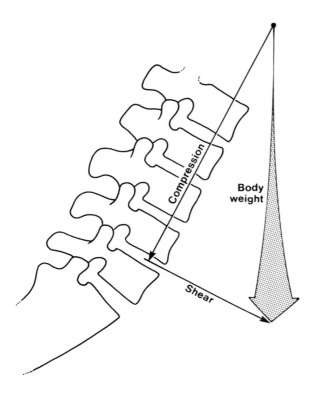

Fig. 7.5 When the lumbar spine is flexed, the weight of the trunk exerts compressive and shearing forces on the intervertebral joints that are proportional to the angle of inclination of the inter-body joint.

ment will tense the joint capsule, and in this regard the tensile strength of the capsule, acting as a ligament, has been measured as 600 N.[9,114]

The other elements that resist the anterior sagittal rotation of flexion are the ligaments of the intervertebral joints. Anterior sagittal rotation results in the separation of the spinous processes and laminae. Consequently, the supraspinous and interspinous ligaments and the ligamenta flava will be tensed, and various types of experiments have been performed to determine the relative contributions of these structures to the resistance of flexion. The experiments have involved either studying the range of motion in cadavers in which various ligaments have been sequentially severed,[532] or determining mathematically the stresses applied to different ligaments on the basis of the separation of their attachments during different phases of flexion.[11]

In young adult specimens, sectioning the supraspinous and interspinous ligaments and ligamenta flava results in an increase of about 5° in the range of flexion.[532] (Lesser increases occur in older specimens, but this difference is discussed in Chapter 12.) Sectioning the zygapophysial joint capsules results in a further 4° of flexion. Transecting the pedicles, to remove the bony locking mechanism of the zygapophysial joints, results in a further 15° increase in range.

In a sense, these observations suggest the relative contributions of various structures to the resistance of flexion. The similar increases in range following the transection of ligaments and capsules suggests that the posterior ligaments and the zygapophysial joint capsules contribute about equally, but their contribution is overshadowed by that of the bony locking mechanism, whose elimination results in a major increase in range of movement. However, such conclusions should be made with caution, for the experiments on which they are based involved sequential sectioning of structures. They do not reveal the simultaneous contributions of various structures, nor possible variations in the contribution by different structures at different phases of movement. Nevertheless, the role of the bony locking mechanism in the stability of the flexed lumbar spine is strikingly demonstrated.

To determine the simultaneous contribution by various structures to the resistance of flexion, mathematical analyses have been performed.[11] The results indicate that in a typical lumbar intervertebral joint, the intervertebral disc contributes about 29% of the resistance, the supraspinous and interspinous ligaments about 19%, the ligamentum flavum about 13%, and the capsules of the zygapophysial joints about 39%. It is emphasised that these figures relate only to the resistance of anterior sagittal rotation, which is the movement that tenses these ligaments. They do not relate to the role played by the bony locking mechanism in preventing anterior translation during flexion.

EXTENSION

In principle, extension movements of the lumbar intervertebral joints are the converse of those that

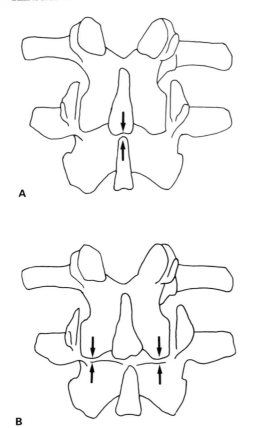

Fig. 7.6 Factors limiting extension. **A**: Posterior sagittal rotation is usually limited by impaction of the tip of an inferior articular process on the underlying lamina. **B**: If impaction occurs unilaterally, any continued extension is transformed into a backwards axial rotation about the impacted joint.

occur in flexion. Basically, the vertebral bodies undergo posterior sagittal rotation and a small posterior translation. However, certain differences are involved because of the structure of the lumbar vertebrae. During flexion, the inferior articular processes are free to move upwards until their movement is resisted by ligamentous and capsular tension. Extension, on the other hand, involves downward movement of the inferior articular processes and the spinous processes, and this movement is limited not by ligamentous tension but by bony impaction.

Bony impaction usually occurs between the spinous processes.[5] As a vertebra extends its spi-

nous process approaches the next lower spinous process. The first limit to extension occurs as the interspinous ligament buckles and becomes trapped between the spinous processes. Further extension is met with further compression of this ligament until the spinous processes virtually come into contact[5] (Fig. 7.6A).

In individuals with wide interspinous spaces, extension may be limited before spinous processes come into contact.[5] Impaction occurs between the tip of one or other of the inferior articular processes of the moving vertebra and the subjacent lamina (Fig. 7.6B). This type of impaction is accentuated when the joint is subjected to the action of the back muscles[14] for in addition to extending the lumbar spine, the back muscles also exert a substantial compression load on it (see Ch. 8). Consequently, during active extension the inferior articular processes are drawn not only into posterior sagittal rotation but also downwards as the entire intervertebral joint is compressed. Under these circumstances the zygapophysial joints become weight-bearing, as explained above (see *Axial compression*).

AXIAL ROTATION

Axial rotation of the lumbar spine involves twisting, or torsion, of the intervertebral discs and impaction of zygapophysial joints, and several studies have addressed the mechanics of discs and zygapophysial joints in rotation and their relative contributions to resistance of this motion.

During axial rotation of an intervertebral joint, all the fibres of the anulus fibrosus that are inclined toward the direction of rotation will be strained. The other half will be relaxed (Ch. 2). Based on the observation that elongation of collagen beyond about 4% of resting length leads to injury of the fibre (Ch. 6), it can be calculated that the maximum range of rotation of an intervertebral disc without injury is about 3°.[240] Beyond this range the collagen fibre will begin to undergo micro-injury.

Experiments on lumbar intervertebral discs have shown that they resist torsion more strongly than bending movements, and the stress-strain curves for torsion rise very steeply in the range 0° to 3° of rotation.[357] Very large forces have to

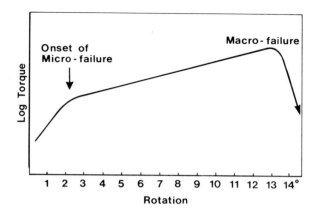

Fig. 7.7 Stress-strain curve for torsion of the intervertebral disc. (Based on Farfan et al.[170])

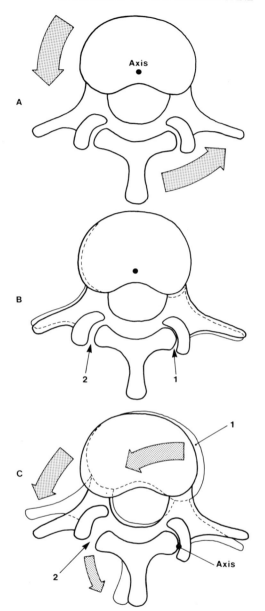

be applied to strain the disc beyond 3° and isolated discs (the posterior elements having being removed) fail macroscopically at about 12° of rotation.[170] Prima facie, this suggests that 12° is the ultimate range for rotation before disc failure occurs, but this relates to overt macroscopic failure. Analysis of the stress-strain curves for intervertebral discs under torsion (Fig. 7.7) reveals an inflection point just before 3° of rotation, which indicates the onset of microscopic failure in the anulus fibrosus.[170] The range between 3° and 12° represents continued micro-failure until overt failure occurs.

In an intact intervertebral joint, the zygapophysial joints, and to a certain extent the posterior ligaments, protect the intervertebral disc from excessive torsion. Because the axis of rotation of a lumbar vertebra passes through the posterior part of the vertebral body,[100] all the posterior elements of the moving vertebra will swing around this axis during axial rotation. As the spinous process moves, the attachments of the supraspinous and interspinous ligaments will be separated, and these ligaments will be placed under tension. Furthermore, one of the inferior articular facets of the upper vertebra will be impacted against its apposing superior articular facet (Fig. 7.8). In the case of left axial rotation it will be the right inferior articular facet that impacts (and vice versa). Once this impaction occurs normal axial rotation is arrested.

Because the joint space of the zygapophysial

Fig. 7.8 The mechanism of left axial rotation of a lumbar intervertebral joint. Two consecutive vertebrae, superimposed on one another, are viewed from above. The upper vertebra is depicted by a dotted line. **A**: Initially, rotation occurs about an axis in the vertebral body. **B**: As the posterior elements swing around, the right inferior articular process of the upper vertebra impacts the superior articular process of the lower vertebra (1). The opposite zygapophysial joint is gapped (2). **C**: Rotation beyond 3° occurs about an axis located in the impacted zygapophysial joint. The intervertebral disc must undergo lateral shear (1), and the opposite zygapophysial joint is gapped and distracted posteriorly (2).

joint is quite narrow, the range of movement before impaction occurs is quite small. Such movement as does occur is accommodated by compression of the articular cartilages which are able to sustain compression because their principal constituents are proteoglycans and water. Water is simply squeezed out of the cartilages, and is gradually re-absorbed when the compression is released.

Given that the distance between a zygapophysial joint and the axis of rotation is about 30 mm, it can be calculated that about 0.5 mm of compression must occur for every 1° of axial rotation. Furthermore, given that the articular cartilages of a lumbar zygapophysial joint are about 2 mm thick (Ch. 3), and that articular cartilage is about 75% water,[225] it can be calculated that to accommodate 3° of rotation, the cartilages must be compressed to about 62% of their resting thickness and must lose more than half of their water. The zygapophysial joints, therefore, provide a substantial buffer during the first 3° of rotation, and the zygapophysial joint must be severely compressed before rotation exceeds the critical range of 3°, beyond which the anulus fibrosus risks torsional injury. Nevertheless, if sufficiently strong forces are applied, rotation can proceed beyond 3°, but then an 'impure' form of rotation occurs as the result of distortion of other elements in the intervertebral joint.

To rotate beyond 3°, the upper vertebra must pivot on the impacted joint, and this joint becomes the site of a new axis of rotation. Both the vertebral body and the opposite inferior articular process will then swing around this new axis. The vertebral body swings laterally and backwards, and the opposite inferior articular process swings backwards and medially (Fig. 7.8C). The sideways movement of the vertebral body will exert a lateral shear on the underlying disc[100,170] which will be additional to any torsional stress already applied to the disc by the earlier rotation. The backward movement of the opposite inferior articular process will strain the capsule of its zygapophysial joint.

During this complex combination of forces and movements, the impacted zygapophysial joint is being strained by compression, the intervertebral disc is strained by torsion and lateral shear, and

the capsule of the opposite zygapophysial joint is being stretched. Failure of any one of these elements can occur if the rotatory force is sufficiently strong, and this underlies the mechanism of torsional injury to the lumbar spine (Ch. 14).

The relative contributions of various structures to the resistance of axial rotation have been determined experimentally, and it is evident that the roles played by the supraspinous and interspinous ligaments, and by the capsule of the tensed (the opposite) zygapophysial joint are not great.[7] The load is borne principally by the impacted zygapophysial joint and the intervertebral disc. Quantitative analysis[170] reveals that the disc contributes 35% of the resistance to torsion, the remaining 65% being exerted by the posterior elements: the tensed zygapophysial joint, the supraspinous and interspinous ligaments, and principally the impacted zygapophysial joint.

LATERAL FLEXION

Lateral flexion of the lumbar spine does not involve simple movements of the lumbar intervertebral joints. It involves a complex, and variable, combination of lateral bending and rotatory movements of the inter-body joints and diverse movements of the zygapophysial joints. Conspicuously, lateral flexion of the lumbar spine has not been subjected to detailed biomechanical analysis, probably because of its complexity, and the greater clinical relevance of sagittal plane movements and axial rotation. However, some aspects of the mechanics of lateral flexion are evident when the range of this movement is considered below.

RANGE OF MOVEMENT

The range of movement of the lumbar spine has been studied in a variety of ways. It has been measured in cadavers,[76,154,170,188,247,249,285,295,421, 467,471,552,557] and in living subjects using either clinical measurement[93,135,214,325,331,335,336,352, 378,379,498,501] or measurements taken from radiographs.[14,144,185,198,231,280,471,505,528,563] Studies of cadavers have the disadvantage that because of post-mortem changes and because cadavers are usually studied with the back musculature removed, the measurements obtained may not accurately reflect the mobility possible in living subjects. However, cadaveric studies have the advantage that motion can be directly and precisely measured and correlated with pathological changes determined by subsequent dissection or histological studies. Clinical studies have the advantage that they examine living subjects, but are limited by the accuracy of the instruments used and the reliability of identifying bony landmarks by palpation. Radiographic studies provide the most accurate measurements of living subjects, but for ethical reasons, they are difficult to perform on large numbers of asymptomatic patients to obtain normatative data.

The total range of motion of the lumbar spine in the sagittal plane and in axial rotation has been determined both in cadavers and in large numbers of living subjects[511] using a specially designed spondylometer.[530] The values obtained for different age groups and sexes are shown in Figures 7.9 and 7.10. In general, the range of sagittal plane movement in cadaveric lumbar spines is between 2° and 10° greater than in the living. The total range of axial rotation in cadavers is quite similar to that recorded in living subjects. Notwithstanding the mean values shown in Figure 7.9, the ranges of values in different age groups for both sagittal and horizontal plane movements are quite wide, although the maximum ranges and mean values decrease with age.

Total ranges of motion are not of any diagnostic value, for aberrations of total movement indicate neither the nature of any disease nor its location. However, total ranges of motion do provide an index of spinal function that reflects the biomechanical and biochemical properties of the lumbar spine. Consequently, their principal value lies in comparing different groups to determine the influence of such factors as age and degeneration, and this is explored later in Chapter 12.

Of greater potential diagnostic significance is the determination of ranges of movement for individual lumbar intervertebral joints, for if focal disease is to affect movement, it is more likely to

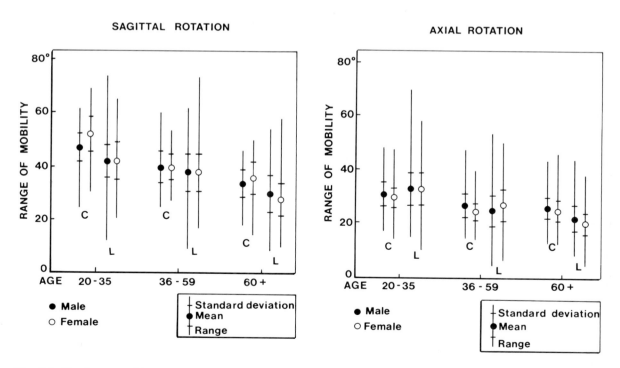

Fig. 7.9 Total ranges of lumbar spine motion in cadavers (C) and living (L) subjects. (Based on Twomey and Taylor.[532]).

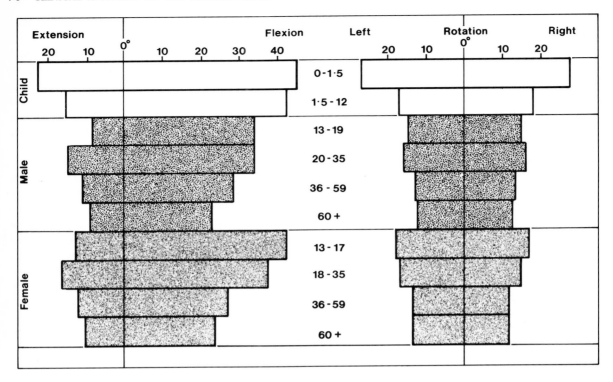

Fig. 7.10 Histograms showing ranges of lumbar spine motion in cadavers of both sexes and at all ages. (Based on Twomey and Taylor.[532]).

be manifest to a greater degree at the diseased segment than in the total range of motion of the lumbar spine.

In cadavers, the range of sagittal rotation of individual lumbar intervertebral joints shows a wide scatter,[243,245] (Fig. 7.11). Although the mean values show an increasing range of mobility from L1 to L5, with L4–5 and L5–S1 having the greatest range of motion in the sagittal plane, this pattern is exhibited by only a minority of patients.[243,245] Most specimens deviate from the pattern expressed by the mean values at at least one intervertebral level. As with total ranges of motion of the lumbar spine, the range of motion of individual segments decreases with age[243,245] (see Ch. 12).

Although there have been many radiographic studies of segmental ranges of motion in living subjects, these have now been superceded by the more accurate technique of biplanar radiography. Conventional radiography has the disadvantage

that it cannot quantify movements not in the plane being studied. Thus, while lateral radiographs can be used to detect movement in the sagittal plane, they do not demonstrate the extent of any simultaneous movements in the horizontal and coronal planes; but such simultaneous movements can affect the radiographic image in the sagittal plane and lead to errors in the measurement of sagittal plane movements.[50,430,433]

The technique of biplanar radiography overcomes this problem by taking radiographs simultaneously through two X-ray tubes arranged at right angles to one another. Analysis of the two simultaneously radiographs allows movements in all three planes to be detected and quantified, allowing a more accurate appraisal of the movements that occur in any one plane.[50,430,433]

There have been two principal results stemming from the use of biplanar radiography. These are the accurate quantification of segmental motion in living subjects, and the demonstration and

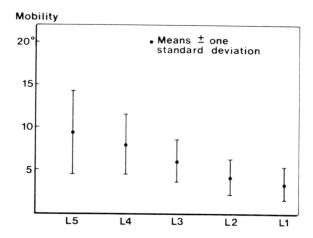

Fig. 7.11 Sagittal plane mobility of lumbar vertebrae in cadavers. (Based on Hilton et al.[245])

quantification of coupled movements.[186,430,432,433] The segmental ranges of motion in the sagittal plane (flexion and extension), horizontal plane (axial rotation) and coronal plane (lateral bending) are shown in Table 7.1. It is notable that, for the same age group and sex (25 to 36 year old males), the total range of sagittal rotation is considerably greater than that detected clinically with a spondylometer (Fig. 7.9). It is also notable that all lumbar joints have the same total range of motion in the sagittal plane, although the middle intervertebral joints have a relatively greater range of flexion, while the highest and lowest joints have a relatively greater range of extension.

As determined by biplanar radiography, the mean values of axial rotation are approximately equal at all levels (Table 7.1), and even the greatest values fall within the limit of 3° which from biomechanical evidence is the range at which micro-trauma to the intervertebral disc would occur. Conspicuously, the values obtained radiographically are noticeably smaller than those obtained both in cadavers and in living subjects using a spondylometer. The reasons for this discrepancy have not been investigated, but may be due to the inability of clinical measurements to discriminate primary and coupled movements.

Coupled movements are movements that occur in an unintended or unexpected direction during the execution of a desired motion, and biplanar radiography reveals the patterns of such movements in the lumbar spine. Table 7.2 shows the ranges of movements coupled with flexion and extension of the lumbar spine and Table 7.3 shows the movements coupled with axial rotation and lateral flexion.

Flexion of lumbar intervertebral joints consistently involves a combination of 8–13° of anterior sagittal rotation and 1–3 mm of forward translation, and these movements are consistently accompanied by axial and coronal rotations of about 1° (Table 7.2). Some vertical and lateral translations also occur but are of small amplitude. Reciprocally, extension involves posterior sagittal rotation and posterior translation, with some axial and coronal rotation, but little vertical or lateral translation (Table 7.2).

Axial rotation and lateral flexion are coupled with one another and with sagittal rotation (Table 7.3). Axial rotation is variably coupled with flexion and extension. Either flexion or extension

Table 7.1 Ranges of segmental motion in males aged 25 to 36 years (Based on Pearcy et al[433] and Pearcy and Tibrewal[432])

| | Mean range (measured in degress, with standard deviation) | | | | | | |
| | Lateral flexion | | Axial rotation | | Flexion | Extension | Flexion and extension |
Level	Left	Right	Left	Right			
L1–2	5	6	1	1	8 ± 5	5 ± 2	13 ± 5
L2–3	5	6	1	1	10 ± 2	3 ± 2	13 ± 2
L3–4	5	6	1	2	12 ± 1	1 ± 1	13 ± 2
L4–5	3	5	1	2	13 ± 4	2 ± 1	16 ± 4
L5–S1	0	2	1	0	9 ± 6	5 ± 4	14 ± 5

Table 7.2 Movements coupled with flexion and extension of the lumbar spine (Based on Pearcy et al[433])

Primary movement and level	Coupled movements					
	Mean (SD) rotations (degrees)			Mean (SD) translations (mm)		
	Sagittal	Coronal	Axial	Sagittal	Lateral	Vertical
Flexion						
L1	8 (5)	1 (1)	1 (1)	3 (1)	0 (1)	1 (1)
L2	10 (2)	1 (1)	1 (1)	2 (1)	1 (1)	1 (1)
L3	12 (1)	1 (1)	1 (1)	2 (1)	1 (1)	0 (1)
L4	13 (4)	2 (1)	1 (1)	2 (1)	0 (1)	0 (1)
L5	9 (6)	1 (1)	1 (1)	1 (1)	0 (1)	1 (1)
Extension						
L1	5 (2)	0 (1)	1 (1)	1 (1)	1 (1)	0 (0)
L2	3 (2)	0 (1)	1 (1)	1 (1)	0 (1)	0 (1)
L3	1 (1)	1 (1)	0 (1)	1 (1)	1 (1)	0 (1)
L4	2 (1)	1 (1)	1 (1)	1 (1)	0 (1)	1 (1)
L5	5 (4)	1 (1)	1 (1)	1 (1)	1 (1)	0 (0)

Table 7.3 Coupled movements of the lumbar spine (Based on Pearcy and Tibrewal[432])

Primary movement and level	Coupled movements					
	Axial rotation degrees (+ve to left)		Flexion/Extension degrees (+ve flexion)		Lateral flexion degrees (+ve to left)	
	mean	range	mean	range	mean	range
Right Rotation						
L1	−1	(−2 to 1)	0	(−3 to 3)	3	(−1 to 5)
L2	−1	(−2 to 1)	0	(−2 to 2)	4	(1 to 9)
L3	−1	(−3 to 0)	0	(−2 to 2)	3	(1 to 6)
L4	−1	(−2 to 1)	0	(−9 to 5)	1	(−3 to 3)
L5	−1	(−2 to 0)	0	(−5 to 3)	−2	(−7 to 0)
Left Rotation						
L1	1	(−1 to 2)	0	(−4 to 4)	−3	(−7 to −1)
L2	1	(−1 to 2)	0	(−4 to 4)	−3	(−5 to 0)
L3	2	(0 to 4)	0	(−3 to 2)	−3	(−6 to 0)
L4	2	(0 to 3)	0	(−7 to 2)	−2	(−5 to 1)
L5	0	(−2 to 2)	0	(−5 to 3)	1	(−0 to 2)
Right Lateral Flexion						
L1	0	(−3 to 2)	−2	(−5 to 1)	−5	(−8 to −2)
L2	1	(−1 to 4)	−1	(−3 to 1)	−5	(−8 to −4)
L3	1	(−1 to 3)	−1	(−3 to 1)	−5	(−11 to 2)
L4	1	(0 to 3)	0	(−1 to 4)	−3	(−5 to 1)
L5	0	(−1 to 2)	2	(−3 to 8)	0	(−2 to 3)
Left Lateral Flexion						
L1	0	(−2 to 2)	2	(−9 to 0)	6	(4 to 10)
L2	−1	(−3 to 1)	−3	(−4 to −1)	6	(2 to 10)
L3	−1	(−4 to 1)	−2	(−4 to 3)	5	(−3 to 8)
L4	−1	(−4 to 3)	−1	(−4 to 2)	2	(−3 to 6)
L5	−2	(−3 to 0)	0	(−5 to 5)	−2	(−6 to 1)

may occur during left or right rotation but neither occurs consistently. Consequently, the mean amount of flexion and extension coupled with axial rotation is zero (Table 7.3). Similarly, lateral flexion may be accompanied by either flexion or extension of the same joint, but extension occurs more frequently and to a greater degree (Table 7.3). So, it might be concluded that lateral flexion is most usually accompanied by a small degree of extension.

The coupling between axial rotation and lateral flexion is somewhat more consistent and describes an average pattern. Axial rotation of the upper three lumbar joints is usually accompanied by lateral flexion to the other side, and lateral flexion is accompanied by contralateral axial rotation (Table 7.3). In contrast, axial rotation of the L5–S1 joint is accompanied by lateral flexion to the same side, and lateral flexion of this joint is accompanied by ipsilateral axial rotation (Table 7.2). The L4–5 joint exhibits no particular bias; in some subjects the coupling is ipsilateral while in others it is contralateral.[432]

While recognising these patterns it is important to note that they represent average patterns. Not all individuals exhibit the same degree of coupling at any segment or necessarily in the same direction as the average; nor do all normal individuals necessarily exhibit the average direction of coupling at every segment. While exhibiting the average pattern of coupling at one level, a normal individual can exhibit contrary coupling at any or all other levels.[430] Consequently, no reliable rules can be formulated to determine whether an individual exhibits abnormal ranges or directions of coupling in the lumbar spine; all that might be construed is that an individual differs from the average pattern, but this may not be abnormal.

The presence of coupling indicates that certain processes must operate during axial rotation to produce inadvertent lateral flexion, and vice versa. However, the details of these processes have not been determined. From first principles, they probably involve a combination of the way zygapophysial joints move and are impacted during axial rotation or lateral flexion; the way in which discs are subjected to torsional strain and lateral shear; the action of gravity; the line of action of the muscles that produce either axial rotation or lateral flexion; the shape of the lumbar lordosis; and the location of the moving segment within the lordotic curve.

Clinical implications

Armed with a detailed knowledge of the range of normal intersegmental motion and the patterns of coupled movements in the lumbar spine, investigators have explored the possibility that patients with back pain or specific spinal disorders might exhibit diagnostic abnormalities of range of motion or coupling. However, the results of such investigations have been disappointing. On biplanar radiography, patients with back pain, as a group, exhibit normal ranges of extension but a reduced mean range of flexion along with greater amplitudes of coupling; those patients with signs of nerve root tension exhibit reduced flexion but normal coupling.[434] However, patients with back pain exhibit such a range of movement that although their mean behaviour as a group differs from normal, biplanar radiography does not allow individual patients to be distinguished from normal with any worthwhile degree of sensitivity.[434] Patients with proven disc herniations exhibit reduced ranges of motion at all segments, but the level of disc herniation exhibits no greater reduction.[518] Increased coupling occurs at the level above a herniation. However, these abnormalities are not sufficiently specific to differentiate between patients with disc herniations and those with low-back pain of other origin.[518] Moreover, discectomy does not result in improvements of range of motion nor does it restore normal coupling.[518]

AXES OF SAGITTAL ROTATION

The combination of sagittal rotation and sagittal translation of each lumbar vertebra that occurs during flexion and extension of the lumbar spine results in each vertebra exhibiting an arcuate motion in relation to the next lower vertebra (Fig. 7.12). This arcuate motion occurs about a centre that lies somewhere below the moving vertebra and can be located by applying elementary geo-

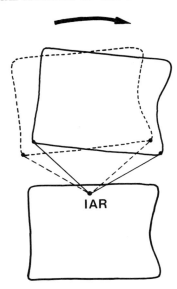

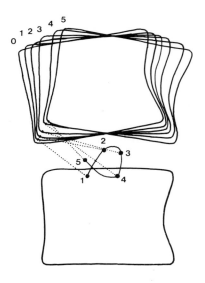

Fig. 7.12 During flexion-extension, each lumbar vertebra exhibits an arcuate motion in relation to the vertebra below. The centre of this arc lies below the moving vertebra and is known as the instantaneous axis of rotation (IAR).

Fig. 7.13 As a vertebra moves from extension to flexion, its motion can be reduced to small sequential increments. Five such phases are illustrated. Each phase of motion has a unique IAR. In moving from position 0 to position 1, the vertebra moved about IAR number 1. In moving from position 1 to position 2 it moved about IAR number 2; and so on. The dotted lines connect the vertebra in each of its five positions to the location of the IAR about which it moved. When the IARs are connected in sequence they describe a locus or a path known as the centrode.

metric techniques to flexion-extension radiographs of the moving vertebrae.[431]

For any arc of movement defined by a given starting position and a given end position of the moving vertebra the centre of movement is known as the **instantaneous axis of rotation** or **IAR**. The exact location of the IAR is a function of the amount of sagittal rotation and the amount of simultaneous sagittal translation that occurs during the phase of motion defined by the starting and end positions selected. However, as a vertebra moves from full extension to full flexion the amount of sagittal rotation versus sagittal translation is not regular; for different phases of motion the vertebra may exhibit relatively more rotation for the same change in translation or vice versa. Consequently, the precise location of the IAR for each phase of motion differs slightly. In essence, the axis of movement of the joint is not constant, and varies in location depending on the position of the joint.

The behaviour of the axis and the path it takes when it moves can be determined by studying the movement of the joint in small increments. If IARs are determined for each phase of motion,

and then plotted in sequence, they depict a locus known as the **centrode** of motion (Fig. 7.13). The centrode is in effect a map of the path taken by the moving axis during the full range of motion of the joint.

In normal cadaveric specimens the centrode is short and is located in a restricted area in the vicinity of the upper end-plate of the next lower vertebra[192,193] (Fig. 7.14A). In specimens with injured or so-called degenerative intervertebral discs, the centrode differs from normal in length, shape and average location[192,193] (Fig. 7.14B). These differences reflect the pathologic changes in the stiffness properties of those elements of the intervertebral joint that govern sagittal rotation and translation. Changes in the resistance to movement cause differences in the IARs at different phases of motion and therefore in the size and shape of the centrode.

Increased stiffness or relative laxity in different structures such as the anulus fibrosus, the

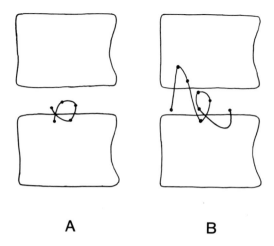

A   B

Fig. 7.14 The centrodes of normal cadaveric intervertebral joints are short and tightly clustered. **B**: Degenerative specimens exhibit longer, displaced and seemingly erratic controdes. (Based on Gertzbein et al.[192,193])

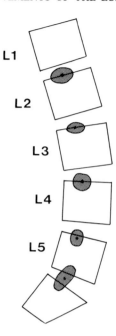

Fig. 7.15 The mean location and distribution of IARs of the lumbar vertebrae. The central dot depicts the mean location while the outer ellipse depicts the two standard deviation range exhibited by 10 normal volunteers. (Based on Pearcy and Bogduk.[431])

zygapophysial joints or the interspinous ligaments will affect sagittal rotation and translation to different extents. Therefore, different types of injury or disease should result in differences, if not characteristic aberrations, in the centrode pattern. Thus, it could be possible to deduce the location and nature of a disease process or injury by examining the centrode pattern it produces. However, the techniques used to determine centrodes are subject to technical errors whenever small amplitudes of motion are studied.[431] Consequently, centrodes can be determined accurately only if metal markers can be implanted to allow exact registration of consecutive radiographic images. Without such markers amplitudes of motion of less than 5° cannot be studied accurately in living subjects. Reliable observations in living subjects can only be made of the IAR for the movement of full flexion from full extension.[431] Such an IAR provides a convenient summary of the behaviour of the joint, and constitutes what can be construed as a reduction of the centrode of motion to a single point.

In normal volunteers, the IARs for each of the lumbar vertebrae fall in tightly clustered zones centred in similar locations for each segment near the superior end-plate of the next lower vertebra[431] (Fig. 7.15). Each segment operates around a very similar point, with little normal variation about the mean location. This indicates that the lumbar spine moves in a remarkably similar way in normal individuals; the forces governing flexion-extension must be similar from segment to segment, and are similar from individual to individual.

In so far as IARs reflect the quality of movement of a segment as opposed to its range of movement, determining the IARs in patients with spinal disorders could possibly provide a more sensitive way of detecting diagnostic movement abnormalities than simply measuring absolute ranges of movement. What remains to be seen is whether IARs in living subjects exhibit detectable aberrations analogous to the changes in centrode patterns seen in cadavers.

8. The lumbar muscles and their fascia

The lumbar spine is surrounded by muscles which for descriptive purposes, and on functional grounds, may be divided into three groups. These are:

1. Psoas major and psoas minor, which cover the anterolateral aspects of the lumbar spine.
2. Intertransversarii laterales and quadratus lumborum, which connect and cover the transverse processes anteriorly.
3. The lumbar back muscles, which lie behind and cover the posterior elements of the lumbar spine.

PSOAS MAJOR AND MINOR

The psoas major is a long muscle which arises from the anterolateral aspect of the lumbar spine and descends over the brim of the pelvis to insert into the lesser trochanter of the femur. It is essentially a muscle of the thigh whose principal action is flexion of the hip. However, under certain circumstances where the thigh is fixed, as in the exercise of 'sit-ups', it can act to flex the lumbar spine.

The psoas major has diverse, but systematic, attachments to the lumbar spine (Fig. 8.1). At each segmental level, it is attached to the medial half or so of the anterior surface of the transverse process, to the intervertebral disc, the margins of the vertebral bodies adjacent to the disc, and to a fibrous arch that connects the upper and lower margins of the lumbar vertebral body. This arch covers the concavity formed by the lateral surfaces of the vertebral body leaving a space between the arch and the bone that transmits the lumbar arteries and veins (see Ch. 10).

The muscle fibres from the L5–S1 intervertebral disc, the margins of the L5 and S1 bodies, the fibrous arch over L5, and the L5 transverse process form the deepest and lowest bundle of fibres within the muscle. These fibres are systematically overlapped by fibres from the disc, vertebral margins, fibrous arch and transverse process at successively higher levels. As a result, the muscle can be seen in cross-section to be layered, with fibres from higher levels forming the outer surface of the muscle and those from lower levels buried sequentially, deeper within its substance.

The psoas minor is an inconstant small muscle belly which arises from the T12–L1 intervertebral disc and forms a very long narrow tendon that inserts into the region of the iliopubic eminence.

INTERTRANSVERSARII LATERALES

The intertransversarii laterales consist of two parts: the intertransversarii laterales ventrales and the intertransversarii laterales dorsales. The ventral intertransversarii connect the margins of consecutive transverse processes, while the dorsal intertransversarii each connect an accessory process to the transverse process below (Fig. 8.2). Both the ventral and dorsal intertransversarii are innervated by the ventral rami of the lumbar spinal nerves,[91] and consequently cannot be classified amongst the back muscles which are all innervated by the dorsal rami (see Ch. 9). On the basis of their attachments and their nerve supply, the ventral and dorsal intertransversarii are considered to be homologous to the intercos-

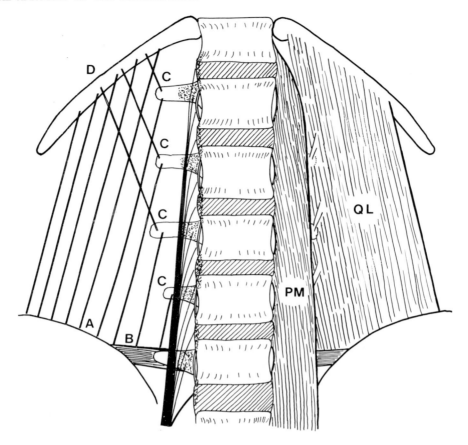

Fig. 8.1 Psoas major (PM) and quadratus lumborum (QL). At each segmental level psoas major attaches to the transverse process, the intervertebral disc and adjacent vertebral margins, and to the tendinous arch covering the vertebral body. The attachments of quadratus lumborum are to the iliac crest (A), the ilio-lumbar ligament (B), the transverse processes (C), and the 12th rib (D).

tal and levator costae muscles of the thoracic region.[91]

The function of the intertransversarii laterales has never been determined experimentally and one can only presume that on the basis of their attachments they act synergistically with the quadratus lumborum in lateral flexion of the lumbar spine.

QUADRATUS LUMBORUM

The quadratus lumborum is a wide, more or less rectangular muscle that covers the lateral two-thirds or so of the anterior surfaces of the L1 to L4 transverse processes and extends laterally a few centimetres beyond the tips of the transverse processes. In detail, the muscle is a complex aggregation of various oblique and longitudinally running fibres that connect the lumbar transverse processes, the ilium and the 12th rib[445] (Fig. 8.1).

Caudally, the muscle arises from the L5 transverse process, the trough formed by the superior and anterior ilio-lumbar ligaments (Ch. 4), and from the iliac crest lateral to the point of attachment of the ilio-lumbar ligament. From this series of attachments the most lateral fibres pass directly towards the lower anterior surface of the 12th rib. More medial fibres pass obliquely upwards and medially to the anterior surfaces of each of the lumbar transverse processes above L5. These oblique fibres intermingle with other

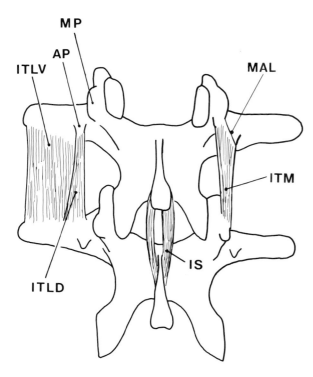

Fig. 8.2 The short, intersegmental muscles. ITLV — intertransversarii laterales ventrales. ITLD — intertransversarii laterales dorsales. ITM — intertransversarii mediales. IS — interspinales. AP — accessory process. MP — mamillary process. MAL — mamillo-accessory ligament.

oblique fibres that run upwards and laterally from each of the lumbar transverse processes to the 12th rib.

The majority of the fibres of the quadratus lumborum are connected to the 12th rib and one of the functions of this muscle is said to be to fix the 12th rib during respiration.[556] The remaining fibres of quadratus lumborum connect the ilium to the upper four lumbar transverse processes, and these fibres are suitably disposed to execute lateral flexion of the lumbar spine.

THE LUMBAR BACK MUSCLES

The lumbar back muscles are those muscles which lie behind the plane of the transverse processes and which exert an action on the lumbar spine. They include muscles that attach to the

lumbar vertebrae and thereby act directly on the lumbar spine, and certain other muscles that, while not attaching to the lumbar vertebrae, nevertheless exert an action on the lumbar spine.

For descriptive purposes and on morphological grounds the lumbar back muscles may be divided into three groups:

1. The short intersegmental muscles — the interspinales and the intertransversarii mediales.
2. The polysegmental muscles that attach to the lumbar vertebrae — the multifidus and the lumbar components of longissimus and iliocostalis.
3. The long polysegmental muscles, represented by the thoracic components of longissimus and iliocostalis lumborum, that in general, do not attach to the lumbar vertebrae but cross the lumbar region from thoracic levels to find attachments on the ilium and sacrum.

The descriptions of the back muscles offered in this chapter, notably those of the multifidus and erector spinae, differ substantially from those given in standard textbooks. Traditionally, these muscles have been regarded as stemming from a common origin on the sacrum and ilium and passing upwards to assume diverse attachments to the lumbar and thoracic vertebrae and ribs. However, in the face of several recent studies of these muscles[56,345,346,348] it is considered more appropriate to view these muscles in the reverse direction — from above downwards. Not only is this more consistent with the pattern of their nerve supply,[66,348] but it clarifies the identity of certain muscles and the identity of the erector spinae aponeurosis, and reveals the segmental biomechanical disposition of the muscles.

Interspinales

The lumbar interspinales are short paired muscles that lie on either side of the interspinous ligament and connect the spinous processes of adjacent lumbar vertebrae (Fig. 8.2). There are four pairs in the lumbar region.

Although disposed to act synergistically with the multifidus to produce posterior sagittal rotation of the vertebra above, the interspinales are quite small and would not contribute appreciably to the force required to move a vertebra. This paradox is similar to that which applies for the intertransversarii mediales and is discussed further in that context.

Intertransversarii mediales

The intertransversarii mediales can be considered to be true back muscles for, unlike the intertransversarii laterales, they are innervated by the lumbar dorsal rami.[66,91] The intertransversarii mediales arise from an accessory process, the adjoining mamillary process and the mamillo-accessory ligament that connects these two processes.[58] They insert into the superior apsect of the mamillary process of the vertebra below (Fig. 8.2).

The intertransversarii mediales lie lateral to the axis of lateral flexion and behind the axis of sagittal rotation. However, they lie very close to these axes and are very small muscles. Therefore, it is questionable whether they could contribute any appreciable force in either lateral flexion or posterior sagittal rotation. It might be argued that perhaps larger muscles might provide the bulk of the power to move the vertebrae, and the intertransversarii could act to 'fine tune' the movement. However, this suggestion is highly speculative, if not fanciful, and does not account for their small size and considerable mechanical disadvantage.

A tantalising alternative suggestion is that the intertransversarii act as large, proprioceptive transducers — their value lies not in the force they can exert, but in the muscle spindles they contain. Placed close to the lumbar vertebral column, the intertransversarii could monitor the movements of the column and provide feedback that influences the action of the surrounding muscles. Such a role has been suggested for the cervical intertransversarii which have been found to contain a high density of muscle spindles.[2,3,99] Indeed, all unisegmental muscles of the vertebral column have between two and six times the density of muscles spindles found in the longer, polysegmental muscles, and there is growing speculation that this underscores the propriocep-

tive function of all short, small muscles of the body.[43,407,436]

Multifidus

Multifidus is the largest and most medial of the lumbar back muscles. It consists of a repeating series of fascicles which stem from the laminae and spinous processes of the lumbar vertebrae and exhibit a constant pattern of of attachments caudally.[348]

The shortest fascicles of the multifidus are the 'laminar fibres' which arise from the caudal end of the dorsal surface of each vertebral lamina and insert into the mamillary process of the vertebra two levels caudad (Fig. 8.3A). The L5 laminar fibres have no mamillary process into which they can insert, and insert instead into an area on the sacrum just above the first dorsal sacral foramen. Because of their attachments, the laminar fibres may be considered homologous to the thoracic rotatores.

The bulk of the lumbar multifidus consists of much larger fascicles that radiate from the lumbar spinous processes. These fascicles are arranged in five overlapping groups such that each lumbar vertebra gives rise to one of these groups. At each segmental level, a fascicle arises from the base and caudolateral edge of the spinous process, and several fascicles arise, by way of a common tendon, from the caudal tip of the spinous process. This tendon is referred to hereafter as 'the common tendon'. Although confluent with one another at their origin, the fascicles in each group diverge caudally to assume separate attachments to mamillary processes, the iliac crest and the sacrum.

The fascicle from the base of the L1 spinous process inserts into the L4 mamillary process, while those from the common tendon insert into the mamillary processes of L5, S1 and the posterior superior iliac spine (Fig. 8.3B).

The fascicle from the base of the spinous process of L2 inserts into the mamillary process of L5, while those from the common tendon insert into the S1 mamillary process, the posterior superior iliac spine, and an area on the iliac crest just caudoventral to the posterior superior iliac spine (Fig. 8.3C).

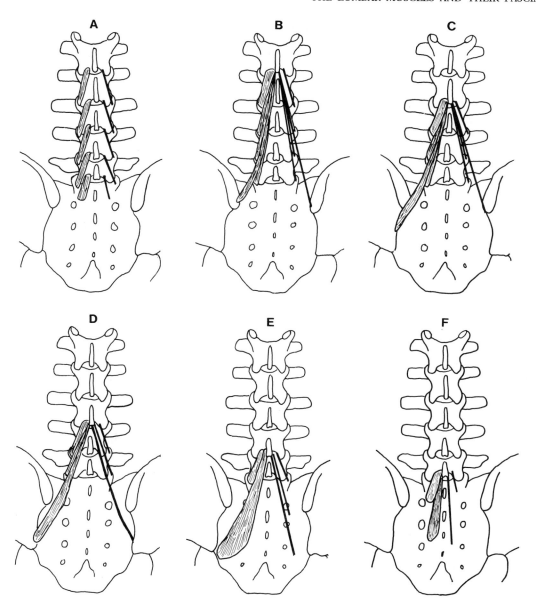

Fig. 8.3 The component fascicles of multifidus. **A**: The laminar fibres of multifidus. **B** to **F**: The fascicles from the L1 to L5 spinous processes respectively.

The fascicle from the base of the L3 spinous process inserts into the mamillary process of the sacrum, while those fascicles from the common tendon insert into a narrow area extending caudally from the caudal extent of the posterior superior iliac spine to the lateral edge of the third sacral segment (Fig. 8.3D). The L4 fascicles insert onto the sacrum in an area medial to the L3 area of insertion, but lateral to the dorsal sacral foramina (Fig. 8.3E), while those from the L5 vertebra insert onto an area medial to the dorsal sacral foramina (Fig. 8.3F).

It is noteworthy that while many of the fascicles of multifidus attach to mamillary processes, some of the deeper fibres of these fascicles attach to the capsules of the zygapophysial joints next to the mamillary processes[329] (Ch. 3). This attachment allows the multifidus to protect the joint capsule from being caught inside the joint during the movements executed by the multifidus.

The key feature of the morphology of the lumbar multifidus is that its fascicles are arranged segmentally. Each lumbar vertebra is endowed with a group of fascicles that radiate from its spinous process, anchoring it below to mamillary processes, the iliac crest and the sacrum. This disposition suggests that the fibres of multifidus are arranged in such a way that their principal action is focused on individual lumbar spinous processes.[348] They are designed to act in concert on a single spinous process. This contention is supported by the pattern of innervation of the muscle. All the fascicles arising from the spinous processes of a given vertebra are innervated by the medial branch of the dorsal ramus that issues from below that vertebra[66,348] (see Ch. 9). Thus, the muscles that directly act on a particular vertebral segment are innervated by the nerve of that segment.

In a posterior view, the fascicles of multifidus are seen to have an oblique, caudolateral orientation. Their line of action, therefore, can be resolved into two vectors: a large vertical vector, and a considerably smaller horizontal vector[345] (Fig. 8.4A).

The small horizontal vector suggests that the multifidus could pull the spinous processes sideways, and therefore produce horizontal rotation. However, horizontal rotation of lumbar vertebrae is impeded by the impaction of the contralateral zygapophysial joints. Horizontal rotation occurs after impaction of the joints only if an appropriate shear force is applied to the intervertebral discs (Ch. 7), but the horizontal vector of multifidus is so small that it is unlikely that multifidus would be capable of exerting such a shear force on the disc by acting on the spinous process. Indeed, electromyographic studies reveal that multifidus is inconsistently active in derotation and that, paradoxically, it is active in both ipsilateral and contralateral rotation.[130] Rotation, therefore, cannot be inferred to be a primary action of multifidus. In this context, multifidus has been said to act only as a 'stabiliser' in rotation,[130,329] but the aberrant movements which it is supposed to stabilise have not been defined (although see below).

The principal action of multifidus is expressed by its vertical vector, and further insight is gained when this vector is viewed in a lateral projection (Fig. 8.4B). Each fascicle of multifidus, at every level, acts virtually at right angles to its spinous process of origin.[345] Thus, using the spinous process as a lever, every fascicle is ideally disposed to produce posterior sagittal rotation of its vertebra. The right-angle orientation, however, precludes any action as a posterior horizontal translator. Therefore, the multifidus can only exert the 'rocking' component of extension of the lumbar spine or control this component during flexion.

Having established that multifidus is primarily a posterior sagittal rotator of the lumbar spine, it is possible to resolve the paradox about its activity during horizontal rotation of the trunk.[345] In the first instance, it should be realised that rotation of the lumbar spine is an indirect action. Active rotation of the lumbar spine occurs only if the thorax is first rotated, and is therefore secondary to thoracic rotation. Secondly, it must be realised that a muscle with two vectors of action cannot use these vectors independently. If the muscle contracts, then both vectors are exerted. Thus, multifidus cannot exert axial rotation without simultaneously exerting a much larger posterior sagittal rotation.

The principal muscles that produce rotation of the thorax are the oblique abdominal muscles. The horizontal component of their orientation is able to turn the thoracic cage in the horizontal plane and thereby impart axial rotation to the lumbar spine. However, the oblique abdominal muscles also have a vertical component to their orientation. Therefore, if they contract to produce rotation they will also simultaneously cause flexion of the trunk, and therefore, of the lumbar spine. To counteract this flexion, and maintain pure axial rotation, extensors of the lumbar spine must be recruited, and this is how multifidus becomes involved in rotation.

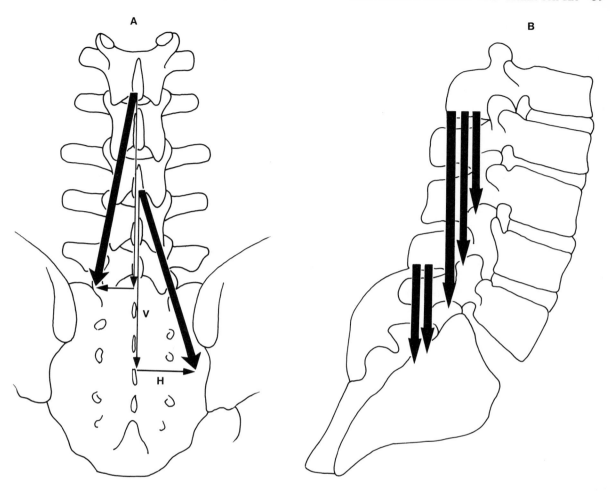

Fig. 8.4 The force vectors of multifidus. **A**: In a postero-anterior view, the oblique line of action of the multifidus at each level (bold arrow) can be resolved into a major vertical vector (V) and a smaller horizontal vector (H). **B**: In a lateral view, the vertical vectors of the multifidus are seen to be aligned at right angles to the spinous processes.

The role of multifidus in rotation is not to produce rotation, but to oppose the flexion effect of the abdominal muscles as they produce rotation. The aberrant motion 'stabilised' by multifidus during rotation is, therefore, the unwanted flexion unavoidably produced by the abdominal muscles.[345]

Apart from its action on individual lumbar vertebrae, the multifidus, because of its polysegmental nature, can also exert indirect effects on any interposed vertebrae. Since the line of action of any long fascicle of multifidus lies behind the lordotic curve of the lumbar spine, such fascicles can act like bowstrings on those segments of the curve that intervene between the attachments of the fascicle. The bowstring effect would tend to accentuate the lumbar lordosis, resulting in compression of intervertebral discs posteriorly and strain of the discs and longitudinal ligament anteriorly. Thus, a secondary effect of the action of multifidus is to increase the lumbar lordosis and the compressive and tensile loads on any vertebrae and intervertebral discs interposed between its attachments.

Lumbar erector spinae

The lumbar erector spinae lies lateral to the multifidus and forms the prominent dorsolateral contour of the back muscles in the lumbar region. It consists of two muscles — the **longissimus thoracis** and the **iliocostalis lumborum**. Furthermore, each of these muscles has two components: a lumbar part, consisting of fascicles arising from lumbar vertebrae, and a thoracic part, consisting of fascicles arising from thoracic vertebrae or ribs.[56,346] These four parts may be referred to respectively as longissimus thoracis pars lumborum, iliocostalis lumborum pars lumborum, longissimus thoracis pars thoracis and iliocostalis lumborum pars thoracis.[346]

In the lumbar region, the longissimus and iliocostalis are separated from each other by the **lumbar intermuscular aponeurosis**, an antero-posterior continuation of the erector spinae aponeurosis.[56,346] It appears as a flat sheet of collagen fibres that extend rostrally from the medial aspect of the posterior superior iliac spine for 6–8 cm. It is formed mainly by the caudal tendons of the rostral four fascicles of the lumbar component of longissimus (Fig. 8.5).

Longissimus thoracis pars lumborum

The longissimus thoracis pars lumborum is composed of five fascicles, each arising from the accessory process and the adjacent medial end of the dorsal surface of the transverse process of a lumbar vertebra (Fig. 8.5).

The fascicle from the L5 vertebra is the deepest and shortest. Its fibres insert directly into the medial aspect of the posterior superior iliac spine. The fascicle from L4 also lies deeply, but lateral to that from L5. Succeeding fascicles lie progressively more dorsally so that the L3 fascicle covers those from L4 and L5, but is itself covered by the L2 fascicle, while the L1 fascicle lies most superficially.

The L1 to L4 fascicles all form tendons at their caudal ends which converge to form the lumbar intermuscular aponeurosis, which eventually attaches to a narrow area on the ilium immediately lateral to the insertion of the L5 fascicle. The lumbar intermuscular aponeurosis thus repre-

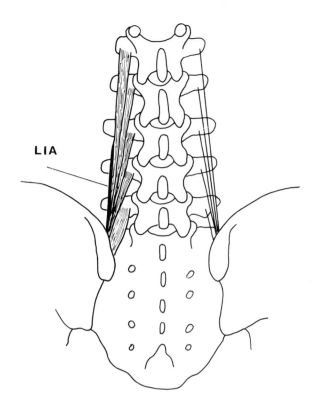

Fig. 8.5 The lumbar fibres of longissimus (longissimus thoracis pars lumborum). On the left, the five fascicles of the intact muscle are drawn. The formation of the lumbar intermuscular aponeurosis (LIA) by the lumbar fascicles of longissimus is depicted. On the right, the lines indicate the attachments and span of the fascicles.

sents a common tendon of insertion, or the aponeurosis, of the bulk of the lumbar fibres of longissimus.

Each fascicle of the lumbar longissimus has both a dorsoventral and a rostrocaudal orientation.[346] Therefore, the action of each fascicle can be resolved into a vertical vector and a horizontal vector, the relative sizes of which differ from L1 to L5 (Fig. 8.6A). Consequently, the relative actions of longissimus differ at each segmental level. Furthermore, the action of longissimus, as a whole, will differ according to whether the muscle contracts unilaterally or bilaterally.

The large vertical vector of each fascicle lies lateral to the axis of lateral flexion and behind the axis of sagittal rotation of each vertebra. Thus, contracting unilaterally the longissimus can

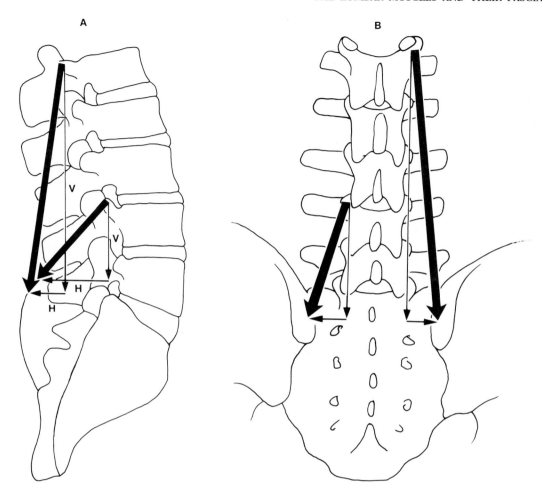

Fig. 8.6 The force vectors of the longissimus thoracis pars lumborum. **A**: In a lateral view, the oblique line of action of each fascicle of longissimus can be resolved into a vertical (V) and a horizontal (H) vector. The horizontal vectors of lower lumbar fascicles are larger. **B**: In a postero-anterior view, the line of action of the fascicles can be resolved into a major vertical vector and a much smaller horizontal vector.

laterally flex the vertebral column, but acting bi-laterally the various fascicles can act, like multifidus, to produce posterior sagittal rotation of their vertebra of origin. However, their attachments to the accessory and transverse processes lie close to the axes of sagittal rotation and therefore, their capacity to produce posterior sagittal rotation is less efficient than that of multifidus which acts through the long levers of the spinous processes.[346]

The horizontal vectors of the longissimus are

directed backwards. Therefore, when contracting bilaterally the longissimus is capable of drawing the lumbar vertebrae backwards. This action of posterior translation can restore the anterior translation of the lumbar vertebrae that occurs during flexion of the lumbar column (Ch. 7). The capacity for posterior translation is greatest at lower lumbar levels where the fascicles of longissimus assume a greater dorsoventral orientation (Fig. 8.6B).

Reviewing the horizontal and vertical actions

of longissimus together, it can be seen that longissimus expresses a continuum of combined actions along the length of the lumbar vertebral column. From below upwards, its capacity as a posterior sagittal rotator increases while reciprocally, from above downwards, the fascicles are better designed to resist or restore anterior translation. It is emphasised that the longissimus cannot exert its horizontal and vertical vectors independently. Thus, whatever horizontal translation it exerts must occur simultaneously with posterior sagittal rotation. The resolution into vectors simply reveals the relative amounts of simultaneous translation and sagittal rotation exerted at different segmental levels.

It might be deduced that because of the horizontal vector of longissimus, this muscle acting unilaterally, could draw the accessory and transverse processes backwards and therefore produce axial rotation. However, in this regard, the fascicles of longissimus are orientated almost directly towards the axis of axial rotation and so are at a marked mechanical disadvantage to produce axial rotation.

Iliocostalis lumborum pars lumborum

The lumbar component of iliocostalis lumborum consists of four overlying fascicles arising from the L1 through to L4 vertebrae. Rostrally, each fascicle attaches to the tip of the transverse process and to an area extending 2–3 cm laterally onto the middle layer of the thoracolumbar fascia (Fig. 8.7).

The fascicle from L4 is the deepest, and caudally it is attached directly to the iliac crest just lateral to the posterior superior iliac spine. This fascicle is covered by the fascicle from L3 that has a similar but more dorsolaterally located attachment on the iliac crest. In sequence, L2 covers L3 and L1 covers L2 with insertions on the iliac crest becoming successively more dorsal and lateral. The most lateral fascicles attach to the iliac crest just medial to the attachment of the 'lateral raphe' of the thoracolumbar fascia (see below). The most medial fibres of iliocostalis contribute to the lumbar intermuscular aponeurosis, but only to a minor extent.

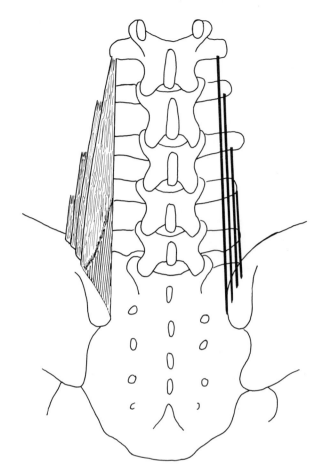

Fig. 8.7 The lumbar fibres of iliocostalis (iliocostalis lumborum pars lumborum). On the left, the four lumbar fascicles of iliocostalis are shown. On the right, their span and attachments are indicated by the lines.

Although an L5 fascicle of iliocostalis lumborum is not described in the literature, it is represented in the ilio-lumbar 'ligament'. In neonates and children this 'ligament' is completely muscular in structure. By the third decade of life the muscle fibres are entirely replaced by collagen, giving rise to the familiar ilio-lumbar ligament.[342] On the basis of sites of attachment and relative orientation the posterior band of the ilio-lumbar ligament would appear to be derived from the L5 fascicle of iliocostalis while the anterior band of the ligament is a derivative of the quadratus lumborum.

A

B

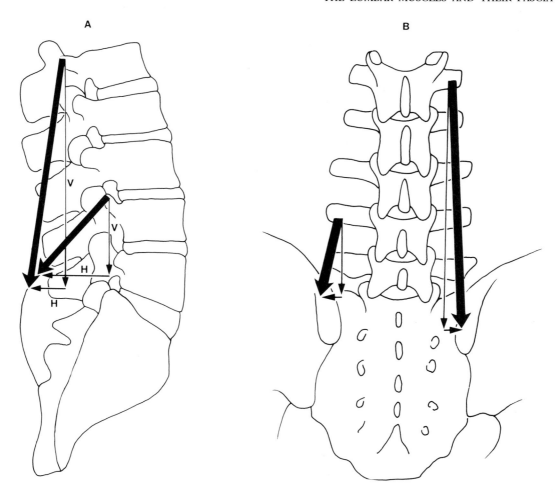

Fig. 8.8 The force vectors of the iliocostalis lumborum pars lumborum. **A**: In a lateral view, the line of action of the fascicles can be resolved into vertical (V) and horizontal (H) vectors. The horizontal vectors are larger at lower lumbar levels. **B**: In a postero-anterior view, the line of action is resolved into a vertical vector and a very small horizontal vector.

The disposition of the lumbar fascicles of iliocostalis is similar to that of the lumbar longissimus, except that the fascicles are situated more laterally. Like that of the lumbar longissimus, their action can be resolved into horizontal and vertical vectors (Fig. 8.8A).

The vertical vector is still predominant, and therefore, the lumbar fascicles of iliocostalis contracting bilaterally can act as posterior sagittal rotators (Fig. 8.8B), but because of the horizontal vector, a posterior translation will be exerted si-multaneously, principally at lower lumbar levels where the fascicles of iliocostalis have a greater forward orientation. Contracting unilaterally, the lumbar fascicles of iliocostalis can act as lateral flexors of the lumbar vertebrae, for which action the transverse processes provide very substantial levers.

Contracting unilaterally, the fibres of iliocostalis are better suited to exert axial rotation than the fascicles of lumbar longissimus, for their attachment to the tips of the transverse processes displaces them from the axis of horizontal rotation and provides them with substantial levers for this action. Because of this leverage, the lower fascicles of iliocostalis are the only intrinsic muscles of the lumbar spine reasonably disposed to produce horizontal rotation. Their effectiveness as rotators, however, is dwarfed by the oblique abdominal muscles that act on the ribs and produce lumbar rotation indirectly by rotating the thoracic cage. However, because iliocostalis cannot exert axial rotation without simultaneously exerting posterior sagittal rotation, the muscle is well suited to co-operate with multifidus to oppose the flexion effect of the abdominal muscles when they act to rotate the trunk.

Longissimus thoracis pars thoracis

The thoracic fibres of longissimus thoracis typically consists of 11 or 12 pairs of small fascicles arising from the ribs and transverse processes of T1 or T2 down to T12 (Fig. 8.9). At each level, two tendons can usually be recognised, a medial one from the tip of the transverse process, and a lateral one from the rib, although in the upper 3 or 4 levels, the latter may merge medially with the fascicle from the transverse process. Each rostral tendon extends 3–4 cm before forming a small muscle belly measuring 7–8 cm in length. The muscle bellies from the higher levels overlap those from lower levels. Each muscle belly eventually forms a caudal tendon that extends into the lumbar region. The tendons run in parallel, with those from higher levels being most medial. The fascicles from the T2 level attach to the L3 spinous process, while the fascicles from the remaining levels insert into spinous processes at progressively lower levels. For example those from T5 attach to L5 and those from T7 to S2 or S3. Those from T8 to T12 diverge from the midline to find attachment to the sacrum along a line extending from the S3 spinous process to the caudal extent of the posterior superior iliac spine.[346] The lateral edge of the caudal tendon of T12 lies alongside the dorsal edge of the lumbar intermuscular aponeurosis formed by the caudal tendon of the L1 longissimus bundle.

The side to side aggregation of the caudal tendons of longissimus thoracis pars thoracis forms

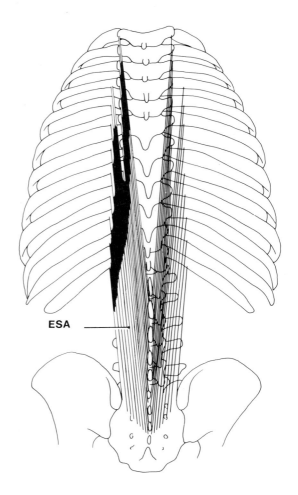

Fig. 8.9 The thoracic fibres of longissimus (longissimus thoracis pars thoracis). The intact fascicles are shown on the left. The darkened areas represent the short muscle bellies of each fascicle. Note the short rostral tendons of each fascicle, and the long caudal tendons, which collectively constitute most of the erector spinae aponeurosis (ESA). The span of the individual fascicles is indicated on the right.

much of what is termed the erector spinae aponeurosis which covers the lumbar fibres of longissimus and iliocostalis, but affords no attachment to them.

The longissimus thoracis pars thoracis is designed to act on thoracic vertebrae and ribs. Nonetheless, when contracting bilaterally it acts indirectly on the lumbar vertebral column, and uses the erector spinae aponeurosis to produce an increase in the lumbar lordosis. However, not all of the fascicles of longissimus thoracis span the entire lumbar vertebral column. Those from the second rib and T2 reach only as far as L3, and only those fascicles arising between the T6 or 7 and the T12 levels actually span the entire lumbar region. Consequently, only a portion of the whole thoracic longissimus acts on all the lumbar vertebrae.

The oblique orientation of the longissimus thoracis pars thoracis, also permits it to laterally flex the thoracic vertebral column and thereby indirectly flex the lumbar vertebral column laterally.

Iliocostalis lumborum pars thoracis

The iliocostalis lumborum pars thoracis consists of fascicles from the lower seven or eight ribs that attach caudally to the ilium and sacrum (Fig. 8.10). These fascicles represent the thoracic component of iliocostalis lumborum, and should not be confused with the iliocostalis thoracis which is restricted to the thoracic region between the upper six and lower six ribs.

Each fascicle of the iliocostalis lumborum pars thoracis arises from the angle of the rib via a ribbon-like tendon measuring some 9–10 cm in length. It then forms a muscle belly of 8–10 cm in length. Thereafter, each fascicle continues as a tendon, contributing to the erector spinae aponeurosis, and ultimately attaching to the posterior superior iliac spine. The most medial tendons, from the more rostral fascicles, often attach more medially, to the dorsal surface of the sacrum, caudal to the insertion of multifidus.

The thoracic fascicles of iliocostalis lumborum have no attachment to lumbar vertebrae. They attach to the iliac crest and thereby span the lumbar region. Consequently, by acting bilaterally, it is possible for them to exert an indirect 'bowstring' effect on the vertebral column causing an increase in the lordosis of the lumbar spine. Acting unilaterally, the iliocostalis lumborum pars thoracis can use the leverage afforded by the ribs to laterally flex the thoracic cage and thereby laterally flex the lumbar vertebral column indirectly. The distance between the ribs and ilium does not shorten greatly during rotation of the trunk, and therefore the iliocostalis

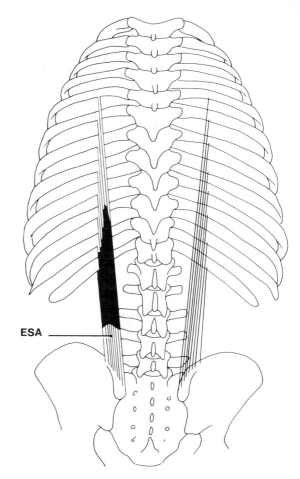

Fig. 8.10 The thoracic fibres of iliocostalis lumborum (iliocostalis lumborum pars thoracis). The intact fascicles are shown on the left, and their span is shown on the right. The caudal tendons of the fascicles collectively form the lateral parts of the erector spinae aponeurosis (ESA).

lumborum pars thoracis can have little action as an axial rotator. However, contralateral rotation greatly increases this distance, and the iliocostalis lumborum pars thoracis can serve to derotate the thoracic cage and, therefore, the lumbar spine.

ERECTOR SPINAE APONEUROSIS

One of the cardinal revelations of recent studies of the lumbar erector spinae[56,346] is that this muscle consists of both lumbar and thoracic fibres. Modern textbook descriptions largely do not recognise the lumbar fibres, especially those of iliocostalis;[56] but moreover, they do not note that the lumbar fibres (of both longissimus and iliocostalis) have attachments quite separate to those of the thoracic fibres. The lumbar fibres of the longissimus and ilicostalis pass between the lumbar vertebrae and the ilium. Thus, through these muscles, the lumbar vertebrae are anchored directly to the ilium. They do not gain any attachment to the erector spinae aponeurosis, which is the implication of all modern textbook descriptions that deal with the erector spinae.

The erector spinae aponeurosis is described as a broad sheet of tendinous fibres that is attached to the ilium, the sacrum, and the lumbar and sacral spinous processes, and which forms a common origin for the lower part of erector spinae. However, as described above, the erector spinae aponeurosis is formed virtually exclusively by the tendons of the longissimus thoracis pars thoracis and iliocostalis pars thoracis.[56,346] The medial half or so of the aponeurosis is formed by the tendons of longissimus thoracis, and the lateral half is formed by the iliocostalis lumborum (Fig. 8.11). The only additional contribution comes from the most superficial fibres of multifidus from upper lumbar levels which contribute a small number of fibres to the aponeurosis[348] (Figs 8.9 and 8.10). Nonetheless, the erector spinae aponeurosis is essentially formed only by the caudal attachments of muscles acting from thoracic levels.

The lumbar fibres of erector spinae do not attach to the erector spinae aponeurosis. Indeed, the aponeurosis is free to move over the surface of the underlying lumbar fibres, and this suggests that the lumbar fibres, which form the bulk of the lumbar back musculature, can act independently from the rest of the erector spinae.

THORACOLUMBAR FASCIA

The thoracolumbar fascia consists of three layers of fascia that envelops the muscles of the lumbar spine, effectively separating them into three compartments. The **anterior layer** of thoracolumbar fascia is quite thin, and is derived from the fascia of quadratus lumborum. It covers the anterior surface of quadratus lumborum, and is attached

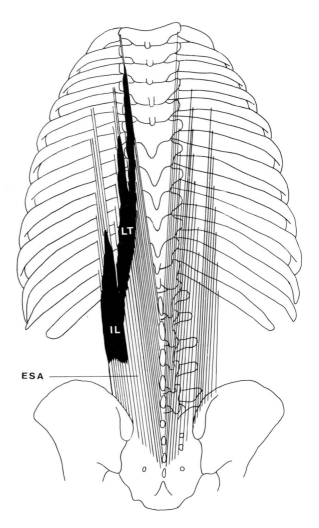

Fig. 8.11 The erector spinae aponeurosis (ESA). This broad sheet is formed by the caudal tendons of the thoracic fibres of longissimus thoracis (LT) and iliocostalis lumborum (IL).

medially to the anterior surfaces of the lumbar transverse processes. In the intertransverse spaces it blends with the intertransverse ligaments, and may be viewed as one of the lateral extensions of the intertransverse ligaments (Ch. 4). Lateral to the quadratus lumborum, the anterior layer blends with the other layers of the thoracolumbar fascia.

The **middle layer** of thoracolumbar fascia lies behind the quadratus lumborum. Medially, it is attached to the tips of the lumbar transverse processes, and is directly continuous with the intertransverse ligaments. Laterally, it gives rise to the aponeurosis of the transversus abdominis. Its actual identity is debatable. It may represent a lateral continuation of the intertransverse ligaments, a medial continuation of the transversus aponeurosis, a thickening of the posterior fascia of the quadratus, or a combination of any or all of these.

The **posterior layer** of thoracolumbar fascia covers the back muscles. It arises from the lumbar spinous processes in the midline posteriorly, and wraps around the back muscles to blend with the other layers of the thoracolumbar fascia along the lateral border of the iliocostalis lumborum. The union of the fasciae is quite dense at this site, and the middle and posterior layers, in particular, form a dense raphe which, for purposes of reference, has been called the **lateral raphe**.[64]

Traditionally, the thoracolumbar fascia has been ascribed no other function than to invest the back muscles and to provide an attachment for the transversus abdominis and the internal oblique muscles.[556] However, in recent years there has been considerable interest in its biomechanical role in the stability of the lumbar spine, particularly in the flexed posture and in lifting. This has resulted in anatomical and biomechanical studies of the anatomy and function of the thoracolumbar fascia, notably its posterior layer.[64,159,212]

The posterior layer of thoracolumbar fascia covers the back muscles from the lumbosacral region through to the thoracic region as far rostrally as the splenius muscle. In the lumbar region, it is attached to the tips of the spinous processes in the midline. Lateral to the erector spinae, between the 12th rib and the iliac crest, it unites with the the middle layer of thoracolumbar fascia in the lateral raphe. At sacral levels, the posterior layer extends from the midline to the posterior superior iliac spine and the posterior segment of the iliac crest.

On close inspection, the posterior layer exhibits a cross-hatched appearance, manifest because it consists of two laminae: a superficial lamina with fibres orientated caudomedially and a deep lamina with fibres oriented caudolaterally.[64]

The superficial lamina is formed by the apo-

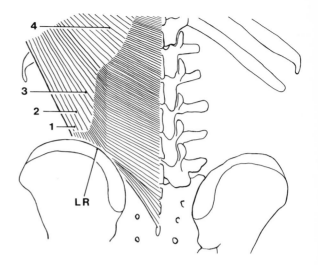

Fig. 8.12 The superficial lamina of the posterior layer of thoracolumbar fascia. 1: Aponeurotic fibres of the most lateral fascicles of latissimus dorsi insert directly into the iliac crest. 2: Aponeurotic fibres of the next most lateral part of latissimus dorsi glance past the iliac crest and reach the midline at sacral levels. 3: Aponeurotic fibres from this portion of the muscle attach to the underlying lateral raphe (LR), and then deflect medially to reach the midline at the L3 to L5 levels. 4: Aponeurotic fibres from the upper portions of latissimus dorsi pass directly to the midline at thoracolumbar levels.

neurosis of latissimus dorsi, but the disposition and attachments of its constituent fibres differs according to the portion of latissimus dorsi from which they are derived (Fig. 8.12). Those fibres derived from the most lateral 2–3 cm of the muscle are short and insert directly into the iliac crest without contributing to the thoracolumbar fascia. Fibres from the next most lateral 2 cm of the muscle approach the iliac crest near the lateral margin of the erector spinae, but then deflect medially, by-passing the crest to attach to the L5 and sacral spinous processes. These fibres form the sacral portion of the superficial lamina. A third series of fibres become aponeurotic just lateral to the lumbar erector spinae. At the lateral border of the erector spinae they blend with the other layers of thoracolumbar fascia in the lateral raphe, but then they deflect medially, continuing over the back muscles to reach the midline at the levels of the L3, 4 and 5 spinous processes. These fibres form the lumbar portion of the superficial lamina of the posterior layer of thoracolumbar fascia.

The rostral portions of the latissimus dorsi cross the back muscles and do not become aponeurotic until some 5 cm lateral to the midline at the L3 and higher levels. These aponeurotic fibres form the thoracolumbar and thoracic portions of the thoracolumbar fascia.

Beneath the superficial lamina, the deep lamina of the posterior layer consists of bands of collagen fibres emanating from the midline, principally from the lumbar spinous processes (Fig. 8.13). The bands from the L4, L5 and S1 spinous processes pass caudolaterally to the posterior superior iliac spine. Those from the L3 spinous process and L3–4 interspinous ligament wrap around the lateral margin of the erector spinae to fuse with the middle layer of thoracolumbar fascia in the lateral raphe. Above L3 the deep lamina progressively becomes thinner, consisting of sparse bands of collagen that dissipate laterally over the erector spinae. A deep lamina is not formed at thoracic levels.

Collectively, the superficial and deep laminae of the posterior layer of thoracolumbar fascia form a retinaculum over the back muscles. Attached to the midline medially and the posterior superior iliac spine and lateral raphe laterally, the fascia covers or ensheaths the back muscles preventing their displacement dorsally. Additionally, the deep lamina alone forms a series of distinct ligaments. When viewed bilaterally, the bands of fibres from the L4 and L5 spinous processes appear like alar ligaments anchoring these spinous processes to the ilia. The band from the L3 spinous process anchors this process indirectly to the ilium via the lateral raphe. Thirdly, the lateral raphe forms a site where the two laminae of the posterior layer fuse not only with the middle layer of thoracolumbar fascia, but also with the transversus abdominis whose middle fibres arise from the lateral raphe (Fig. 8.13). The posterior layer of thoracolumbar fascia thereby provides an indirect attachment for the transversus abdominis to the lumbar spinous processes. The mechanical significance of these three morphological features is explored below in the section on functions of the back muscles and their fascia.

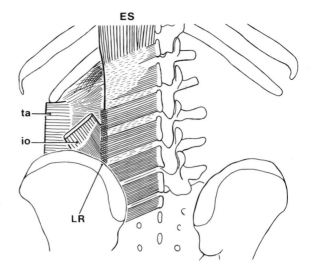

Fig. 8.13 The deep lamina of the posterior layer of thoracolumbar fascia. Bands of collagen fibres pass from the midline to the posterior superior iliac spine and to the lateral raphe (LR). Those bands from the L4 and L5 spinous processes form alar-like ligaments that anchor these processes to the ilium. Attaching to the lateral raphe laterally are the aponeurosis of transversus abdominis (ta), and a variable number of the most posterior fibres of internal oblique (io). ES — erector spinae.

FUNCTIONS OF THE BACK MUSCLES AND THEIR FASCIA

Each of the lumbar back muscles is capable of several possible actions. No action is unique to a muscle and no muscle has a single action. Instead, the back muscles provide a pool of possible actions that may be recruited to suit the needs of the vertebral column. Therefore, the functions of the back muscles need to be considered in terms of the observed movements of the vertebral column. In this regard, three types of movements can be addressed: (1) minor active movements of the vertebral column, (2) postural movements, and (3) major movements in forward bending and lifting. In this context 'postural movements' refers to movements, usually subconscious, that occur to adjust and maintain a desired posture when this is disturbed, usually by the influence of gravity.

Minor active movements

In the upright position, the lumbar back muscles play a minor, or no active role in executing movement, for gravity provides the necessary force. During extension, the back muscles contribute to the initial tilt, drawing the line of gravity backwards,[181,382] but are unnecessary for further extension. Muscle activity is recruited when the movement is forced or resisted[417] but is restricted to muscles acting on the thorax. The lumbar multifidus, for example, shows little or no involvement.[383]

The lateral flexors can bend the lumbar spine sideways, but once the centre of gravity of the trunk is displaced, lateral flexion can continue under the influence of gravity. However, the ipsilateral lateral flexors are used to direct the movement, and the contralateral muscles are required to balance the action of gravity and control the rate and extent of movement. Consequently, lateral flexion is accompanied by bilateral activity of the lumbar back muscles, but the contralateral muscles are relatively more active, as it is they which must balance the load of the laterally flexing spine.[23,83,181,382,418,447] If a weight is held in the hand on the side to which the spine is laterally flexed, a greater load is applied to the spine, and the contralateral back muscles show greater activity to balance this load.[23,418]

Maintenance of posture

The upright vertebral column is well stabilised by its joints and ligaments, but it is still liable to displacement by gravity or when subject to assymetrical weight-bearing. The back muscles serve to correct such displacements, and depending on the direction of any displacement, the appropriate back muscles will be recruited.

During standing at ease, the back muscles may show slight continuous activity,[15,18,20,31,83,84,124,130,181,281,282,301,382,417,447,541] intermittent activity,[180,181,417,447,541] or no activity,[31,281,282,301,541] and the amount of activity can be influenced by changing the position of the head or allowing the trunk to sway.[181]

The explanation for these differences probably lies in the location of the line of gravity in relation to the lumbar spine in different individuals.[31,301,298,417,541] In about 75% of individuals the line of gravity passes in front of the centre of the L4 vertebra, and therefore, essentially in front of the lumbar spine.[31,301] Consequently, gravity will exert a constant tendency to pull the thorax and lumbar spine into flexion. To preserve an upright posture, a constant level of activity in the posterior sagittal rotators of the lumbar spine will be needed to oppose the tendency to flexion. Conversely, when the line of gravity passes behind the lumbar spine, gravity tends to extend it, and back muscle activity is not required. Instead abdominal muscle activity is recruited to prevent the spine extending under gravity.[31,301]

Activities that displace the centre of gravity of the trunk side-ways will tend to cause lateral flexion. To prevent undesired lateral flexion, the contralateral lateral flexors will contract. This occurs when weights are carried in one hand.[181,281] Carrying equal weights in both hands does not displace the line of gravity, and back muscle activity is not increased substantially on either side of the body.[181,281]

During sitting, the activity of the back muscles is similar to that during standing,[18,20,27] but in supported sitting, as with the elbows resting on the knees, there is no activity in the lumbar back muscles,[181,447] and with arms resting on a desk, back muscle activity is substantially decreased.[18,20] In reclined sitting, the back rest supports the weight of the thorax lessening the need for muscular support. Consequently, increasing the reclination of the back rest of a seat decreases lumbar back muscle activity.[18,20,389,390]

Major active movements

Forward flexion and extension of the spine from the flexed position are movements during which the back muscles have their most important function. As the spine bends forward, there is an increase in the activity of the back muscles,[15,23,83,130,180,181,206,305,382,383,414,427,447] and this increase is proportional to the angle of flexion and the size of any load carried.[21,23,418,479] The movement of forward flexion is produced by gravity, but the extent and the rate at which it proceeds is controlled by the eccentric contraction of the back muscles. Movement of the thorax on the lumbar spine is controlled by the long thoracic fibres of longissimus and iliocostalis. The long tendons of insertion allow these muscles to act around the convexity of the increasing thoracic kyphosis and anchor the thorax to the ilium and sacrum. In the lumbar region, the multifidus and the lumbar fascicles of longissimus and iliocostalis act to control the anterior sagittal rotation of the lumbar vertebrae. At the same time the lumbar fascicles of longissimus and iliocostalis also act to control the associated anterior translation of the lumbar vertebrae.

At a certain point during forward flexion, the activity in the back muscles ceases, and the vertebral column is braced by the locking of the zygapophysial joints and tension in its posterior ligaments (Ch. 7). This phenomenon is known as **critical point**.[180,297,298,382] However, critical point does not occur in all individuals, or in all muscles.[130,181,447,541] When it does occur, it does so when the spine has reached about 90% maximum flexion, even though at this stage, the hip flexion that occurs in forward bending is still only 60% complete.[297,298] Carrying weights during flexion causes the critical point to occur later in the range of vertebral flexion.[297,298]

The physiological basis for critical point is still obscure. It may be due to reflex inhibition initiated by proprioceptors in the lumbar joints and ligaments, or in muscle stretch and length receptors.[297] Whatever the mechanism, the significance of critical point is that it marks the transition of spinal load-bearing from muscles to the ligamentous system.

Extension of the trunk from the flexed position is characterised by high levels of back muscle activity.[130,180,181,382,427] In the thoracic region, the iliocostalis and longissimus, acting around the thoracic kyphosis, lift the thorax by rotating it backwards. The lumbar vertebrae are rotated backwards principally by the lumbar multifidus, causing their superior surfaces to be progressively tilted upwards to support the rising thorax.

Compressive loads of the back muscles

Because of the downward direction of their action, as the back muscles contract they exert a longitudinal compression of the lumbar vertebral column, and this compression raises the pressure in the lumbar intervertebral discs. Any activity that involves the back muscles, therefore, is associated with a rise in nuclear pressure. As measured in the L3–4 intervertebral disc, the nuclear pressure correlates with the degree of myoelectric activity in the back muscles.[17,23,390,418,419]. As muscle activity increases, disc pressure rises.

Disc pressures and myoelectric activity of the back muscles have been used extensively to quantify the stresses applied to the lumbar spine in various postures and by various activities.[18,24–27,388–390,394,395] From the standing position, forward bending causes the greatest increase in disc pressure. Lifting a weight in this position raises disc pressure even further, and the pressure is greatly increased if a load is lifted with the lumbar spine both flexed and rotated. Throughout these various manoeuvres, back muscle activity increases in proportion to the disc pressure.

One of the prime revelations of combined discometric and electromyographic studies of the lumbar spine during lifting relates to the comparative stresses applied to the lumbar spine by different lifting tactics. In essence, it has been shown that, on the basis of changes in disc pressure and back muscle activity, there are no differences between using a 'stoop' lift or a 'leg' lift, i.e. lifting a weight with a bent back versus lifting with a straight back.[22,23,389,390] The critical factor is the distance of the load from the body. The further the load is from the chest the greater the stresses on the lumbar spine, and the greater the disc pressure and back muscle activity.[22]

Strength of the back muscles

The strength of the back muscles has been determined in experiments on normal volunteers.[372] Two measures of strength are available: the absolute maximum force of contraction in the upright posture and the moment generated on the lumbar spine. The absolute maximum strength of the back muscles as a whole is about 4000 N. Acting on the short moment arms provided by the spinous processes and pedicles of the lumbar vertebrae this force converts to an extensor moment of 200 Nm. These figures apply to average males under the age of 30; young females exhibit about 60% of this strength, while individuals over the age of 30 are about 10–30% weaker respectively.[372]

Lifting

In biomechanical terms, the act of lifting constitutes a problem in balancing moments. When an individual bends forwards to execute a lift flexion occurs at the hip joint and in the lumbar spine. Indeed most of the forward movement seen during trunk flexion occurs at the hip joint.[297] The flexion forces are generated by gravity acting on the mass of the object to be lifted and on the mass of the trunk above the level of the hip joint and lumbar spine (Fig. 8.14). These forces exert flexion moments on both the hip joint and the lumbar spine. In each case the moment will be the product of the force and its perpendicular distance from the joint in question. The total flexion moment acting on each joint will be the sum of the moments exerted by the mass to be lifted and the mass of the trunk. For a lift to be executed these flexion moments have to be overcome by a moment acting in the opposite direction. This could be exerted by longitudinal forces acting downwards behind the hip joint and vertebral column or by forces acting upwards in front of the joints pushing the trunk upwards.

There are no doubts as to the capacity of the hip extensors to generate large moments and overcome the flexion moments exerted on the hip joint even by the heaviest of loads that might be lifted.[163,165] However, the hip extensors are only able to rotate the pelvis backwards on the femurs; they do not act on the lumbar spine. Thus, regardless of what happens at the hip joint the lumbar spine still remains subject to a flexion moment that must be overcome in some other way. Without an appropriate mechanism the lumbar spine would stay flexed as the hips extended;

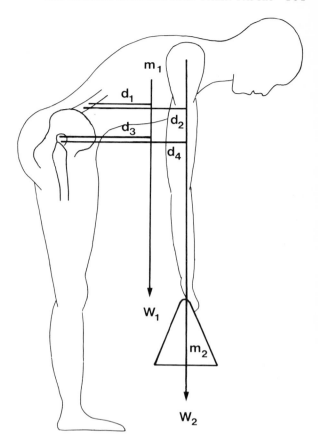

Fig. 8.14 The flexion moments exerted on a flexed trunk. Forces generated by the weight of the trunk and the load to be lifted act vertically in front of the lumbar spine and hip joint. The moments they exert on each joint are proportional to the distance between the line of action of each force and the joint in question. The mass of the trunk (m_1) exerts a force (W_1) that acts a measurable distance in front of the lumbar spine (d_1) and the hip joint (d_3). The mass to be lifted (m_2) exerts a force (W_2) that acts a measurable distance form the lumbar spine (d_2) and the hip joint (d_4). The respective moments acting on the lumbar spine will be W_1d_1 and W_1d_3; those on the hip joint will be W_2d_2 and W_2d_4.

indeed as the pelvis rotated backwards, flexion of the lumbar spine would be accentuated as its bottom end was pulled backwards with the pelvis while its top end remained stationary under the load of the flexion moment. A mechanism is required to allow the lumbar spine to resist this deformation or to cause it to extend in unison with the hip joint.

Despite much investigation and debate, the exact nature of this mechanism remains unresolved. In various ways the back muscles, intra-abdominal pressure, the thoracolumbar fascia and the posterior ligamentous system have been believed to participate.

For light lifts the flexion moments generated are relatively small. In the case of a 70 kg man lifting a 10 kg mass in a fully stooped position, the upper trunk weighs about 40 kg and acts about 30 cm in front of the lumbar spine while the arms holding the mass to be lifted lie about 45 cm in front of the lumbar spine. The respective flexion moments are therefore $40 \times 9.8 \times 0.30 = 117.6$ Nm and $10 \times 9.8 \times 0.45 = 44.1$ Nm, a total of 161.7 Nm. This load is well within the capacity of the back muscles (200 Nm, see above). Thus, as the hips extend, the lumbar back muscles are capable of resisting further flexion of the lumbar spine and indeed, could even actively extend it, and the weight would be lifted.

Increasing the load to be lifted to over 30 kg increases the flexion moment to 132.2 Nm, which when added to the flexion moment of the upper trunk, exceeds the capacity of the back muscles. To remain within the capacity of the back muscles such loads must be carried closer to the lumbar spine, i.e. they must be borne with a much shorter moment arm. Even so, decreasing the moment arm to about 15 cm limits the load to be carried to about 90 kg. The back muscles are simply not strong enough to raise greater loads. Such realisations have generated concepts of several additional mechanisms that serve to aid the back muscles in overcoming large flexion moments.

In 1957 Bartelink[42] raised the proposition that intra-abdominal pressure could aid the lumbar spine in resisting flexion by acting upwards on the diaphragm — the so-called intra-abdominal balloon mechanism. Bartelink himself was circumspect and reserved in raising this conjecture, but the concept was rapidly popularised particularly amongst physiotherapists. Even though it was never validated, the concept seemed to be treated as proven fact. It received early endorsement in orthopaedic circles,[383] and intra-abdominal pressure was adopted by ergonomists and others as a measure of spinal stress and safe-lifting standards.[117–120,497,525,527] In more contemporary studies, intra-abdominal pressure has been monitored during various spinal movements and lifting tasks.[22,23,368]

Reservations about the validity of the abdominal balloon mechanism have arisen from several quarters. Studies of lifting tasks reveal that unlike myoelectric activity, intra-abdominal pressure does not correlate well with the size of the load being lifted or the applied stress on the vertebral column as measured by intradiscal pressure.[17,327,419] Indeed, deliberately increasing intra-abdominal pressure by a Valsalva manoeuvre does not relieve the load on the lumbar spine but actually increases it.[392] Clinical studies have shown that although abdominal muscles are weaker than normal in patients with back pain, intra-abdominal pressure is not different.[235] Furthermore, strengthening the abdominal muscles both in normal individuals[234] and in patients with back pain[236] does not influence intra-abdominal pressure during lifting.

The most strident criticism of the intra-abdominal balloon theory comes from bioengineers and others who maintain that (1) to generate any significant antiflexion moment the pressure required would exceed the maximum hoop tension of the abdominal muscles;[166,171,210] (2) such a pressure would be so high as to obstruct the abdominal aorta[166] (a reservation raised by Bartelink himself[42]); and (3) because the abdominal muscles lie in front of the lumbar spine and connect the thorax to the pelvis, whenever they contract to generate pressure they must also exert a flexion moment on the trunk, which would negate any antiflexion value of the intra-abdominal pressure.[46,163,165,210]

These reservations inspired an alternative explanation of the role of the abdominal muscles during lifting. Farfan, Gracovetsky and colleagues[163,210–212] noted the criss-cross arrangement of the fibres in the posterior layer of thoracolumbar fascia and surmised that if lateral tension was applied to this fascia it would result in an extension moment being exerted on the lumbar spinous processes. Such tension could be exerted by the abdominal muscles that arise from the thoracolumbar fascia, and the trigonometry of the fibres in the thoracolumbar fascia was such that they could convert lateral tension into an appreciable extension moment — the so-called 'gain' of the thoracolumbar fascia.[210] The role of the abdominal muscles during lifting was thus to brace, if not actually extend, the lumbar spine by pulling on the thoracolumbar fascia. Any rises in intra-abdominal pressure were thereby only coincidental, occurring because of the contraction of the abdominal muscles acting on the thoracolumbar fascia.

Subsequent anatomic studies revealed several liabilities of this model.[64] First, the posterior layer of thoracolumbar fascia is well developed only in the lower lumbar region, but nevertheless its fibres are appropriately orientated to enable lateral tension exerted on the fascia to produce extension moments at least on the L2 to L5 spinous processes (Fig. 8.15). However, dissection reveals that of the abdominal muscles internal oblique offers only a few fibres that irregularly attach to the thoracolumbar fascia; transversus abdominis is the only muscle that consistently attaches to the thoracolumbar fascia, but only its very middle fibres do so. The size of these fibres is such that even upon maximum contraction the force they exert is very small. Calculations revealed that the extensor moment they could exert on the lumbar spine amounted to less than 6 Nm.[347] Thus, the contribution that abdominal muscles might make to antiflexion moments is trivial, a conclusion also borne out by subsequent, independent modelling studies.[370]

A totally different model of lifting was elaborated by Farfan and Gracovetsky.[163,210,212] Noting the weakness of the back muscles these authors proposed that extension of the lumbar spine was not required to lift heavy loads or loads with long moment arms. They proposed that the lumbar spine should remain fully flexed in order to engage, i.e. maximally stretch, what they referred to as the 'posterior ligamentous system', namely the capsules of the zygapophysial joints, the interspinous and supraspinous ligaments, and the posterior layer of thoracolumbar fascia, the latter acting passively to transmit tension between the lumbar spinous processes and ilium.

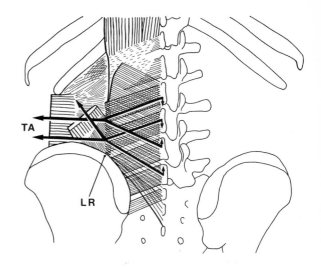

Fig. 8.15 The mechanics of the thoracolumbar fascia. From any point in the lateral raphe (LR), lateral tension in the posterior layer of thoracolumbar fascia is transmitted upwards through the deep lamina of the posterior layer, and downwards through the superficial layer. Because of the obliquity of these lines of tension, a small downward vector is generated at the midline attachment of the deep lamina, and a small upward vector is generated at the midline attachment of the superficial lamina. These mutually opposite vectors tend to approximate or oppose the separation of the L2 and L4, and L3 and L5 spinous processes. Lateral tension on the fascia can be exerted by the transversus abdominis (TA), and to a lesser extent by the few fibres of internal oblique when they attach to the lateral raphe.

Under such conditions the active energy for a lift was provided by the powerful hip extensor muscles. These rotated the pelvis backwards. Meanwhile, the external load acting on the upper trunk kept the lumbar spine flexed. Tension would develop in the posterior ligamentous system which bridged the thorax and pelvis. With the posterior ligamentous system so engaged, as the pelvis rotated backwards the lumbar spine would be passively raised while remaining in a fully flexed position. In essence, the posterior sagittal rotation of the pelvis would be transmitted through the posterior ligaments first to the L5 vertebra, then to L4 and so on, up through the lumbar spine into the thorax. All that was required was that the posterior ligamentous system be sufficiently strong to withstand the passive tension generated in it by the movement of the pelvis at one end and the weight of the trunk and external load at the other. The lumbar spine would thereby be raised like a long, rigid arm rotating on the pelvis and raising the external load with it.

Contraction of the back muscles was not required if the ligaments could take the load. Indeed, muscle contraction was distinctly undesirable, for any active extension of the lumbar spine would disengage the posterior ligaments and preclude them from transmitting tension. The back muscles could be recruited only once the trunk had been raised sufficiently to shorten the moment arm of the external load reducing its flexion moment to within the capacity of the back muscles.

The attraction of this model was that it overcame the problem of the relative weakness of the back muscles by dispensing with their need to act, which in turn was consistent with the myoelectric silence of the back muscles at full flexion of the trunk and the recruitment of muscle activity only once the trunk had been elevated and the flexion moment arm had been reduced. Support for the model also came from surgical studies which reported that if the midline ligaments and thoracolumbar fascia were conscientiously reconstructed after multi-level laminectomies, the postoperative recovery and rehabilitation of patients were enhanced.[107]

However, while attractive in a qualitative sense, the mechanism of the posterior ligamentous system was not validated quantitatively. The model requires that the ligaments be strong enough to sustain the loads applied. In this regard, data on the strength of the posterior ligaments are scant and irregular, but sufficient data are available to permit an initial appraisal of the feasibility of the posterior ligament model.

The strength of spinal ligaments varies considerably, but average values can be calculated. Table 8.1 summarises some of the available data. It is evident that the strongest posterior 'ligaments' of the lumbar spine are the zyga-pophysial joint capsules and the thoracolumbar fascia forming the midline 'supraspinous ligament'. However, when the relatively short moment arms over which these ligaments act are considered, it transpires that the maximum moment they can

Table 8.1 Strength of the posterior ligamentous system

Ligament	Reference	Average force at failure (N)	Moment arm (m)	Maximum moment (Nm)
PLL	385	90	0.02	1.8
LF	385	244	0.03	7.3
ZJC	385 114	680 672	0.04	27.2
ISL	385	107	0.05	5.4
TLF	385	500	0.06	30.0
Total				51.7

PLL — posterior longitudinal ligament. LF — ligmentum flavum. ZJC — zygapophysial joint capsules (bilaterally). ISL — interspinous ligament. TLF — the posterior layer of thoracolumbar fascia and the erector spinae aponeurosis that forms the so-called supraspinous ligament. Average force at failure has been calculated using raw data provided in the references cited. The moment arms are estimates based on inspection of a respresentative vertebra measuring the perpendicular distance between the location of the IAR and the sites of attachment of the various ligaments.

sustain is relatively small. Even the sum total of all their moments is considerably less than that required for heavy lifting and is some four times less than the maximum strength of the back muscles. Of course, it is possible that the data quoted may not be representative of the true mean values of the strength of these ligaments, but it does not seem likely that the literature quoted underestimated their strength by a factor of four or more. Under these conditions, it is evident that the posterior ligamentous system alone is not strong enough to perform the role required of it in heavy lifting. The posterior ligamentous system is not strong enough to replace the back muscles as a mechanism to prevent flexion of the lumbar spine during lifting. Some other mechanism must operate.

One such mechanism is that of the **hydraulic amplifier** effect.[211] It was originally proposed by racovetsky, Farfan and Lamy[211] that because the thoracolumbar fascia surrounded the back muscles as a retinaculum it could serve to brace these muscles and enhance their power. The engineering basis for this effect is complicated, and the concept remained unexplored until very recently. A mathematical proof has been published which suggests that by investing the back muscles the thoracolumbar fascia enhances the strength of the back muscles by some 30%.[263] This is an appreciable increase and an attractive mechanism for enhancing the antiflexion capacity of the back muscles. However, the validity of this proof is still being questioned on the grounds that the principles used, while applicable to the behaviour of solids, may not be applicable to muscles; and the concept of the hydraulic amplifier mechanism still remains under scrutiny.

Quite a constrasting model has been proposed to explain the mechanics of the lumbar spine in lifting. It is based on an arch theory and maintains that the behaviour, stability and strength of the lumbar spine during lifting can be be explained by viewing the lumbar spine as an arch braced by intra-abdominal pressure.[32,37] This intriguing concept, however, has not met with any degree of acceptance and indeed, has been challenged from some quarters.[4]

In summary, despite much effort over recent years the exact mechanism of heavy lifting still remains unexplained. The back muscles are too weak to extend the lumbar spine against large flexion moments; the intra-abdominal balloon has been refuted; the abdominal mechanism and thoracolumbar fascia has been refuted and the posterior ligamentous system appears too weak to replace the back muscles. Engineering models of the hydraulic amplifier effect and the arch model are still subject to debate.

What remains to be explained is what provides the missing force to sustain heavy loads, and why is intra-abdominal pressure so consistently generated during lifts if it is neither to brace the thoracolumbar fascia or to provide an intra-abdominal balloon? At present these questions can only be addressed by conjecture, but certain concepts appear worthy of consideration.

With regard to intra-abdominal pressure, one concept that has been overlooked in studies of lifting is the role of the abdominal muscles in controlling axial rotation of the trunk. Investigators have focused their attention on movements in the sagittal plane during lifting and have ignored the fact that when bent forward to address an object to be lifted the trunk is liable to axial rotation. Unless the external load is perfectly balanced and lies exactly in the midline, it will cause the trunk to twist to the left or right. Thus, to keep the weight in the midline and in the sagittal plane the lifter must control any twisting effect. The oblique abdominal muscles are the principal rotators of the trunk and would be responsible for this bracing. In contracting to control axial rotation, the abdominal muscles would secondarily raise intra-abdominal pressure. This pressure rise is therefore an epiphenomenon and would reflect not the size of any external load but its tendency to twist the flexed trunk.

With regard to loads in the sagittal plane, the passive strength of the back muscles has been neglected in discussions of lifting. From the behaviour of isolated muscle fibres it is known that as a muscle elongates its maximum contractile force diminishes, but its passive elastic tension rises; so much so that in an elongated muscle the total passive and active tension generated is at least equal to the maximum contractile capacity of the muscle at resting length. Thus, although they become electrically silent at full flexion, the back muscles are still capable of providing passive tension equal to their maximum contractile strength. This would allow the silent muscles to supplement the engaged posterior ligamentous system. With the back muscles providing some 200 Nm and the ligaments some 50 Nm or more, the total antiflexion capacity of the lumbar spine rises to about 250 Nm which would allow some 30 kg to be safely lifted at 90° trunk flexion. Larger loads could be sustained by proportionally shortening the moment arm. Consequently, the mechanism of lifting may well be essentially as proposed by Farfan and Gracovetsky,[163,211,212] save that the passive tension in the back muscles constitutes the major component of the 'posterior ligamentous system'.

9. Nerves of the lumbar spine

The lumbar spine is associated with a variety of nerves, the central focus of which are the lumbar **spinal nerves**. These lie in the intervertebral foramina and are connected to the spinal cord by the **spinal nerve roots** which occupy the vertebral canal. Peripherally (i.e. outside the vertebral column), the spinal nerves divide into their branches: the **ventral** and **dorsal rami**. Running along the anterolateral aspects of the lumbar vertebral column are the lumbar **sympathetic trunks** which communicate with the ventral rami of the lumbar spinal nerves.

LUMBAR SPINAL NERVES

The lumbar spinal nerves lie in the intervertebral foramina and are numbered according the vertebra beneath which they lie. Thus, the L1 spinal nerve lies below the L1 vertebra in the L1–2 intervertebral foramen; the L2 spinal nerve lies below the L2 vertebra, and so on. Centrally, each spinal nerve is connected to the spinal cord by a dorsal and a ventral root. Peripherally, each spinal nerve divides into a larger ventral ramus and a smaller dorsal ramus. The spinal nerve roots join the spinal nerve in the intervertebral foramen, and the ventral and dorsal rami are formed just outside the intervertebral foramen. Consequently, the spinal nerves are quite short. Each is no longer than the width of the intervertebral foramen in which it lies (Fig. 9.1).

The medial (or central) end of the spinal nerve may be difficult to define for it depends on exactly where the dorsal and ventral roots of the nerve converge to form a single trunk. Sometimes, the spinal nerve may be very short, less than 1 mm, in which case the roots distribute

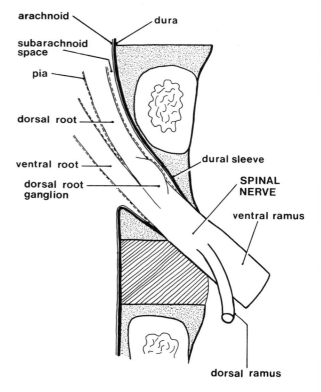

Fig. 9.1 A sketch of a lumbar spinal nerve, its roots and meningeal coverings. The nerve roots are invested by pia mater, and covered by arachnoid and dura as far as the spinal nerve. The dura of the dural sac is prolonged around the roots as their dural sleeve, which blends with the epineurium of the spinal nerve.

their fibres directly to the ventral and dorsal rami without really forming a spinal nerve. Otherwise, the roots generally form a short trunk whose length measures a few millimetres from the point of junction of the nerve roots to the point of division of the ventral and dorsal rami.

LUMBAR NERVE ROOTS

The **dorsal root** of each spinal nerve transmits sensory fibres from the spinal nerve to the spinal cord. The **ventral root** largely transmits motor fibres from the cord to the spinal nerve, but may also transmit some sensory fibres. The ventral roots of the L1 and L2 spinal nerves additionally transmit preganglionic, sympathetic, efferent fibres.

The spinal cord terminates in the vertebral canal opposite the level of the L1–2 intervertebral disc, although it may end as high as T12–L1 or as low as L2–3.[340] Consequently, to reach the spinal cord, the lower lumbar (and sacral) nerve roots must run within the vertebral canal where they are largely enclosed in the dural sac (Fig. 9.2). Within the dural sac, the lumbar nerve roots run freely, mixed with the sacral and coccygeal nerve roots to form the **cauda equina**, and each

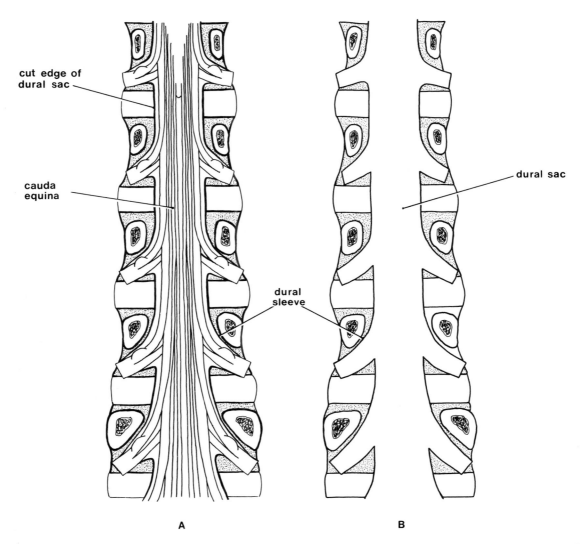

Fig. 9.2 A sketch of the lumbar nerve roots and the dural sac. **A**: The posterior half of the dural sac has been removed to reveal the lumbar nerve roots as they lie within the dural sac, forming the cauda equina. **B**: The intact dural sac is depicted, as it lies on the floor of the vertebral canal.

root is covered with its own sleeve of pia mater that is continuous with the pia mater of the spinal cord. All the roots of the cauda equina are bathed in cerebrospinal fluid which percolates through the subarachnoid space of the dural sac.

For the greater part of their course, the nerve fibres within each nerve root are gathered into a single trunk, but near the spinal cord they are separated into smaller bundles called **rootlets** that eventually attach to the spinal cord. The size and number of rootlets for each nerve root is variable, but in general they are 0.5–1 mm in diameter and number between 2 and 12 for each root.[68] The rootlets of each ventral root attach to the ventrolateral aspect of the cord, while those of the dorsal roots attach to the dorsolateral sulcus of the cord, and along the ventral and dorsal surface of the cord the rootlets form an uninterrupted series of attachments (Fig. 9.3).

A pair of spinal nerve roots leaves the dural sac just above the level of each intervertebral foramen. They do so by penetrating the dural sac in an inferolateral direction, taking with them an extension of dura mater and arachnoid mater referred to as the **dural sleeve** (Fig. 9.2). This sleeve encloses the nerve roots as far as the intervertebral foramen and spinal nerve where the dura mater merges with, or becomes, the epineurium of the spinal nerve (Fig. 9.1). The pia mater of each of the nerve roots also extends as far as the spinal nerve, as does an extension of the subarachnoid space (Fig. 9.1). Thus, the nerve roots are ensheathed with pia mater and bathed in cerebrospinal fluid as far as the spinal nerve.

Immediately proximal to its junction with the spinal nerve, the dorsal root forms an enlargement, the **dorsal root ganglion**, which contains the cell bodies of the sensory fibres in the dorsal root. The ganglion lies within the dural sleeve of the nerve roots and occupies the upper, medial part of the intervertebral foramen, but may lie further distally in the foramen if the spinal nerve is short.

The angle at which each pair of nerve roots leaves the dural sac varies from above downward. The L1 and L2 roots leave the dural sac at an obtuse angle, but the dural sleeves of the lower nerve roots form increasingly acute angles with

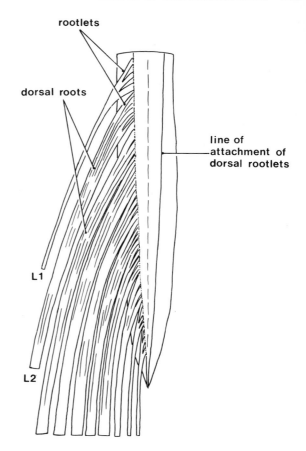

Fig. 9.3 An illustration of the lower end of the spinal cord and the pattern of attachment of the dorsal nerve roots and dorsal nerve rootlets.

the lateral margins of the dural sac (Fig. 9.2). The angles formed by the L1 and L2 roots are about 80° and 70° respectively, while the angles of the L3 and L4 roots are each about 60° and that of the L5 roots is 45°.[67]

The level of origin of the nerve root sleeves also varies from above downwards. In general, the sleeves arise opposite the back of their respective vertebral bodies. Thus, the L1 sleeve arises behind the L1 body; the L2 sleeve behind the L2 body, and so on. However, successively lower sleeves arise increasingly higher behind their vertebral bodies until the sleeve of the L5 nerve roots arises behind the L4–5 intervertebral disc.[67]

Relations of the nerve roots

The relations of the nerve roots are of critical importance in the pathology of nerve root compression, for space-occupying lesions of any of the tissues intimately, or even distantly, related to the nerve roots may encroach upon them. In this regard, the majority of structures related to the nerve roots have already been described (Ch. 5), although the anatomy of the spinal blood vessels is described in detail in Chapter 10.

The most intimate relations of the nerve roots are the meninges. The roots of the cauda equina are enclosed in the dural sac, and bathed in cerebrospinal fluid. Beyond the dural sac, individual pairs of roots are ensheathed by pia, arachnoid and dura in the nerve root sleeves (Figs 9.1 and 9.4). The relevance of this relationship is that tumours or cysts of the dura or arachnoid can at times form space-occupying lesions that compress the roots. Running within the root sleeves are the radicular arteries and veins (see Ch. 10), and the relevance of this relationship is described in Chapter 13.

As a whole, the dural sac rests on the floor of the vertebral canal (Ch. 5). The anterior relations of the dural sac are, therefore, the backs of the vertebral bodies and the intervertebral discs, and covering these structures is the posterior longitudinal ligament (Fig. 9.4). Running across the floor of the vertebral canal, and therefore anterior to the dural sac, are the anterior spinal canal arteries (see Ch. 10) and the sinuvertebral nerves (see below). Posteriorly, the dural sac is related to the roof of the vertebral canal: the laminae and ligamenta flava (Ch. 5).

A space intervenes between the dural sac and the osseo-ligamentous boundaries of the vertebral canal, and this space is referred to as the **epidural space**. This space, however, is quite narrow, for the dural sac is applied very closely to the osseo-ligamentous boundaries of the vertebral canal. It is almost a 'potential space', and the term 'epidural region' has been advocated as an alternative description to avoid the connotation of a wide, empty space[426] (Fig. 9.4).

The epidural space is principally filled by a thin layer of areolar connective tissue which varies from diaphanous to pseudomembranous in struc-

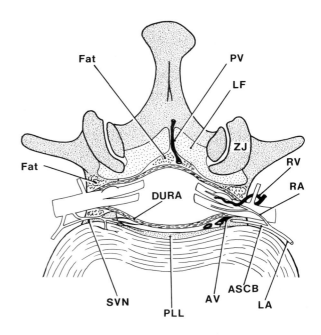

Fig. 9.4 A transverse section through the vertebral canal and intervertebral foramina to demonstrate the relations of the lumbar nerve roots. The roots are enclosed in their dural sleeve, which is surrounded by epidural fat in the intervertebral foramina. Radicular veins (RV) and radicular arteries (RA) run with the nerve roots. Anteriorly the roots are related to the intervertebral disc and posterior longitudinal ligament (PLL), separated from them by the sinuvertebral nerves (SVN), elements of the anterior internal vertebral venous plexus (AV), and the anterior spinal canal branches (ASCB) of the lumbar arteries (LA). Posteriorly, the roots are separated from the ligamentum flavum (LF) and zygapophysial joints (ZJ) by elements of the posterior internal vertebral venous plexus (PV), and epidural fat which lodges in the recess between the ligamentum flavum of each side.

ture.[426] Running within this areolar tissue are the anterior and posterior internal vertebral venous plexuses (see Ch. 10), and located within it are collections of fat. The epidural fat is not distributed uniformly throughout the epidural space, but is concentrated around the nerve roots in the intervertebral foramina, and in collections wrapped in areolar tissue and lodged in the midline recesses between the ligamenta flava at each segmental level.[426]

Individual pairs of nerve roots, enclosed in their dural sleeves course to their intervertebral foramina along the radicular canals (Ch. 5). Consequently, they are related laterally to a pedicle, and ventrally, from above downwards they cross the back of a vertebral body to enter the upper portion of their intervertebral foramen. Dorsally, they are covered by a lamina and its ligamenta flava which separate the root sleeve from the overlying zygapophysial joints (Ch. 5).

Within the vertebral canal, the dural sac and the nerve root sleeves are tethered to the vertebral column.[426,492] At each segmental level, dural ligaments arise from the anterior aspect of the dural sac and attach to the posterior longitudinal ligament. These are flanked by further ligaments that arise from the anterolateral aspects of the dural sac and attach to the lateral edge of the posterior longitudinal ligament. These ligaments are variably developed at the L1 to L4 levels, but are well-developed at L5.[492] Posteriorly, the dural sac is attached to the roof of the vertebral canal by occasional, weak pseudo-ligamentous connections.[426]

The nerve root sleeves are tethered both within the vertebral canal and in the intervertebral foramen. At the proximal end of the root sleeve, ligaments connect the dura to the posterior longitudinal ligament and the periosteum of the adjacent pedicle.[441,492] In the intervertebral foramen, the root sleeve is surrounded by circumferential layers of connective tissue that indirectly bind the nerve roots and spinal nerve to the margins of the foramen, but mainly to the capsule of the zygapophysial joint dorsally.[441,492] At the outer end of the intervertebral foramen, the spinal nerve may be related to a transforaminal ligament when one is present (Ch. 4). As a rule, the spinal nerve lies below most forms of transforaminal ligaments, but emerges above the inferior transforaminal variety[207] (Ch. 4).

The relative size of the spinal nerve and nerve roots within the intervertebral foramen varies from level to level and is important with respect to the risk of spinal nerve and nerve root compression. As an approximate rule, the cross-sectional area of an intervertebral foramen increases from L1–2 to L4–5, but the L5–S1 foramen is conspicuously smaller than the rest,[231] but paradoxically, the L5 spinal nerve is the largest of the lumbar nerves.[231] Consequently, the L5 spinal nerve occupies about 25–30% of the available area in an intervertebral foramen, while the other lumbar nerves occupy between 7 and 22%, making the L5 nerve the most susceptible to foraminal stenosis.

Anomalies of the nerve roots

The clinically most significant anomalies of the lumbar nerve roots are aberrant courses and anastomoses between nerve roots,[82,153,291,369,403,448,457] and the morphology of these anomalies is summarised in Figure 9.5.

Type 1 anomalies are aberrant courses. Two pairs of nerve roots may arise from a single dural sleeve (Type 1A), or a dural sleeve may arise from a low position on the dural sac (Type 1B). Type 2 anomalies are those in which the number of roots in an intervertebral foramen varies. A foramen may be unoccupied by a nerve (Type 2A), in which case the foramen above or below contains two sets of roots, or a foramen may contain a supernumerary set of roots (Type 2B). Type 3 anomalies are extra-dural anastomoses between roots in which a bundle of nerve fibres leaves one dural sleeve to enter an adjacent one. This type of anomaly may be superimosed on a Type 2 anomaly.

These anomalies, per se, do not produce symptoms. Patients with conjoined or aberrant nerve roots may pass their entire life without developing symptoms. However, doubled nerve roots occupy far more of the available space in the radicular canal or the intervertebral foramen than a single root. Therefore, if a space-occupying lesion develops, it is more likely to compress a double nerve root, and produce symptoms sooner, than if a normal single root was present. Thus, although root anomalies do not render patients more likely to develop disorders of the lumbar spine, they do render them more likely to develop symptoms in the presence of space-occupying lesions.

The other clinical significance of anomalous roots relates to the interpretation of clinical signs. Clinical examination might indicate compression of a particular nerve root, but if that root has an anomalous course, the structural lesion causing the compression may not be located at the expected site. For example, signs of L4 nerve root compression most often suggest compression in

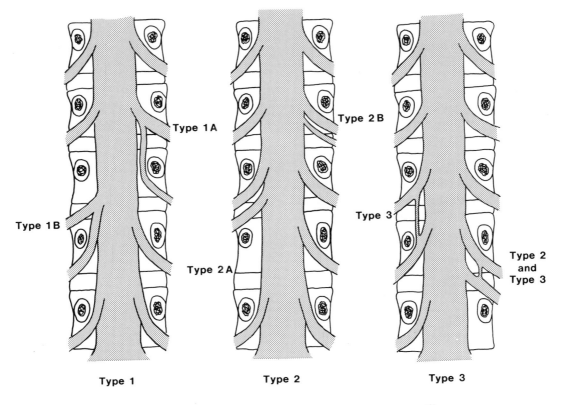

Fig. 9.5 Extra-dural anomalies of the lumbar nerve roots. (Based on Neidre and MacNab.[403])

the L4 radicular canal or in the L4–5 intervertebral foramen; but in the case of an anomalous L4 root being compressed, the lesion could be at the L3, or perhaps the L5 vertebral level, depending on the type of anomaly. Alternatively, in the case of doubled nerve roots, a single compressive lesion could produce signs suggestive of two lesions compressing two consecutive nerve roots.

Fortunately, symptomatic nerve root anomalies are not common, and such confusing considerations do not regularly complicate clinical practice. The incidence of anomalies has been estimated at about 8.5%,[231] but when symptomatic, the major types are readily recognised in myelograms.[68] Nonetheless, nerve root anomalies should be borne in mind and considered as a possibility in patients with unusual distributions of neurological signs.

The surgical significance of nerve root anomalies relates to the mobility of anomalous nerve roots, the care necessary when operating in their vicinity, and the types of procedures that can be carried out to decompress them. These issues are explored in the surgical literature.[68,403]

Another feature of nerve roots that is not an anomaly, but rather a variation, is intrathecal anastomoses. Within the dural sac, bundles of nerve fibres may pass from one nerve root to the next, and such communications have an incidence of 11–30%.[116] They usually occur close to the spinal cord, and may vary in size from small filaments to substantial bundles.[116] Since they occur proximal to the regions where nerve roots are liable to compression, these anastomoses are not of diagnostic clinical significance, but they are of relevance to neurosurgeons operating on the proximal ends of nerve roots.[116,420]

DORSAL RAMI

The L1 to L4 dorsal rami are short nerves that arise almost at right angles from the lumbar spinal nerve.[70] Each nerve measures about 5 mm in length,[66] and is directed backwards towards the upper border of the subjacent transverse process. The L5 dorsal ramus differs, in that it is longer and travels over the top of the ala of the sacrum[66] (Fig. 9.6).

As they approach their transverse processes, the L1–4 dorsal rami divide into 2 or 3 branches (Fig. 9.6). A **medial** branch and a **lateral** branch are always represented at every level. The variable, third branch is the **intermediate** branch. Although this branch is always represented it frequently arises from the lateral branch instead of the dorsal ramus itself.[66] The L5 dorsal ramus forms only a medial branch and a branch that is equivalent to the intermediate branches of the other lumbar dorsal rami.

The lateral branches of the lumbar dorsal rami are principally distributed to the iliocostalis lumborum muscle, but those from the L1, L2 and L3 levels can emerge from the dorsolateral border of this muscle to become cutaneous. Cutaneous branches of these pierce the posterior layer of thoracolumbar fascia and descend inferolaterally across the iliac crest to innervate the skin of the buttock, over an area extending from the iliac crest to the greater trochanter.[279] When crossing the iliac crest, these nerves run parallel to one another with those from lower levels lying most medial.

Variations occur in the regularity with which branches of the L1, L2 and L3 dorsal rami become cutaneous.[354] Most commonly only the L1 lateral branch becomes cutaneous. This occurs in some 60% of individuals. Both L1 and L2 become cutaneous in about 27% of cases, and all three levels furnish cutaneous branches in only 13% of cases. Regardless of its segmental origin, the lowest and most medial nerve that crosses the iliac crest does so approximately 7 to 8 cm from the midline.[354]

The intermediate branches of the lumbar dorsal rami have only a muscular distribution, to the lumbar fibres of the longissimus muscle, and within this muscle they form an intersegmental

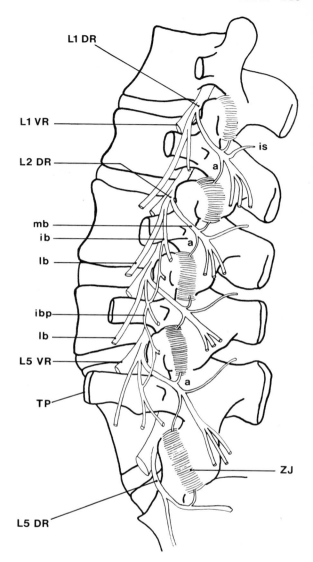

Fig. 9.6 A sketch of a left posterior view of the lumbar spine showing the branches of the lumbar dorsal rami. (Based on Bagduk et al.[66]) VR — ventral ramus. DR — dorsal ramus. mb — medial branch. ib — intermediate branch. lb — lateral branch. ibp — intermediate branch plexus. is — interspinous branch. a — articular branch. ZJ — zygapophysial joint.

plexus[66,70] (Fig. 9.6). The intermediate branch of the L5 dorsal ramus supplies the lowest fibres of longissimus which arise from the L5 transverse process and attach to the medial aspect of the iliac crest (Ch. 8).

It is the medial branches that are of paramount clinical relevance because of their distribution to the zygapophysial joints. The medial branches of the L1 to L4 dorsal rami run across the top of their respective transverse processes and pierce the dorsal leaf of the intertransverse ligament at the base of the transverse process (Ch. 4, Fig. 4.7). Each nerve then runs along bone at the junction of the root of the transverse process with the root of the superior articular process (Fig. 9.6). Hooking medially around the base of the superior articular process, each nerve is covered by the mamillo-accessory ligament (Ch. 4). Finally, it crosses the vertebral lamina, where it divides into multiple branches that supply the multifidus muscle, and interspinous muscle and ligament, and two zygapophysial joints.

Each medial branch supplies the zygapophysial joints above and below its course[59,66,70,323,329,438] (Fig. 9.6). Histological studies have shown that capsules of the lumbar zygapophysial joints are richly innervated with encapsulated, unencapsulated and free nerve endings,[59,251,272] and are therefore endowed with the appropriate sensory apparatus to transmit proprioceptive and nociceptive information. Nerve fibres are also distributed to the intra-articular inclusions found within these joints.[200,201,203]

The medial branch of the L5 dorsal ramus has a similar course and distribution to those of the L1 to L4 dorsal rami, except that instead of crossing a transverse process, it crosses the ala of the sacrum. It runs in the groove formed by the junction of the ala and the root of the superior articular process of the sacrum before hooking medially around the base of the lumbosacral zygapophysial joint. It sends an articular branch to this joint before ramifying in multifidus.

The muscular distribution of the medial branches of the lumbar dorsal rami is very specific. Each medial branch supplies only those muscles that arise from the lamina and spinous process of the vertebra with the same segmental number as the nerve.[66,348] Thus, for example, the L1 medial branch supplies only those fibres from the L1 vertebra; the L2 nerve supplies only those muscles from the L2 vertebra, and so on. This relationship can be stated more formally as 'the muscles arising from the spinous process and lamina of a lumbar vertebra are innervated by the medial branch of the dorsal ramus that issues immediately below that vertebra'. The same applies for the interspinous ligaments. This relationship indicates that the principal muscles that move a particular segment are innervated by the nerve of that segment (Ch. 8).

Variations have been reported in the number and nature of branches of the lumbar dorsal rami that innervate the lumbar zygapophysial joints. Lazorthes and Juskiewenski[323] reported that occasionally an articular branch may arise from the dorsal ramus proper and innervate the ventral aspect of the adjacent joint. A similar branch was described by Auteroche,[35] who also described multiple articular branches arising from the spinal nerve, the lateral branch of the dorsal ramus, and from the entire length of the medial branch. Such a plethora of articular nerves has not been observed in any other study.[66,70,323,329,438] The study by Auteroche was based solely on dissection using magnifying glasses; the nature of the putative articular branches was not confirmed histologically. Under such conditions it is possible to mistake collagen fibres for articular nerves. Studies using a dissecting microscope and histological corroboration do not support his generous description of articular branches. Similarly, ascending articular branches from the root of the medial branch as described by Paris[422] have not been confirmed histologically, nor have they been seen in previous studies,[66,70,323,329,438] and indeed have been explicitly denied in subsequent studies.[344]

VENTRAL RAMI

The ventral rami of the lumbar spinal nerves emerge from the intervertebral foramen by piercing the ventral leaf of the intertransverse ligament (Ch. 4). Therefore, they enter the space in front of the ligaments, and lie within the substance of the psoas major muscle. Within the muscle they enter into the formation of plexuses. The L1 to L4 ventral rami form the lumbar plexus, and the L4 and L5 ventral rami join to form the lumbosacral trunk which enters the lumbosacral plexus. Because these plexuses are not particularly relevant to the pathology or physiology of lumbar spinal disorders, their anatomy will not be further explored. They are adequately decribed in other textbooks of anatomy.[556]

The one exception to this exclusion relates to the course of the L5 ventral ramus. This nerve crosses the ala of the sacrum, below the L5 transverse process, and in this location can be trapped between these two bones. This phenomen has been called the 'far out syndrome' and is described fully elsewhere.[568]

The principal relevance of the lumbar ventral rami to lumbar spine disorders lies in their communication with the grey rami communicantes and the innervation of the lumbar intervertebral discs. This is described in the following section.

SYMPATHETIC NERVES

The lumbar sympathetic trunks descend through the lumbar region along the anterolateral borders of the lumbar vertebral column. Each trunk is applied to the vertebral column next to the medial edge of the attachment of the psoas major muscle. The number of ganglia on the trunks varies from one to six,[69] but most commonly four are present.[259]

Branches of the lumbar sympathetic trunks are distributed to abdominal and pelvic blood vessels and viscera, and some direct branches pass into the psoas major muscle,[259] but the principal branches are the rami communicantes to the lumbar ventral rami. White rami communicantes are distributed to the L1 and L2 ventral rami, and grey rami communicantes are distributed to every lumbar ventral ramus. The number of rami communicantes to each lumbar nerve varies from one to three, and exceptionally may be as high as five.[259]

In general, the rami communicantes reach the ventral rami by passing through the tunnels deep to the tendinous arches of the psoas muscle that cover the concave lateral surfaces of the lumbar vertebral bodies (Ch. 8). These tunnels direct them to the lower borders of the transverse processes where the rami communicantes join the ventral rami just outside the intervertebral foramina. Rami communicantes may also reach the ventral rami by penetrating the substance of psoas.[65,259]

The efferent fibres of the rami communicantes are principally destined to be distributed to the blood vessels and skin in the territories supplied by the lumbar spinal nerves, but in the vicinity of the lumbar spine, rami communicantes are involved in the formation of the lumbar sinuvertebral nerves and in the innervation of the lumbar intervertebral discs.

SINUVERTEBRAL NERVES

The sinuvertebral nerves are recurrent branches of the ventral rami that re-enter the intervertebral foramina to be distributed within the vertebral

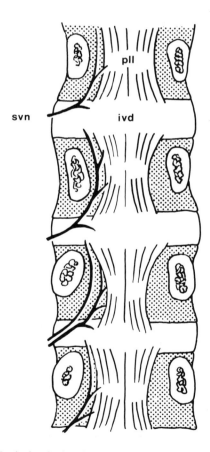

Fig. 9.7 A sketch showing the course and skeletal distribution of the lumbar sinuvertebral nerves (svn). Each nerve supplies the intervertebral disc (ivd) at its level of entry into the vertebral canal, the disc above, and the intervening posterior longitudinal ligament (pll). In about one-third of cases, the nerve at a particular level may be represented by more than one filament.

canal.[59,65,293,322,438,562] They are mixed nerves, each being formed by a somatic root from a ventral ramus and an autonomic root from a grey ramus communicans.

In the intervertebral foramina the lumbar sinuvertebral nerves run across the back of the vertebral body, just below the upper pedicle. Within the vertebral canal, each nerve forms an ascending branch which passes rostrally, parallel to the posterior longitudinal ligament, to which it sends branches, and ends in the next higher intervertebral disc which it also supplies. A shorter, descending branch ramifies in the disc and ligament at the level of entry of the parent nerve (Fig. 9.7).

In addition to this skeletal distribution, each lumbar sinuvertebral nerve is distributed to the blood vessels of the vertebral canal and to the ventral aspect of the dura mater. In the dura mater each sinuvertebral nerve forms ascending and descending meningeal branches.[137,293] The descending branches are the longer, extending up to two segments caudally, while the ascending branch ascends up to one segment.[293] The dura mater is in fact covered with a dense plexus of nerves on its ventral surface.[216] This plexus extends around the lateral aspect of the dural sac but attenuates dorsally. The paramedian portion of the dorsal aspect of the dural sac is distinctly devoid of nerve fibres.[137,216]

INNERVATION OF THE LUMBAR INTERVERTEBRAL DISCS

Whether or not the lumbar intervertebral discs receive an innervation has long been a controversial issue. Early studies failed to demonstrate nerve fibres or nerve endings within the discs,[267,283,562] and the results of these studies have been used to promulgate the conclusion that the lumbar discs lack an innervation.[16,316,571] However, other studies identified nerve fibres in the superficial layers of the anulus fibrosus,[139,251,272,473] and in a painstaking study, Malinsky[355] demonstrated a variety of free and complex endings in the outer third of the anulus.

Malinsky's studies[355] demonstrated that in the prenatal period, nerves are abundant in the anulus fibrosus, where they form simple free endings; and that they increase in number in older fetuses. During the post-natal period, various types of non-encapsulated receptors occur, and in adult material five types of nerve terminations can be found: simple and complex free nerve endings, 'shrubby' receptors, others that form loops and mesh-like formations, and clusters of parallel free nerve endings. On the surface of the anulus fibrosus, various types of encapsulated and complex unencapsulated receptors occur. They are all relatively simple in structure in neonates, but more elaborate forms occur in older and mature specimens.

Within a given disc, Malinsky[355] reported that receptors are not uniformly distributed. The greatest number of endings occurs in the lateral region of the disc, and nearly all the encapsulated receptors are located in this region. Following post-natal development, there is a relative decrease in the number of receptors in the anterior region, such that in adults the greatest number of endings occurs in the lateral regions of the disc, a smaller number in the posterior region, and the least number anteriorly.

Malinsky's findings have been confirmed in studies by Rabischong et al[455] and by Yoshizawa et al.[574] The latter workers studied specimens of intervertebral discs removed at operation for anterior and posterior lumbar interbody fusion. They found abundant nerve endings with various morphologies throughout the outer half of the anulus fibrosus. The varieties of nerve endings found included free terminals, often ending in club-like or bulbous expansions or complex sprays; and less commonly, terminals forming convoluted tangles or glomerular formations that were occasionally demarcated by a 'capsule-like' condensation of adjacent tissue.

The sources of the nerve endings in the lumbar discs are the lumbar sinuvertebral nerves, and branches of the lumbar ventral rami and the grey rami communicantes.[65,510] As described previously, each lumbar sinuvertebral nerve supplies the disc at its level of entry into the vertebral canal and the disc above (Fig. 9.7). The posterolateral corner of each lumbar disc receives branches from the lumbar ventral rami that arise just outside the intervertebral foramina (Figs 9.8 and 9.9), and this region of the disc also receives

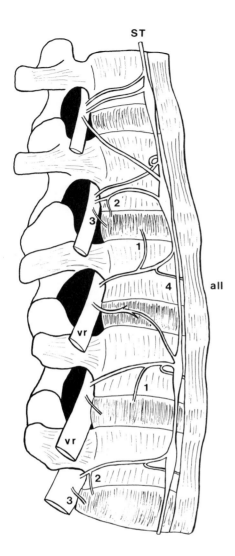

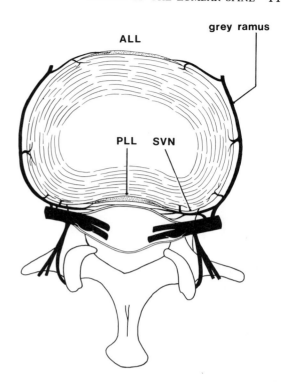

Fig. 9.9 The nerve supply of a lumbar intervertebral disc depicted in a transverse view of the lumbar spine. Branches of the grey rami communicantes and the sinuvertebral nerves (SVN) are shown entering the disc and the anterior and posterior longitudinal ligaments (ALL, PLL). Branches from the sinuvertebral nerves also supply the anterior aspect of the dural sac and dural sleeve.

Fig. 9.8 A sketch of the nerve supply of the lumbar intervertebral discs outside the vertebral canal. Laterally, the discs receive branches (1) from the grey rami communicantes of the sympathetic trunk (ST). Posterolaterally, they receive branches (2, 3) from the grey rami communicantes and the ventral rami (vr) as they emerge form the intervertebral foramina. The anterior longitudinal ligament (all) is innervated by recurrent branches (4) from the grey rami.

a branch from the grey ramus communicans just before it connects with the ventral ramus (Figs 9.8 and 9.9). The lateral aspects of the lumbar discs are innervated by branches of the grey rami communicantes (Figs 9.8 and 9.9).

The sinuvertebral nerves also innervate the posterior longitudinal ligament, while the anterior longitudinal ligament is innervated by branches of the grey rami communicantes (Figs 9.7, 9.8 and 9.9). Histological studies have established the presence of nerve endings in these ligaments,[251,283,473] and a recent study has revealed that many of these endings contain substance P, a putatative transmitter substance involved in nociception.[306]

The fact that the lumbar intervertebral discs and their adjacent ligaments are innervated by branches of the sympathetic nervous system does not necessarily mean that afferent fibres from these structures return to the central nervous system via the sympathetic trunk. Rather, it has been suggested that somatic afferent fibres from the

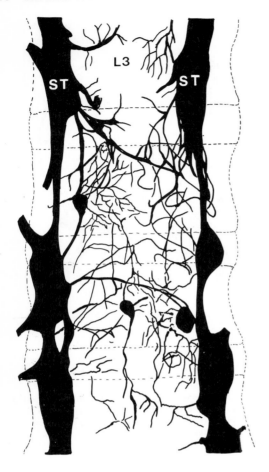

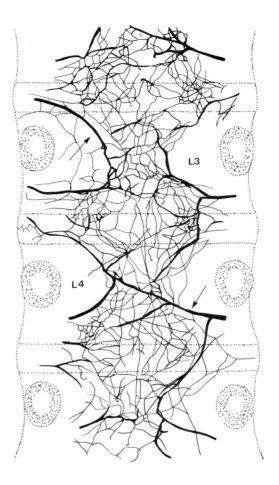

Fig. 9.10 A sketch of the nerve plexus accompanying the anterior longitudinal ligament at the levels of the L3 and lower vertebrae, as seen in whole mounts of human fetuses. (Based on Groen et al.[217]) ST — lumbar sympathetic trunk.

Fig. 9.11 A sketch of the nerve plexus accompanying the posterior longitudinal ligament at the levels of the L3 and lower vertebrae, as seen in whole mounts of human fetuses. (Based on Groen et al.[217]) The large fibres arrowed represent what would on dissection be found to be the sinuvertebral nerves.

discs and ligaments simply use the course of the rami communicantes to return to the ventral rami.[65]

The presence of nerve endings in the lumbar intervertebral discs raises the question as to their function. Any free endings associated with blood vessels in the disc may reasonably be ascribed a vasomotor or vaso-sensory function,[65,355] but because the anulus fibrosus contains so few blood vessels (see Ch. 10) this is unlikely to be the function for the majority of the nerve fibres in

the anulus fibrosus. For the encapsulated receptors on the surface of the disc, Malinsky[355] postulated a proprioceptive function. Theoretically, this would be a valid, useful role for these receptors, but the only study that has addressed this contention failed to find any evidence in its favour.[315] However, this study was performed on cats, which are not a suitable model, for the cat is a quadrapedal animal whose vertebral column is not used for weight-bearing, and may not be endowed with receptors and reflexes that would

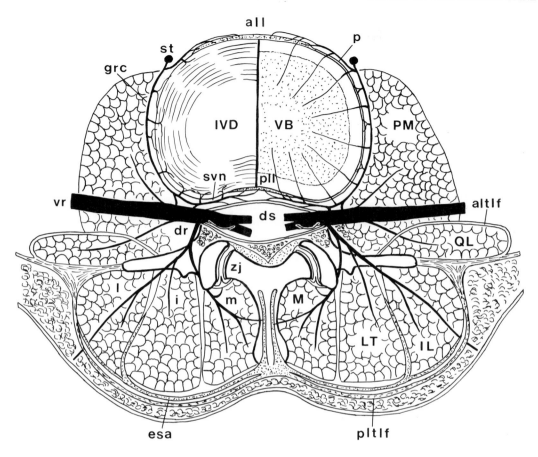

Fig. 9.12 Innervation of the lumbar spine. A cross-sectional view incorporating the level of the vertebral body (VB) and its perisoteum (p) on the right and the intervertebral disc (IVD) on the left. PM — psoas major. QL — quadratus lumborum. IL — iliocostalis lumborum. LT — longissimus thoracis. M — multifidus. altlf — anterior layer of thoracolumbar fascia. pltlf — posterior layer of thoracolumbar fascia. esa — erector spinae aponeurosis. ds — dural sac. zj — zygapophysial joint. pll — posterior longitudinal ligament. all — anterior longitudinal ligament. vr — ventral ramus. dr — dorsal ramus. m — medial branch. i — intermediate branch. l — lateral branch. svn — sinuvertebral nerve. grc — grey ramus communicans. st — sympathetic trunk.

be appropriate for an upright vertebral column. Therefore, a proprioceptive role for the intervertebral disc has not been excluded.

In other tissues of the body, isolated free nerve endings are ascribed a nociceptive function, and it is presumable that they play a similar role in the lumbar intervertebral discs. Although there is no explicit evidence that disc pain can be ascribed to a particular type of nerve ending in the disc, there is abundant evidence that the disc can be painful, and the issue of disc pain is addressed in Chapter 13.

MICROSCOPIC NEUROLOGY

The preceding descriptions of the sinuvertebral nerves and the innervation of the lumbar discs constitute only part of the real picture. The nerves described above are only those visible under a dissecting microscope. Recent studies using whole mounts of human fetuses stained for acetylcholinesterase reveal that the anterior elements of the lumbar spine are endowed with an extensive plexus of nerve fibres.[217] A plexus bridging the two lumbar sympathetic trunks covers the anterior longitudinal ligament (Fig. 9.10), while an extensive plexus accompanies the posterior longitudinal ligament (Fig. 9.11). This latter plexus is derived from the sinuvertebral nerves which at microscopic levels consist of numerous, fine filaments. These plexuses supply superficial branches that innervate the periosteum of the vertebral body, and long, penetrating branches that enter the intervertebral discs and vertebral bodies, the latter following blood vessels as far as the centre of the bone.

Amongst the microscopic filaments within the plexus of the posterior longitudinal ligament certain larger fibres can be discerned; these correspond to the sinuvertebral nerves described in dissection studies (Fig. 9.11), but in number and total volume they are only a proportion of the total number of nerve fibres that innervate the vertebral bodies and intervertebral discs. Similarly, dissectable grey rami communicantes represent only the larger connections between the sympathetic trunks and the ventral rami. The intervertebral discs are thus innervated not only by the dissectable branches from the sinuvertebral nerves, the ventral rami and the grey rami communicantes but extensively by the anterior and posterior longitudinal plexuses.

SUMMARY

The lumbar spine receives an extensive innervation (Fig. 9.12). Posteriorly the branches of the lumbar dorsal rami are distributed to the back muscles and the zygapophysial joints. Anteriorly the ventral rami supply the psoas major and quadratus lumborum. The vertebral bodies and intervertebral discs are surrounded by extensive plexuses of nerves that accompany the longitudinal ligaments and which are derived from the lumbar sympathetic trunks. Within the posterior plexus larger filaments constitute the sinuvertebral nerves. Short branches innervate the vertebral periosteum, and long penetrating branches enter the vertebral body from all aspects of its circumference. Nerves enter the outer third of the anulus fibrosus from the longitudinal plexuses anteriorly, laterally and posteriorly. The posterior plexus innervates the dura mater and nerve root sleeves along their anterior and lateral aspects.

10. Blood supply of the lumbar spine

The blood supply of the lumbar spine is derived from the lumbar arteries, and its venous drainage is through the lumbar veins. The topographical anatomy of these vessels is described below, and more detailed descriptions of their distribution to the vertebral bodies, the spinal nerve roots and intervertebral discs are provided under separate headings.

THE LUMBAR ARTERIES

A pair of lumbar arteries arises from the back of the aorta in front of each of the upper four lumbar vertebrae.[108,459] Occasionally, the arteries at a particular level may arise as a single common trunk which rapidly divides into right and left branches. At the L5 level, the fifth lumbar arteries arise from the median sacral artery, but otherwise they resemble the other lumbar arteries.

Each lumbar artery passes backwards around its related vertebral body (Fig. 10.1), lying in the concavity formed by the lateral surface of the vertebral body where it is covered by the tendinous arch of the psoas muscle. Upon reaching the level of the intervertebral foramen, the artery divides into several branches (Fig. 10.2).

Lateral branches pass through the psoas and quadratus lumborum muscles eventually to supply the abdominal wall. Others pass with the ventral ramus and dorsal ramus of the spinal nerve supplying the paravertebral muscles innervated by these nerves. A substantial posteriorly directed branch passes below the transverse process, running perpendicular to the lateral border of the pars interarticularis of the lamina, to enter the back muscles[108,127] (Fig. 10.2). In addition

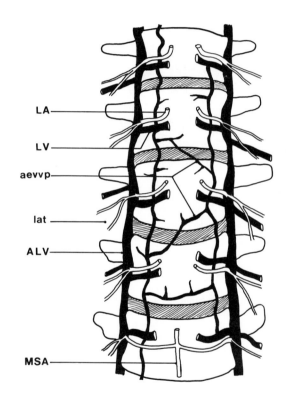

Fig. 10.1 An anterior view of the lumbar spine showing its intrinsic blood vessels. LA: lumbar artery. LV: lumbar vein. ALV: ascending lumbar vein. MSA: median sacral artery. lat: lateral branches of the lumbar arteries. aevvp: elements of the anterior external vertebral venous plexus.

to supplying the back muscles, the posterior branches of the lumbar arteries form anastomoses around the zygapophysial joints, which they supply, and plexuses that surround and supply the laminae and spinous processes.[108]

Opposite the intervertebral foramen, three me-

121

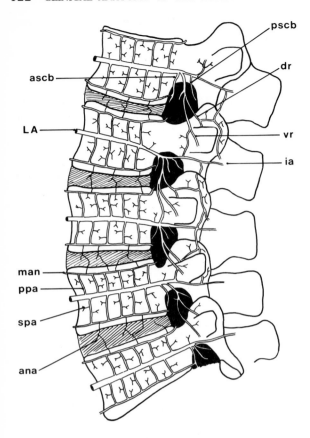

Fig. 10.2 A lateral view of the lumbar spine showing the lumbar arteries and their branches. LA: lumbar artery. ascb: anterior spinal canal branch. pscb: posterior spinal canal branch. dr: branches accompanying dorsal ramus of spinal nerve. vr: branches accompanying ventral ramus of spinal nerve. ia: posterior branch related to the pars interarticularis of the lamina. man: metaphysial anastomosis. ppa: primary periosteal artery. spa: secondary periosteal artery. ana: anastomosis over the surface of the intervertebral disc.

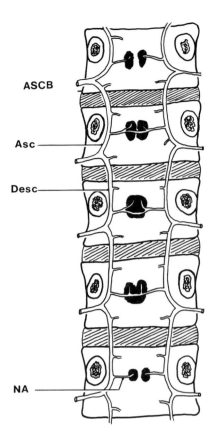

Fig. 10.3 A sketch of the anterior spinal canal branches (ASCB) of the lumbar arteries, their ascending (Asc) and descending (Desc) branches, and the nutrient arteries (NA) to the vertebral bodies.

dially directed branches arise from the lumbar artery (Fig. 10.2). These are the anterior spinal canal branch, the posterior spinal canal branch, and the radicular branch.[108,127] The radicular branches are described in detail later. The anterior spinal canal branch at each level enters the intervertebral foramen and bifurcates into ascending and descending branches. The ascending branch crosses the intervertebral disc and circumvents the base of the pedicle above to anastomose with the descending branch from the next higher segmental level. In this way a series of arterial arcades is formed across the back of the lumbar vertebral bodies, i.e. along the floor of the vertebral canal (Fig. 10.3).

The posterior spinal canal branches also form arcades in a similar way but on the internal surface of the roof of the vertebral canal, i.e. along the laminae and ligamenta flava. Secondary branches of this arcade pass to the epidural fat and dural sac, and well-defined branches pass into the laminae and into the base of each spinous process. The branch to each lamina enters near its junction with the pedicle and bifurcates into branches that ascend and descend within the bone into the superior and inferior articular processes. The branch to each spinous process penetrates the bone as far as its tip.

THE LUMBAR VEINS

Several veins surround and drain the lumbar spine. These are the lumbar veins, the ascending lumbar veins and several vertebral venous plexuses. The lumbar veins accompany the lumbar arteries in their course around the vertebral bodies, and drain into the inferior vena cava (Fig. 10.1). Opposite the intervertebral foramina the lumbar veins on each side communicate with the ascending lumbar vein: a long channel that runs in front of the bases of the transverse processes (Fig. 10.4). Inferiorly on each side, the ascending lumbar vein communicates with the common iliac vein, while superiorly, the right ascending lumbar vein becomes the azygous vein, and the left ascending lumbar vein becomes the hemiazygous vein.

Over the anterolateral aspects of the lumbar spine, a variable series of vessels interconnect the lumbar veins to form the **anterior external vertebral venous plexus** (Fig. 10.4). Within the vertebral canal, two other plexuses are formed. One covers the floor of the vertebral canal, and is known as the **anterior internal vertebral venous plexus** (Fig. 10.5). The other lines the roof of the vertebral canal and is called the **posterior internal vertebral venous plexus**. Within the vertebral canal these plexuses extend superiorly to thoracic levels, and inferiorly to sacral levels, and at each intervertebral foramen the two internal vertebral venous plexuses communicate with the ascending lumbar veins.

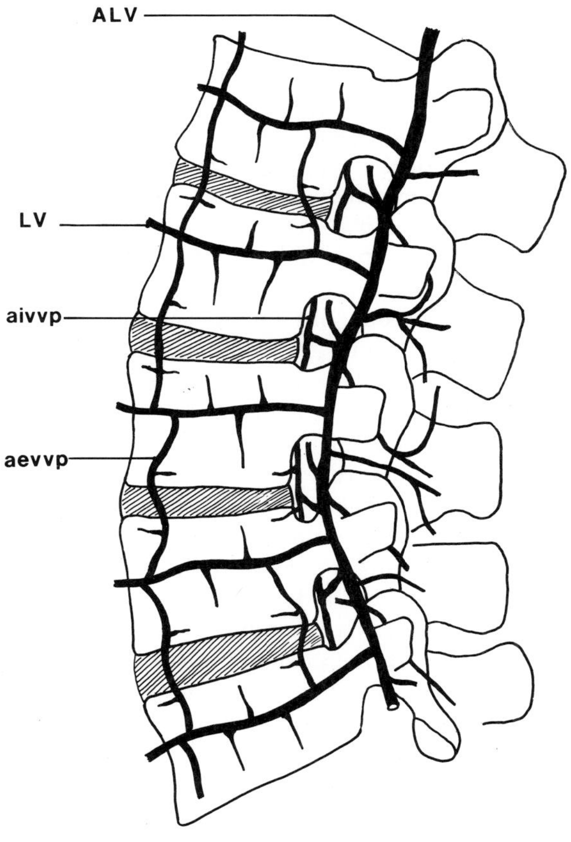

Fig. 10.4 A lateral view of the lumbar spine showing the tributaries of the lumbar veins. ALV: ascending lumbar vein. LV: lumbar vein. aivvp: elements of the anterior internal vertebral venous plexus. aevvp: elements of the anterior external vertebral venous plexus.

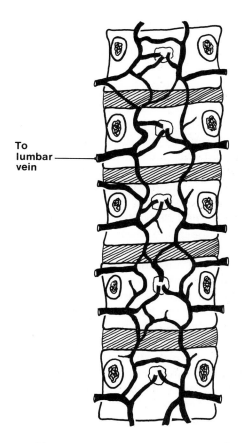

Fig. 10.5 The anterior internal vertebral venous plexus.

Depending on local pressure changes, blood from the internal vertebral venous plexuses may drain to the ascending lumbar veins or may drain within the vertebral canal upwards to thoracic levels and higher, or downwards to sacral levels. Space-occupying lesions in the vertebral canal may, therefore, re-direct flow in any of these directions, and raised intra-abdominal pressure may globally prevent drainage into the ascending lumbar veins, and force blood to drain through the vertebral canal to thoracic levels.

Veins from the back muscles and from the external aspects of the posterior elements of the lumbar vertebrae drain towards the intervertebral foramina where they join the lumbar veins or the ascending lumbar veins. Internally, the posterior elements are drained by the posterior internal vertebral venous plexus. The venous drainage of the vertebral bodies and the spinal nerve roots is described below in conjunction with the arterial supply of these structures.

BLOOD SUPPLY OF THE VERTEBRAL BODIES

As each lumbar artery crosses its vertebral body it gives off some 10–20 ascending and descending branches called the **primary periosteal arteries**.[459] Branches of these vessels supply the periosteum and outermost walls of the vertebral body (Figs 10.2 and 10.6). Similar periosteal branches arise from the arcade of the anterior spinal canal arteries to supply the posterior wall of the vertebral body (Figs 10.2 and 10.6).

At the upper and lower ends of each vertebral body, terminal branches of the primary periosteal arteries form an anastomotic ring called the metaphysial anastomosis.[459] This ring runs parallel to the superior or inferior border of the vertebral body and surrounds its anterior and lateral aspects (Figs 10.2 to 10.6).

Branches from the metaphysial anastomosis and others from the lumbar arteries and the anterior spinal canal arteries penetrate and supply the internal parts of the vertebral body. The penetrating branches of the anterior spinal canal arteries pierce the middle of the posterior surface of the vertebral body, and are known as the **nutrient arteries** of the vertebral body. They divide into ascending and descending branches that supply the central core of the vertebral body (Fig. 10.6). Penetrating branches of the lumbar arteries, called the **equatorial arteries**, pierce the anterolateral surface of the vertebral body at its midpoint and divide into ascending and descending branches that join those of the nutrient arteries to supply the central core of the vertebra.

The peripheral parts of the upper and lower ends of the vertebral body are supplied by penetrating branches of the metaphysial anastomosis called **metaphysial arteries**. Several metaphysial arteries pierce the anterior and lateral surfaces of the vertebral body at its upper and lower ends, and each artery supplies a wedge-shaped region that points towards the central core of the vertebral body (Fig. 10.6).

In the region of the vertebral end-plate, terminal branches of the metaphysial arteries and the nutrient arteries form dense capillary plexuses in the subchondral bone deep to the end-plate and in the base of the end-plate cartilage.[108,109] Details of the morphology of this plexus are not known in the human, but in the dog, certain differences occur in different regions. Over the nucleus pulposus the capillary terminations are sessile and discoid 'like the suckers on the tentacle of an octopus',[106] while over the anulus fibrosus the capillary terminals are less dense, smaller and simpler in appearance.[106] The functional significance of these differences, however, still remains obscure.

The principal veins of the vertebral body are the **basivertebral veins**. These are a series of long veins running horizontally through the middle of the vertebral body (Fig. 10.7). They drain primarily posteriorly, forming one or two large veins that pierce the posterior surface of the vertebral body to enter the anterior internal vertebral venous plexus. Anteriorly, the basivertebral veins drain to the anterior external vertebral venous plexus.

Within the vertebral body the basivertebral veins receive vertically running tributaries from the upper and lower halves of the vertebral body. In turn these veins receive oblique tributaries from the more peripheral parts of the vertebral

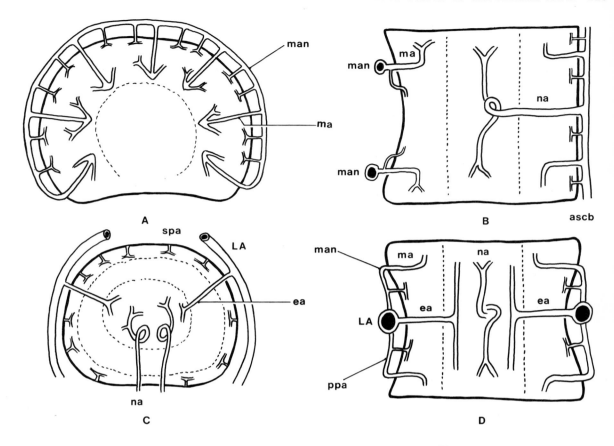

Fig. 10.6   The intra-osseous arteries of the lumbar vertebral bodies. (Based on Ratcliffe.[459]) **A**: Transverse section of upper or lower end of vertebral body showing the metaphysial anastomosis (man) and the sectors supplied by the metaphysial arteries (ma). **B**: Midline, sagittal section showing the central distribution of the nutrient artery, and the peripheral distribution of the metaphysial arteries (ma) and the penetrating branches of the anterior spinal canal branches (ascb). **C**: Transverse section through the middle of the vertebral body showing the central distribution of the nutrient arteries (na) augmented by equatorial branches (ea) of the lumbar artery (LA), and the superficial distribution of the secondary periosteal arteries (spa). **D**: Frontal section through the middle of the vertebral body showing the central distribution of the nutrient arteries (na) and the equatorial arteries (ea), and the peripheral distribution of the metaphysial anastomosis (man), metaphysial arteries (ma), and the primary periosteal arteries (ppa) that arise from the lumbar artery (LA).

body. A large compliment of vertical veins runs through the central core of the vertebral body and are involved in the drainage of the end-plate regions.

In the region immediately adjacent to each vertebral end-plate, the capillaries of the subchondral bone drain into a system of small veins that lies parallel to the disc/bone interface (Fig. 10.7). This is the **subchondral post-capillary venous network**.[108,109] Short vertical veins

drain this network into a larger venous system that again lies parallel to the vertebral end-plate (Fig. 10.7). This is the **horizontal subarticular collecting vein system**.[108,109] The veins in this system are arranged in a radial pattern that converges centrally opposite the nucleus pulposus. Here the veins turn towards the centre of the vertebral body and form the vertical veins that drain through the central core of the body to the basivertebral veins. Peripheral elements of the

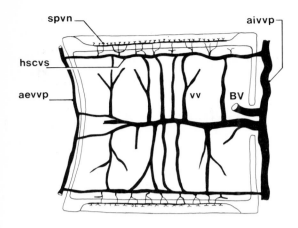

Fig. 10.7 The intra-osseous veins of the lumbar vertebral bodies. (Based on Crock et al.[109]). spvn: subchondral post-capillary venous network. hscvs: horizontal subchondral collecting vein system. vv: vertical veins within the vertebral body. BV: the basivertebral veins. aivvp: anterior internal vertebral venous plexus. aevvp: anterior external vertebral venous plexus.

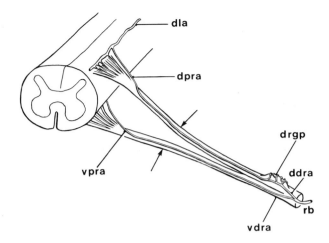

Fig. 10.8 The arterial supply of a typical lumbar nerve root. The dorsal nerve rootlets are supplied by tiny branches of the dorsolateral artery of the spinal cord (dla). The nerve roots are supplied by the dorsal and ventral proximal radicular arteries (dpra, vpra) and the dorsal and ventral distal radicular arteries (vdra, ddra) which are branches of the radicular branch (rb) of the lumbar artery. The proximal and distal arteries anastomose at the junction of the middle and medial thirds of the nerve root (arrows). The dorsal root ganglion is supplied by a plexus of small arteries (drgp).

horizontal subarticular collecting vein system drain to the anterior external and anterior internal vertebral venous plexuses.

BLOOD SUPPLY OF THE SPINAL NERVE ROOTS

The lumbar spinal nerve roots receive their blood supply from two sources. Proximally, they are fed by vessels from the conus medullaris of the spinal cord. Distally, in the intervertebral foramina, they receive the radicular branches of the lumbar arteries.[129,424,425]

At their attachment to the conus medullaris, virtually each of the ventral and dorsal rootlets is supplied by a fine branch derived from the extramedullary longitudinal vessels of the conus (Fig. 10.8), but the distribution of these small branches is limited to a few centimetres along the rootlets.[424] The rest of the proximal ends of the dorsal and ventral roots are supplied by the proximal, ventral and dorsal radicular arteries (Fig. 10.8).

The dorsal proximal radicular arteries arise from the dorsolateral longitudinal vessels of the conus (derived from the posterior spinal arteries), and the ventral proximal radicular arteries arise from the 'accessory anterolateral longitudinal channels' (derived from the anterior spinal artery).[424] Each proximal radicular artery travels with its root, but is embedded in its own pial sheath, until several millimetres from the surface of the spinal cord, it penetrates the root.[424] Upon entering the root, the radicular artery follows one of the main nerve bundles along its entire length, and gives off collateral branches that enter and follow other nerve fascicles. Within a root there may be one to three substantial vessels that could be named as the proximal radicular artery.

At each intervertebral foramen, the radicular branch of the lumbar artery enters the spinal nerve and then divides into branches that enter the ventral and dorsal roots (Fig. 10.8). These vessels may be referred to as the distal radicular arteries, to distinguish them from the proximal radicular arteries arising form the conus medullaris. Each distal radicular artery passes proximally along its root, giving off collateral branches, until it meets and anastomoses with its

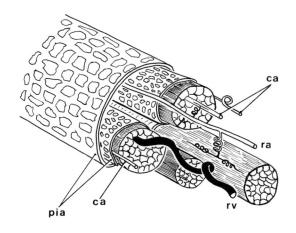

Fig. 10.9 A sketch of the distribution of radicular vessels in a nerve root (based on Parke and Watanabe.[424]) The radicular artery (ra) runs with the nerve bundles in the nerve root, accompanied by several collateral arteries (ca) in adjacent nerve bundles. The arteries anastomose with one another through coiled junctions. The radicular vein (rv) has a sinuous course separate to that of the arteries.

respective proximal radicular artery. En route, the dorsal distal radicular artery forms a plexus around the dorsal root ganglion.[425]

Within each root, collateral branches of the proximal and distal radicular arteries communicate with one another through transverse branches (Fig. 10.9), and a particular feature of these branches in the adult is that they are coiled.[424] Similarly, their parent vessels are coiled proximal and distal to the origin of each of these transverse communicating branches (Fig. 10.9). These coils appear to be designed to accommodate the stretching of the nerve root that occurs during movements of the lumbar spine.[425] They are less developed in neonates because of the relatively shorter length of the lumbar spinal nerve roots, and hence, a lesser propensity for them to stretch.

The point of anastomosis between the proximal and the distal radicular arteries lies in the proximal half of each root.[425] Consequently, the proximal radicular artery supplies the proximal one-third or so of the root, while the distal two-thirds are supplied by the distal radicular artery. Arterial supply, however, is neither the only nor the principal source of nutrition for the roots. Only some 35% of the glucose absorbed by a

root comes from the radicular arteries. The rest is absorbed directly from the surrounding cerebrospinal fluid.[424]

The veins of the nerve roots may be divided into proximal and distal radicular systems, but are fewer in number than the corresponding arteries and run courses separate to those of the arteries.[424] The veins tend to lie deep in the nerve bundle and assume a spiralling course (Fig. 10.9). The proximal veins drain towards the spinal cord, while the distal veins drain towards the intervertebral foramina where they join the tributaries of the lumbar veins and the ascending lumbar veins.

NUTRITION OF THE INVERTEBRAL DISC

The intervertebral disc is not an inert structure. The cartilage cells in the nucleus pulposus and the fibroblasts in the anulus fibrosus are biologically active, albeit at a low-grade level, but this activity is essential for the constant synthesis and replacement of proteoglycans and collagen.[360,490,539,540] To sustain this activity these cells require nutrition.[359] However, the intervertebral discs receive no major arterial branches.

The only vessels that actually enter the discs are small branches from the metaphysial arteries which anastomose over the outer surface of the anulus fibrosus (Fig. 10.2), but these branches are restricted to only the very outermost fibres of the anulus.[360] Consequently, for their nutrition, intervertebral discs are dependent on diffusion, and this diffusion takes place from the two closest available systems of vessels: those in the outer anulus, and the capillary plexuses beneath the vertebral end-plates.

To reach the nucleus pulposus, nutrients like oxygen, sugar and other molecules must diffuse across the matrix of the vertebral end-plate or through the anulus fibrosus. Subsequently, nutrients to the nucleus must permeate the proteoglycan matrix of the nucleus. The rate of diffusion of nutrients through these media is dependent on three principal factors: (1) the concentration gradient of any particular substance; (2) the resistance to diffusion offered by the end-plate or the anulus fibrous; and (3) the resistance to diffusion offered by the proteoglycans of the nucleus.[359]

In this respect, the permeability of the anulus fibrosus and the vertebral end-plates differs. Virtually the entire anulus fibrosus is quite permeable to most substances, but only the central portions of the vertebral end-plates are permeable.[359,539,540] However, because the surface area of the end-plates is greater than that of the anulus, the relative contributions to disc nutrition from the anulus and the end-plates is approximately the same. This conclusion, however, holds only for uncharged molecules which are unaffected by other processes.[359,539,540] The diffusion of charged molecules is affected by the chemical properties of the nucleus pulposus.

The resistance to diffusion of charged molecules offered by the nucleus pulposus is a property of the high concentration of the negatively charged carboxyl and sulphate radicals in its mucopolysaccharides.[359,539] Uncharged molecules like glucose or oxygen permeate readily through the proteoglycan matrix of the nucleus, but negatively charged substances, like sulphate ions and chloride ions, meet great resistance once they cross the end-plates and reach the matrix.

On the other hand, positively charged ions like sodium and calcium, pass readily from the end-plates into the matrix.

Because the concentration of mucopolysaccharides in the anulus fibrosus is less than that in the nucleus pulposus, the anulus offers less resistance to the diffusion of negatively charged molecules, and most negatively charged solutes that reach the nucleus do so via the anulus.[359]

Although it is generally regarded that diffusion is the principal mechanism by which nutrients reach the inner parts of the intervertebral disc,[255,540] there has been some work to suggest that compression of the intervertebral disc tends to squeeze water out of it, and when the compression is released the water returns. It is maintained by some authorities that this flux of water is capable of carrying nutrients with it.[311] In particular, it has been shown in animal experiments that spinal movements, over a long period of time, exert a positive nutritional effect on the disc.[254] It is presumable that a similar phenomenon occurs in humans, but the extent to which exercise might benefit human discs, or whether it forestalls disc degeneration, still remains to be shown.

11. Embryology and development

After 15 days of development, the human embryo is in the form of a flat, ovoid disc which consists of two layers of cells: the **ectoderm** dorsally, and the **endoderm** ventrally (Fig. 11.1). The ectoderm is that layer which principally will give rise to the skin and spinal cord. The endoderm forms the alimentary tract.[226]

At the caudal end of the embryo, the cells of the ectoderm become rounded and heap up, forming an elevation known as the **primitive streak**.[226] Cells from the primitive streak migrate laterally and forwards, insinuating between the ectoderm and endoderm to form a third layer in the embryo called the **mesoderm** (Figs 11.1 and 11.2). Just in front of the primitive streak, another thickening develops, known as **Hensen's node**. From this node, a cord of cells, known as the **notochord**, migrates forwards between the ectoderm and endoderm (Fig. 11.2). By about 28 days, the notochord fully demarcates the midline of the embryo,[226] and induces the formation of the vertebral column around it. Dorsal to the notochord, the ectoderm forms the **neural tube** which differentiates into the brain and spinal cord.

On each side of the notochord, the mesoderm of the embryo is thickened to form a longitudinal mass known as the **paraxial** mesoderm. By the 21st day of development the paraxial mesoderm starts to be marked by transverse clefts across its dorsal surface. These clefts separate the paraxial mesoderm into segments called **somites** (Fig. 11.3). The first somites appear in the region of the head, and others appear successively caudally.

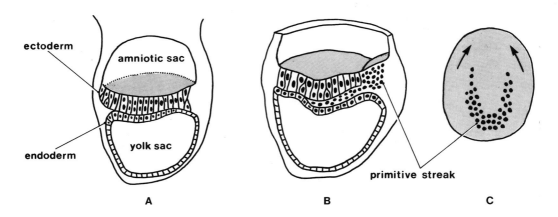

Fig. 11.1 Schematic illustrations of the development of the mesodermal layer of early human embryos. **A**: A sagittal section of an early embryo consisting of only ectoderm and endoderm. The amniotic sac lies dorsal to the embryonic plate and the yolk sac is suspended from the endodermal layer. **B**: Ectodermal cells at the caudal end of a 15 day embryo have heaped up to form the primitive streak which gives rise to the mesodermal cells. **C**: Top view of the embryo in Fig. 11.1B, showing the forward migration of the mesodermal cells, either side of the midline, underneath the ectodermal layer.

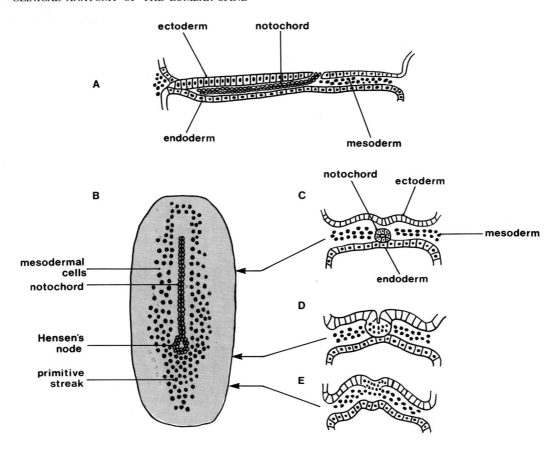

Fig. 11.2 Schematic illustrations of the further development of the mesoderm. **A**: A sagittal section of an embryo showing the notochord having extended forwards between the ectoderm and endoderm, and behind it the mesoderm of the primitive streak. **B**: A top view of the same embryo showing the notochord and mesoderm viewed through the ectoderm over the top of the embryo. **C,D** and **E**: Transverse sections of the embryo through the notochord, Hensen's node, and the primitive streak.

By about the 30th day of embryonic development, a total of 42–44 somites are formed.[226]

The clefts demarcating tsomites are actually indentations, so the segmentation they create is apparent only along the dorsal aspect of the paraxial mesoderm. Deeply, beneath the surface of the embryo, the paraxial mesoderm remains a single, longitudinally continuous mass.[549] Using the transverse clefts as a guide, however, the further development of each somite can be traced.

The 42–44 somites of the human embryo can be named as 4 occipital, 8 cervical, 12 thoracic, 5 lumbar, 5 sacral and 8–10 coccygeal somites. The 1st occipital and the last 7–8 coccygeal somites regress and give rise to no permanent structures.[226] The remaining three occipital somites are involved in the formation of the occipital region of the skull and the tongue. The other somites form the vertebral column and the trunk.

The cells in the somites are originally epithelial in nature, but gradually they change into loosely arranged tissue called **mesenchyme** (Fig. 11.4). In transverse section, each somite is roughly triangular in outline, presenting ventral and dorsolateral borders, and a medial border facing the neural tube (Fig. 11.5).

Within the somite, two clusters of cells develop. Those cells in the ventral and medial regions of the somite rapidly multiply and form

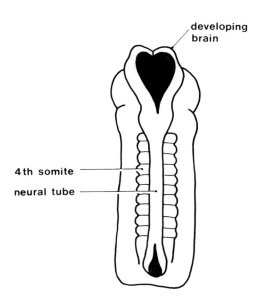

Fig. 11.3 A dorsal view of an embryo with 10 somites.

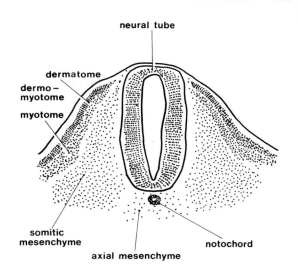

Fig. 11.5 Transverse section of an early somite, showing the relationship of the mesenchyme to the neural tube and notochord, and its differentiation into the somitic mesenchyme and the dermo-myotome.

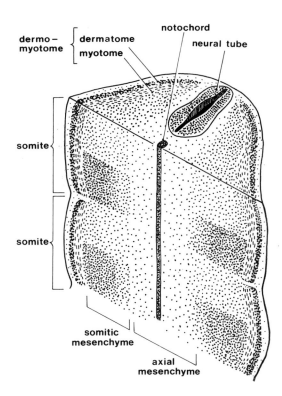

Fig. 11.4 Combined coronal and transverse sections of the somites of an embryo. The somitic mesenchyme has differentiated into dense caudal halves and lighter cranial halves.

a mass that, in the past, has been referred to as the sclerotome, but for reasons outlined elsewhere[549] the term **somitic mesenchyme** is used in this text. These cells are exclusively involved in the formation of the vertebral column. The remaining cells, along the dorsolateral border of the somite, give rise to the musculature and skin of the trunk and are collectively referred to as the **dermo-myotome**.

The further development of the somitic mesenchyme and the dermo-myotome is similar for every somite. Therefore, the development of the lumbar region, as described below, is in principle the same as that seen in the cervical and thoracic regions, the principal differences lying only in the particular segments of the vertebral column that are eventually formed.

THE FATE OF THE SOMITIC MESENCHYME

The somitic mesenchyme undergoes several changes that eventually result in the formation of a primitive model of the vertebral column, and this phase of development of the vertebral column is known as the **mesenchymal** phase.

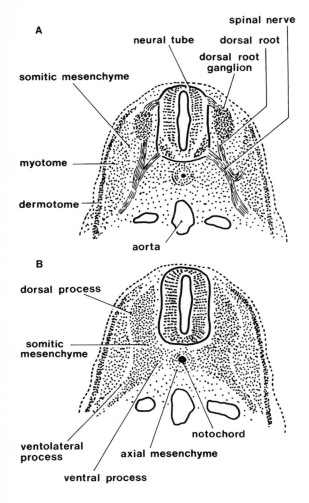

Fig. 11.6 Transverse sections through (**A**) the less dense cranial half of a somite, and (**B**) the denser caudal half. In **A**, the somitic mesenchyme surrounds the developing spinal nerve. In **B**, the axial mesenchyme surrounds the notochord, and the somitic mesenchyme has formed dorsal, ventrolateral and ventral processes. (Based on Verbout.[549]).

The notochord lies between the aorta ventrally, and the neural tube dorsally. The neural tube is flanked by the somitic mesenchyme, but the somitic mesenchyme initially does not extend as far medially as the notochord. The notochord is surrounded separately by a continuous column of very loose-meshed mesenchyme called the **axial mesenchyme**[549] (Fig. 11.5). The density of the axial mesenchyme gradually increases as these cells multiply and surround the notochord (Figs 11.6 and 11.7). Meanwhile, a separate series of events occurs in the somitic mesenchyme.

In the caudal half of each somite the density of nuclei increases, giving it a darker staining appearance (Figs 11.4 and 11.7B). The cranial half of the somite remains less dense, and is invaded by the developing spinal nerve (Figs 11.6A and 11.7C). The nerve grows laterally to invade the dermo-myotome, and as the nerve increases in length and thickness, the cells of the cranial half of the somite come to be arranged in concentric layers around the nerve.[549] In time, the developing nerve occupies most of the entire cranial half of the somite, which itself gives rise to little but perineural tissue. It is the denser, caudal half of each somite that participates in the formation of the vertebral column.

In the caudal half of each somite, two processes develop: a dorsal process, and a ventrolateral process.[549] The dorsal process spreads dorsally to surround the neural tube, and will give rise to the neural arch (Fig. 11.6B). Hence, it is also referred to as the **arcual** process. The ventrolateral process extends laterally, and gives rise to the costal element of the future vertebrae. Hence, it is also referred to as the **costal** process (Fig. 11.6B). In the lumbar region, the costal elements of each vertebra are represented in the form of the transverse processes.

As the axial mesenchyme increases in density, its cells assume a concentric orientation around the notochord. These cells will form the greater part of the future vertebral body, and that portion of the body which they form is referred to as the **centrum** (Fig. 11.7). Opposite the lower half of the cranial portion of the adjacent somite, a zone of higher density develops in the axial mesenchyme (Fig. 11.7). This zone forms the predecessor to the future intervertebral disc.[549]

While these events take place in the axial mesenchyme, a third process develops in the somitic mesenchyme. This process, known as the ventral, or **chordal** process, extends towards the notochord to blend with the axial mesenchyme just caudal to the zone of the future intervertebral disc.[549] In this way, the chordal process connects the somitic mesenchyme with the centrum of the vertebral body, and the vertebral body is eventu-

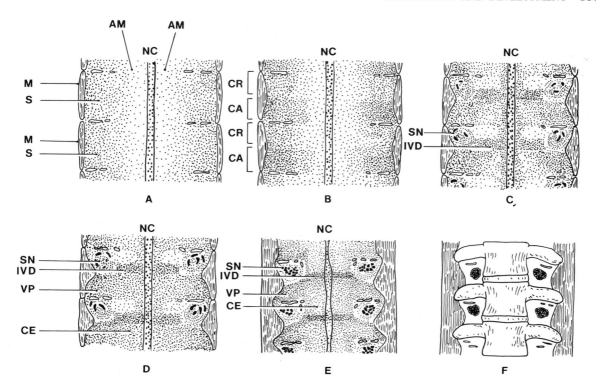

Fig. 11.7 The appearance of coronal sections of consecutive somites, showing the stages of development of the lumbar vertebrae. **A**: Early mesenchymal stages. M — myotome. S — somitic mesenchyme. AM — axial mesenchyme. NC — notochord. **B**: The somites have differentiated into dense caudal (CA) and less dense cranial (CR) halves. **C**: The cranial somitic mesenchyme has condensed around the developing spinal nerve (SN), and the future intervertebral disc (IVD) is marked as a zone of increased density in the axial mesenchyme opposite the lower end of the cranial half of the somite. **D**: The ventrolateral process of the somitic mesenchyme (VP) extends between consecutive myotomes, and the ventral process blends with the axial mesenchyme to form the centrum (CE). **E**: Mesenchymal cells have transformed into a cartilaginous model of the future vertebra, and the notochord is being squeezed out of the centrum. **F**: The relative location of the definitive osseous vertebrea. (Based on Verbout.[549])

ally formed by the centrum and the terminal portions of the chordal processes from each side.

The dorsal processes of the somitic mesenchyme continue to extend around the sides of the neural tube, and just lateral to the developing dorsal root ganglion, the dorsal processes of adjacent somites blend with one another at the sites of the future zygapophysial joints.[549] Elsewhere, the neural arches of adjacent segments are bridged by less dense condensations of mesenchyme that will give rise to the ligaments of the neural arch.

By this stage of development, the shape of the future vertebra is outlined by mesenchymal tissue. Condensations of the axial mesenchyme have surrounded the notochord and have moulded the vertebral body. The future intervertebral disc has condensed in the axial mesenchyme opposite the lower half of the cranial portion of the somitic mesenchyme. The cranial half of each somite has condensed around the developing spinal nerve, and will form only perineural tissue. The condensed caudal half of the somitic mesenchyme has formed three processes. A ventral process blends with the axial mesenchyme below the intervertebral disc, while a dorsal process embraces the side of the neural tube. Together, the ventral and dorsal processes outline the future neural arch. The ventrolateral process radiates from the neural arch on each side to outline the future transverse process. At this stage of development, the left and right dorsal processes do not yet meet behind the neural tube, and are united only by a membrane.[415,416] The neural arch is completed dorsally at a later stage of development.

The succeeding phases of development of the vertebrae involve the replacement of the mesenchymal model, first by cartilage, and then by bone, and these phases are described later, after the description of the development of the dermomyotome.

FATE OF THE DERMO-MYOTOME

Initially, two types of cells are evident in the dermo-myotome. Epithelial cells cover the dorsolateral surface of the somite and can be recognised as the **dermatome**. Deep to these lie mesenchymal cells, collectively known as the **myotome**. Gradually, the cells of the dermatome lose their epithelial character and become incorporated into the myotomal mass, but they remain attached to the overlying ectoderm, and give rise to the dermis and subcutaneous tissue.[226] The cells of the myotome give rise to muscular tissue.

The myotomal mass maintains its ventrolateral location in relation to the somitic mesenchyme. Opposite the condensed caudal half of the somite it is gradually displaced laterally by the developing ventrolateral process. Opposite the looser cranial half of the somite, it bulges towards the somite, but is also indented by the developing spinal nerve[549] (Fig. 11.7).

As the spinal nerve divides into a ventral and dorsal ramus at about the 40th day of development,[416] the myotome splits into two portions.[226] The division occurs along a plane depicted by the developing transverse processes, and the two portions are separated by a septum that forms the future intertransverse ligaments (Fig. 11.8). The dorsal portion of the myotome is known as the **epimere**, or **epaxial** portion, and is innervated by the dorsal ramus of the spinal nerve. The ventral portion is known as the **hypomere**, or **hypaxial** portion, and is innervated by the ventral ramus of the spinal nerve.

In the lumbar region, the hypomere will develop into those muscles ventral to the

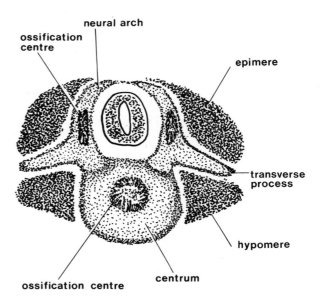

Fig. 11.8 A schematic illustration of a transverse section of a cartilaginous lumbar vertebra showing the ossification centres in the centrum and neural arches, and the disposition of the myotomes into epimeres and hypomeres.

intertransverse ligaments. The lumbar myotomes largely give rise to the intertransversarii laterales, and the quadratus lumborum and psoas muscles. Most of the muscles of the abdominal wall develop from the hypomeres of the lower thoracic somites, but the L1 hypomere contributes to the lower portions of these muscles.

The epimeres throughout the vertebral column divide further into medial and lateral divisions[226,569] which are supplied by the medial and lateral branches of the dorsal rami, respectively. In the lumbar region, the medial division forms the multifidus muscle, while the lateral division forms the iliocostalis and longissimus muscles.

CHONDRIFICATION

As the mesenchymal models of the vertebrae are being completed, some of the mesenchymal cells change character and become cartilaginous. This occurs at about the 6th week of gestation[416] and heralds the onset of the **cartilaginous** phase of vertebral development.

A pair of chondrification centres appear in the centrum of each vertebra. They rapidly fuse into one centre that expands to chondrify the entire centrum.[226] Chondrification centres also appear in each half of the neural arch. These expand dorsally through the dorsal process of the somitic mesenchyme on each side, and meet one another behind the neural tube to complete the neural arch. From the site of union, a cartilaginous spinous process develops dorsally. The neural arch centres also extend laterally to chondrify the transverse process; and ventrally along the ventral process of the somitic mesenchyme, to blend with the chondrifying centrum.

As a consequence of these events, a cartilaginous model of the future vertebra is laid down, but even as chondrification of the vertebral column is being completed, these cartilaginous models start to be replaced by definitive, osseous vertebrae (Fig. 11.8).

OSSIFICATION

Ossification is the third phase of development of the vertebral column. It commences during the 9th to 10th weeks of intrauterine life,[556] but is not completed until adolescent life. The first process of ossification is called **primary** ossification, and occurs at sites where blood vessels invade the cartilaginous models of the future vertebrae.

The cartilaginous neural arches are invaded from behind to form a primary ossification centre in each half of the neural arch (Fig. 11.8). The cartilaginous vertebral body is invaded by blood vessels through its anterior and posterior surfaces. Some authorities maintain that these two sets of blood vessels give rise respectively to separate ventral and dorsal ossification centres, which rapidly fuse to form a single ossification centre in the middle of the future vertebral body,[139] but others maintain that this phenomenon is only a variation that occurs in about 5% of cases.[39,95] Another variant is two centres lying lateral to one another,[39] but the most common pattern is to have one, single centre.[39]

The onset of ossification differs according to vertebral level and the part to be ossified. Primary ossification centres in the neural arches first appear at cervico-thoracic levels, followed by upper cervical and then thoraco-lumbar levels. Centres in the neural arches then appear progressively in

cranial and caudal directions from these levels.[38] Primary centres in the vertebral bodies first appear at lower thoracic and upper lumbar levels, and then progressively appear at levels above and below these.[38] In this way, ossification centres are established in the bodies and neural arches of the lumbar vertebrae by the 12th–14th week of gestation.

In the centrum of the vertebral body, the primary ossification centre expands radially and towards the intervertebral discs above and below. It reaches the anterior aspect of the centrum by about 22 weeks antenatal life, and the posterior aspect by about 25 weeks,[508] but ossification does not reach the superior and inferior surfaces of the vertebral body which remain cartilaginous, and form the growth-plates of the vertebral body. In the neural arches, ossification extends in all directions from the primary centre: ventrally towards the vertebral body, laterally into the transverse process, and dorsally around the neural tube.

At birth, the lumbar vertebrae are still not completely ossified (Figs 11.9 and 11.10). The bulk of the centrum is ossified and in lateral radiographs has the appearance of an ovoid block of bone with convex upper and lower surfaces.[72,80,478] Large vascular channels penetrate the anterior and posterior aspects of the centrum,[139] and on radiographs of neonatal spines, these appear as areas of translucency.[478] The upper and lower surfaces of the vertebral body are still covered by the thick cartilage plates, and the combined height of these plates and the intervertebral disc is approximately the same as the height of the ossified lumbar vertebral bodies.[72,80,478] The pedicles and the proximal parts of the laminae and transverse processes are ossified, but the spinous processes and the distal parts of the transverse processes are still cartilaginous. The articular processes are ossified for the most part, but their distal ends remain cartilaginous.

After birth, ossification of the vertebrae continues as the vertebrae increase in size with growth. Ossification of the vertebral body extends radially and in the direction of the end-plates. Further details of vertebral body growth are described separately in a later section.

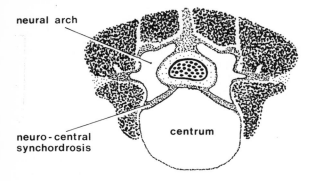

neural arch

neuro-central
synchordrosis

centrum

Fig. 11.9 A schematic illustration of a neonatal lumbar vertebra showing the extent of ossification of the centrum and the neural arches.

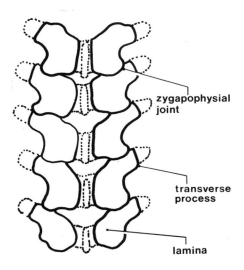

zygapophysial
joint

transverse
process

lamina

Fig. 11.10 A sketch of a dorsal view of a neonatal lumbar spine showing the extent of ossification of the neural arches.

Ossification continues to spread slowly through the neural arch and its processes. The laminae are fully ossified and unite dorsal to the spinal cord during the first post-natal year.[223,556] At this same time the bulk of the spinous process is ossified,[478] but its dorsal edge remains cartilaginous until puberty, as do the tips of the transverse processes and the ends of the articular processes.

At puberty, **secondary** ossification centres appear in the cartilaginous tips of the spinous process, the tips of the transverse processes, and in the cartilaginous mamillary processes.[85,556] Secondary ossification centres may appear in the tips of the inferior articular processes, but this phenomenon does not occur regularly, and is described further in the later section on the zygapophysial joints.

The secondary ossification centres of each lumbar vertebra are separated from the rest of the vertebra by a narrow interval of cartilage, and remain separated during the final periods of spinal growth. Gradually, this intervening cartilage is replaced by bone, and the secondary centres fuse with the rest of the vertebra by about the 25th year of life.[556]

THE FATE OF THE NOTOCHORD

During the mesenchymal phase of development of the vertebral column, the notochord persists as a central axis through the middle of the future vertebral bodies and intervertebral discs. The deepest mesenchymal cells gradually assume a concentric arrangement around the notochord forming a **perichordal sheath**.

As chondrification of the vertebral bodies proceeds, the cells of the notochord appear to be squeezed out of the vertebral body into the intervertebral discs[102,139,292] (Fig. 11.7), and the notochord is progressively narrowed until it forms little more than a streak of tissue on the vertebral body, known as the **mucoid streak**. Expansion of the ossification centre of the vertebral centrum destroys the mucoid streak, and in general, any vestige of the notochord in the vertebral body is obliterated.[139]

In about 7% of cases, ossification does not completely obliterate the region of the notochord, and a vertical canal may persist in the vertebral body.[507] These canals are most frequently filled with fibrocartilage or fibrous tissue, but rarely, pockets of notochordal cells may persist in parts of the canal.[507]

In the developing intervertebral disc, the fate of the notochord is entirely different, for instead of being obliterated, it participates in the formation of the nucleus pulposus.

DEVELOPMENT OF THE INTERVERTEBRAL DISC

In the primitive mesenchymal intervertebral disc, the cells gradually come to be arranged in concentric layers, lying in parallel rows between one vertebra and the next.[429] This arrangement foreshadows the future concentric structure of the lamellae of the anulus fibrosus (Fig. 11.11A).

Towards the centre of the disc, the cells are irregularly arranged around the notochord, and gradually the cells closer to the notochord take on the appearance of embryonic cartilage[429] (Fig. 11.11B). At about 55 days of development, the notochord expands in the centre of the disc, its cells being separated into strands and groups,

called the **chorda reticulum**, embedded in an amorphous mucoid substance (Fig. 11.11B). The expanded notochord is surrounded by embryonic cartilage, and around the perimeter of the disc, collagen fibres appear to form the anulus fibrosus.

Collagen fibres are deposited in the anulus fibrosus as early as the 10th week of gestation,[241] and their orientation is the same as that in the adult.[239] Their ends are inserted into the cartilage plates that cover the superior and inferior aspects of the vertebral bodies. Fibres in the anulus fibrosus are quite evident in the 4th month and are well developed by 5 to 6 months.[139] Accompanying the development of the anulus fibrosus, the anterior and posterior longitudinal ligaments

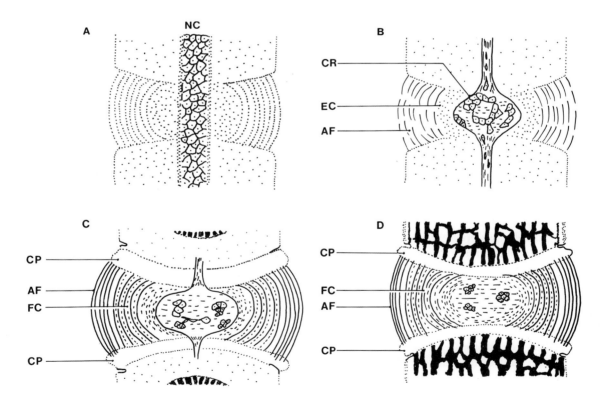

Fig. 11.11 Stages in the development of the intervertebral disc. (Based on Peacock.[429]) **A**: A mesenchymal disc in which the central cells surround the notochord (NC), and the peripheral cells are arranged in a radial pattern indicative of the future lamellae of the anulus fibrosus. **B**: The notochord has expanded and its cells form the chorda reticulum (CR). Mesenchymal cells surrounding the notochord have transformed into embryonic cartilage (EC), and the peripheral cells have formed the orientated collagen fibres of the anulus fibrosus (AF). **C**: The disc consists of an expanded notochord with fewer cells, surrounded by fibrocartilage (FC) and the collagenous anulus fibrosus which attaches to the cartilaginous plates of the vertebrae (CP). **D**: A neonatal disc.

condense out of the perivertebral mesenchyme during the 7th to 9th weeks.[139]

In the centre of the intervertebral disc, the notochord continues to expand radially, and the perichordal cartilage assumes a looser arrangement.[429] The cartilage cells closer to the anulus fibrosus undergo a transition to fibrocartilage whose collagen fibres are arranged in parallel sheets like the fibre of the anulus fibrosus (Fig. 11.11C).

At birth, the notochordal area is formed essentially by an amorphous mucoid material that contains only a few small groups of notochordal cells. The notochordal area is surrounded by a capsule of fibrocartilage, and beyond this lies the collagenous anulus fibrosus. At this stage, the structure of the anulus resembles that seen in the adult (Fig. 11.11D).

After birth, some of the notochordal cells may persist in the disc, but eventually all notochordal cells undergo necrosis during infancy.[101,373] After the age of 4 years, no viable notochordal cells remain, and the centre of the disc contains only the notochordal mucoid material and the perichordal fibrocartilage.

From this account, it is evident that the anulus fibrosus develops in situ from the mesenchyme of the primitive intervertebral disc, while the nucleus pulposus has a dual origin. Its central part is derived from the notochord, while its peripheral part is formed by fibrocartilage derived from the mesenchyme of the primitive disc. After birth, notochordal cells disappear leaving only fibrocartilage and a proteoglycan matrix in the nucleus.

In the neonate and infant, the nucleus pulposus is wedge-shaped in median section with its main mass located posteriorly in the disc.[508] By 2 years of age this shape is reversed, and the main mass lies anteriorly.[508] From the 4th to 8th years of life, the nucleus assumes an elliptical shape and occupies the centre of the disc. This final change in position occurs as the child masters upright weight-bearing and gait, and accompanies the development of the lumbar lordosis and a rapid increase in height of the lumbar vertebrae and discs.[508]

Between the ages of 2 and 7 years, the lumbar discs change their shape from a biconcave disc bounded by convex bony surfaces to a biconvex disc bounded by concave surfaces,[508] and throughout childhood the lumbar discs undergo a major increase in height. The L4–5 disc, for example, increases from 3 mm in height to about 10 mm, between birth and the age of 12.

GROWTH OF THE VERTEBRAL BODIES

After birth, the lumbar vertebral bodies lose their rounded, ovoid appearance and become rectangular in profile. However, they are still largely covered by cartilage. Superiorly and inferiorly they are capped by cartilage that form the growth plates of the vertebrae and which will eventually form the end-plates of the intervertebral discs. Posterolaterally on each side, the centrum is covered by a layer of cartilage that separates the centrum from the ossified ventral process of the neural arch, now the pedicle of the vertebra. Technically, this junction between the neural arch and the centrum forms a joint, which is known as the **neurocentral joint** or more accurately as the **neurocentral synchondrosis**.

The neurocentral joints persist into childhood, but gradually the cartilage is ossified and the pedicles fuse with the centrum by about the age of 6 years.[478] In fusing with the centrum, the pedicles contribute to the formation of the vertebral body, which is, therefore, formed largely by the ossified centrum but also by the ventral ends of the neural arches.

Horizontal growth

Horizontal growth of the vertebral body occurs by periosteal ossification,[72,80,304] and from birth to the age of 7 years, the antero-posterior diameter of a typical lumbar vertebral body increases from 3 mm to about 22 mm[72] or 27 mm.[508] During the same period, the lateral diameter increases from 7 mm to about 36 mm.[508] By the age of 17 years, the antero-posterior diameter reaches 34 mm.[72] Between the ages of 5–13 years, the transverse diameter of the lumbar vertebral bodies in males increases by about 26% at the L1 and L3 levels, and by 30% at L5. In females, the corresponding increases are bout 15% and 22%.[512] From puberty to adulthood the transverse diameters increase by 5–10% in both males and females. The mean values for the L1, L3 and L5 vertebrae increase from, 38, 42 and 48 mm to 42, 44 and 52 mm respectively.[512]

Longitudinal growth

Longitudinal growth of the vertebral bodies occurs as a result of the proliferation and ossification of the cartilages remaining on the superior and inferior surfaces of the vertebral body.[52,80] These cartilages cover the entire superior and inferior surfaces, but also overlap onto the anterior, lateral and posterior margins of the vertebral body[131,139,478] (Fig. 11.12). On their discal aspect these cartilages blend with the developing intervertebral disc. They are directly confluent with the fibrocartilage of the developing nucleus, and they anchor the fibres of the anulus fibrosus (Fig. 11.12). On the vertebral aspect of each plate, the cartilage cells are arranged in vertical columns,[52,102] and ossification occurs by the same process seen in the metaphyses of long bones.[225]

The cells furthest away from the cartilage plate are surrounded by calcified matrix and undergo ossification, whereupon they are incorporated into the vertebral body. Longitudinal growth occurs as these cells are replaced by division of cells closer to the main body of the cartilage plate. Growth continues as long as this replacement continues, and the rate of growth appears to be equal at both the upper and lower growth plates.[208,304]

Between birth and the age of 5 years, a typical lumbar vertebra increases in height from 5 mm to about 15 mm [508,512] or 18 mm.[72] From the age of 5 to the age of 13, it increases to about 22 mm, and reaches 25 mm by adulthood.[512] Other studies estimate the sizes of the vertebrae at the age of 13 and at adulthood to be 26 mm and 34 mm respectively.[72] The average vertical dimensions of all the lumbar vertebrae and intervertebral discs at various ages are shown in Table 11.1. The dramatic increase in size during childhood is readily apparent. During adolescence, females exhibit somewhat smaller average dimensions than males, but approach male dimensions more closely by adulthood.

The extent of longitudinal growth of the central region of the vertebral body appears to be genetically determined, but the longitudinal growth of the peripheral portions is dependent on activity asociated with weight-bearing in the erect posture.[508] With assumption of the lumbar lordosis, the nucleus pulposus comes to be located in the centre of each intervertebral disc,[508]

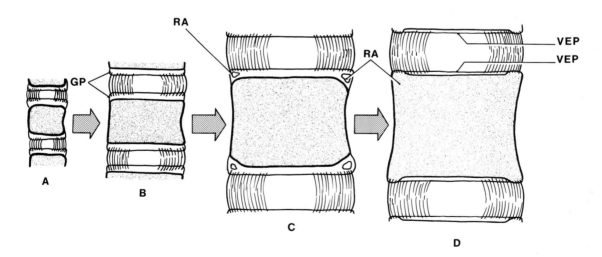

Fig. 11.12 Stages in the growth of the vertebral bodies. **A:** The vertebral bodies, discs and growth plates (GP) of a one year old infant. **B:** The same structures in a pre-pubertal child. **C:** The appearance of the ring apophyses (RA) in adolescence. **D:** Ossification of the ring apophyses and the formation of the vertebral end-plates (VEP) in adulthood.

Table 11.1 Vertical dimension of lumbar vertebrae and intervertebral discs

Age (in years)	Mean vertical dimension (mm)*				
	0–1.5	1.5–12	13–19	20–35	
			25.2	25.3	male
L1 Body	7.9	14.4	22.8	24.9	females
			7.1	6.0	
L1–2 Disc	2.6	5.7	7.0	6.2	
			25.1	25.8	
L2 Body	8.0	15.0	22.4	25.3	
			10.4	10.4	
L2–3 Disc	3.5	7.6	10.4	10.0	
			25.2	25.7	
L3 Body	7.9	14.8	22.3	25.6	
			10.7	11.0	
L3–4 Disc	4.0	7.9	11.3	10.5	
			25.1	25.5	
L4 Body	7.6	14.5	22.6	25.0	
			11.8	11.5	
L4–5 Disc	4.0	8.5	10.4	11.1	
			23.7	24.1	
L5 Body	7.2	14.5	22.1	24.1	
			11.2	10.7	
L5–S1 Disc	3.6	8.2	9.8	10.8	

* Based on direct measurements of the mid-vertical diameters of the vertebral bodies and intervetebral discs in 204 cadavers. (Twomey L, unpublished data)

and this location of the nucleus acts as a stimulus for growth of the more peripheral parts of the vertebral body.[508] It is as if the peripheral parts grow to attempt to surround the nucleus, and this differential growth accounts for the relatively concave shape of the superior and inferior surfaces of the developing vertebral bodies.

Longitudinal growth of the vertebral bodies continues throughout childhood and adolescence, but gradually the rate of growth slows down, and is completed between the ages of 18 and 25.[85] As ossification ceases, the growth plates get thinner, and the vertebral surface of the growth plate is sealed off from the vertebral body by both a calcified layer of cartilage, and the development of the subchondral bone plate at each end of the vertebral body. The hyaline and fibrocartilage remaining on the surfaces of the body then become the vertebral end-plate of the intervertebral disc.

During vertebral growth the cartilaginous growth-plates are nourished by blood vessels that ascend and descend along the outer surfaces of the vertebral body and enter the peripheral edges of the growth plates. They then run within the

growth plate towards its centre, raising ridges in the cartilage over the upper and lower surfaces of the vertebral body. These ridges radiate from the centre of the growth plate to its perimeter, and are more marked anteriorly. As growth slows down, the vessels in these ridges are gradually obliterated, and the ridges disappear.[131]

Ring apophysis

During the growth period, a separate series of events involve the perimeter of the cartilaginous growth plates, but do not contribute to growth. These events relate to the formation of the ring apophyses of the vertebrae (Ch. 1). In the edges of the cartilaginous plates, where they overlap the anterior, lateral and posterior margins of the vertebral body, foci of calcification appear, at the ages of 6–8 years in girls, and 7–9 years in boys.[478] These foci are subsequently ossified as a result of vascular infiltration. At first, many such foci surround the upper and lower margins of the vertebral body, but by about the age of 12 years they coalesce to form a single rim, or a ring. This ring surrounds the entire perimeter of the vertebral body but is better developed anteriorly and laterally. It remains separated from the rest of the vertebral body by a thin layer of hyaline cartilage, but eventually fuses with the vertebra, sometime between the ages of 14–15[478] or 16–21[81,555] (Fig. 11.12).

At no time does the ring apophysis contribute to growth, but its fusion with the rest of the vertebral body signals the cessation of longitudinal growth. One effect of the ring apophysis is that because it develops as a result of ossification of the margins of the cartilage growth plate, it incorporates those fibres of the anulus fibrosus that inserted into the perimeter of the plate (Fig. 11.12D). This explains why the peripheral fibres of the adult anulus have a bony attachment while the more central fibres are inserted into the vertebral end-plate.

DEVELOPMENT OF THE ZYGAPOPHYSIAL JOINTS

Compared to the embryology and development of the vertebral bodies, the development of the lumbar zygapophysial joints has received scant attention. There are few descriptions in the English language literature, although some major studies have been published in the continental literature.[218,343,519,520] Notwithstanding this relative neglect there are some fascinating and clinically relevant aspects of the development of these joints.

The lumbar zygapophysial joints develop from the mesenchyme of the neural arches. Rudimentary mesenchymal articular processes appear at about 32 days of development,[415] and the mesenchymal processes of consecutive vertebrae eventually meet one another at about 50 days.[343] The future joint space is initially surrounded and filled with mesenchyme, but as the articular processes chondrify, this tissue gradually recedes to form the articular capsule, any intra-articular structures, and a joint space. Chondrification commences at about 50 days,[415] and ossification by about 100 days.

Although definitive joints are formed by the 9th month of gestation,[343,520] at birth the articular processes are incompletely ossified. They are flat and spatular-like, and their tips are still covered by cartilage.[223] The superior articular process is rudimentary and is about half the length of the inferior articular process, but undergoes extensive development during the first two years of life.

At birth, the lumbar zygapophysial joints are all orientated in a coronal plane, like the joints of the thoracic vertebrae, but during post-natal growth their orientation changes to that seen in adults by about the age of 11 years[264,343,412,520] (Fig. 11.13). Rotation is achieved by differential rates and extents of ossification of the articular processes.[461]

At birth, bone occurs in the medial and basal parts of both inferior and superior articular processes. Further ossification occurs in three directions: towards the apex of each articular process along the medial margins of the joint, towards the joint surface leaving a joint cartilage, and around the lateral aspects of each articular process[461] (Fig. 11.14). Medial growth occurs rapidly but ceases at half a year of age. After this age the medial margin of the joint is resorbed and remodelled as the neural arch expands to assume adult proportions.[461,462] Lateral ossifica-

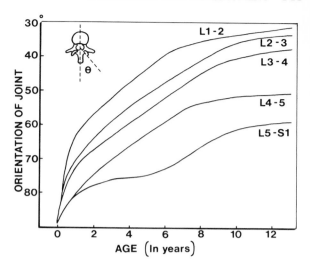

Fig. 11.13 The orientation of the lumbar zygapophysial joints as a function of age during growth. (Based on Lutz.[343]).

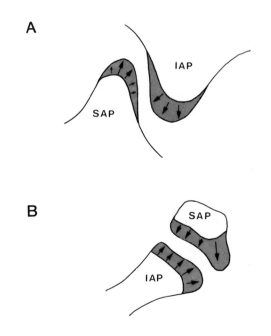

Fig. 11.14 The directions of ossification of the articular processes. **A**: lateral view. **B**: top view. (Based on Reichmann.[461]) SAP — superior articular process. IAP — inferior articular process. In the neonate only the basal regions of each articular process are ossified. Their tips are covered by cartilage into which ossification extends.

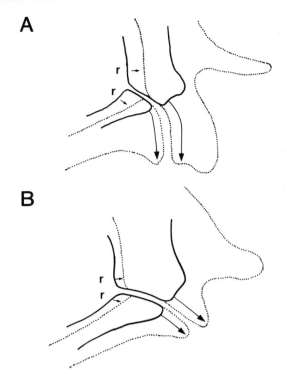

Fig. 11.15 Relative directions of growth of a zygapophysial joint as seen in transverse sections. **A**: upper lumbar levels. **B**: lower lumbar levels. The darker outline represents the size and configuration of the neonatal joint. The lighter outline represents the size and configuration established by later childhood. The larger arrows indicate the direction of growth of the articular processes. The smaller arrows indicate areas where bone is resorbed (r) to allow the neural canal to enlarge with growth. (Based on Reichmann.[461])

tion is more protracted as further cartilage is laid down as ossification proceeds. With medial ossification completed, continued lateral ossification brings about the apparent rotation of the joint (Fig. 11.15). The joints are fully ossified by about 7 to 9 years of age, by which age the adult orientation is virtually fully established (Fig. 11.13).

Variations in the extent of developmental rotation account for the variations in orientation of the lumbar zygapophysial joints seen in adults (Ch. 3). Joints with a more pronounced posterior, lateral growth would exhibit curvatures (Fig. 11.15A); those with a more pronounced lateral growth and less dorsal growth would tend to remain planar (Fig. 11.15B).

The cause of joint 'rotation' is unknown. It may be a genetically determined property of the lumbar zygapophysial joints, but other explanations have been suggested. Because it occurs as the child learns to stand erect and begins to use the multifidus muscle in everyday activities, some authors[412] attribute rotation of the lumbar zygapophysial joints to the action of multifidus (Ch. 8). By pulling on the mamillary processes the multifidus swings the lateral extremity of the superior articular process to a more dorsal position, thereby rotating the plane of the joint or imparting a curvature to it.

The articular processes continue to grow until about the age of 20,[328] and infrequently, secondary ossification centres (epiphyses) may appear in the tip of the inferior articular processes at puberty. The exact incidence of these centres is unknown, but when formed, these centres fuse with the main part of the inferior articular process between 15–21 years of age.[221,371,478]

SIGNIFICANCE

Details of the development of the lumbar vertebral bodies and zygapophysial joints have been emphasised above not so much for academic purposes but to illustrate that the developing lumbar spine is plastic. The adult shape of the vertebrae and their joints is not established at birth; nor are the spines of children miniature versions of those of adults. The vertebrae are continually growing and moulding to the forces habitually exerted on them. The final adult form is as much a product of the postures and activities assumed during childhood as it is a product of genetic programming. The implications of this relationship with respect to preventing possibly deleterious aberrations of the shape of vertebrae and joints have still to be explored.

DEVELOPMENTAL ANOMALIES

The developmental anomalies of the lumbar spine are vast and varied, and, in general, are thoroughly described in major textbooks of spinal morphology and radiology,[147,223,366,478] and research papers specifically addressing this issue.[71,444,491,566,567]

Systematically, lumbar vertebral anomalies can be classified into:

1. Agenesis, or failure of development, of one or more parts of a vertebra.
2. Failure of union of parts.
3. Changes in number or identity.

Part or all of a vertebral body may fail to be formed. When this occurs, the body assumes a wedge-shape, with the orientation of the wedge dependent on which part of the body fails. Failure of the anterior half of the body leads to anterior wedging. Failure of the posterior part causes posterior wedging, and lateral failure leads to lateral wedging. The embryological basis for these deformities is described in detail elsewhere.[478]

Individual components of the neural arches may fail to develop. In particular a pedicle may be absent or not ossified,[121,349,575] and articular processes, mostly inferior articular processes, may fail to develop.[28,287,302]

The most common form of non-union is spina bifida, in which the laminae of a vertebra, most commonly L5, fail to unite dorsally behind the cauda equina. This may simply be failure of ossification of an otherwise united cartilaginous neural arch, but spina bifida can be associated with minor and quite major abnormalities of the dural sac, cauda equina and spinal cord.[71,147,478]

The secondary ossification centres of the inferior articular processes may fail to unite with the articular process, or may be late in so doing. Under these circumstances the isolated ossicle formed by the secondary centre may mimic a fractured articular process.[41,463] United epiphyses occur in asymptomatic[41,173,187,404,463] and symptomatic[41,187,294,404,440,463] individuals, and it is not clear under what circumstances they can cause symptoms. It seems possible that if they were detached from the articular process, they could interfere with the mechanics of the zygapophysial joint like a loose body;[223] and compression of the underlying spinal nerve roots by a dislocated epiphysis has been described.[449] Estimates of the incidence of united epiphyses vary from 1.5%[173,449] to 14%.[258]

Alterations in vertebral number and identity affect principally the lumbosacral region where the last lumbar vertebra may become incorporated into the sacrum (sacralisation), thereby reducing the number of lumbar vertebrae to four; or conversely the first sacral vertebra may be mobile (lumbarisation) in which case the number of lumbar vertebrae increases to six. Various intermediate states of these same processes occur, with vertebrae showing features of partial lumbarisation or sacralisation.[71,478,491,567] None of these anomalies, per se, are the cause of symptoms,[493] unless some other disease process or injury is superimposed.

Articular tropism

One of the consequences of the rotation that the lumbar zygapophysial joints undergo is that the extent of rotation of the left and right joints at any segmental level may not be equal. Thus, the joints may be asymmetrically orientated, a condition referred to as **articular tropism**. The incidence of tropism is about 20% at all lumbar levels,[258,491] but may be as high as 30% at the lumbosacral level,[71] with 20% of lumbosacral zygapophysial joints showing an asymmetry greater than 10°.[37]

Early views suggested that articular tropism predisposed to the development of osteoarthritis in the more asymmetrical joint and to consequent narrowing of the related intervertebral foramen.[454] Others felt that asymmetry allowed unequal rotation of the intervertebral joint[554] and rendered it more susceptible to 'ligamentous injury'[37,566] (although exactly which ligaments were likely to be injured was not specified). Contemporary evidence indicates that the significance of articular tropism relates to failure of the joints to protect the intervertebral disc from torsional injury.

Biomechanical studies have shown that asymmetrical zygapophysial joints do not equally resist postero-anterior shear stresses applied to the intervertebral joint. The unequal load-sharing causes the intervertebral joint to rotate whenever it is subjected to shear stress, as in weight-bearing or flexion (Ch. 7). The upper vertebra in the joint rotates towards the side of the more coronally orientated joint.[113] Consequently, the anulus fibrosus is subjected to inordinate stresses during weight-bearing and flexion movements of the lumbar spine. Repeated insults sustained in this way could damage the anulus fibrosus.

Post-mortem studies support this contention. Radial fissures in the anulus fibrosus are a sign of torsional injury to the intervertebral disc (see Ch. 14), and post-mortem studies reveal that over 80% of unilateral fissures occur in intervertebral joints whose zygapophysial joints are assymetrical by more than 10°, and in 80% of these cases the fissure points towards the side of the more obliquely (coronally) orientated joint.[172] Furthermore, articular tropism occurs in as many as 90% of patients presenting with low-back pain and sciatica, with the symptoms occurring on the side of the more obliquely set joint.[169]

12. Age changes of the lumbar spine

Textbook descriptions imply that the structure of the lumbar spine conforms to some sort of standard or even ideal form, and that a standard description is applicable to all individuals. However, such descriptions only reflect the average, healthy, young, adult spine. Yet even then the lumbar spine is subject to variations; for example, in the shape and orientation of the zygapophysial joints (Ch. 3), the shape of the lumbar lordosis (Ch. 5), and the possible ranges of movement (Ch. 7). What is considered the 'normal' lumbar spine is only a composite of the mean values, or most common form, of these and other possible variables.

In this regard, 'normal' is defined as the structure most commonly exhibited by individuals in a population. However, when defined in this way, normality is greatly influenced by age. As individuals age, their lumbar spines undergo changes that are fairly uniformly reflected by the population. Thus, what is 'normal' for a young, adult population may not be 'normal' for an older population. Moreover, if changes uniformly exhibited by an older population are not associated with symptoms, then they cannot be regarded as pathological. They are simply part of the natural, biological process of ageing. Each age group, therefore, defines its own normal standards, and in order that clinicians neither confuse age changes with pathological changes, nor misconstrue them as such, they should be aware of what constitutes the natural changes with age in the lumbar spine.

In this regard, the fundamental age changes of the lumbar spine occur at the biochemical level. In turn, these affect the micro-biomechanical and overt biomechanical properties of the spine, which ultimately are reflected in the morphology of different components of the lumbar spine and its patterns of movement.

BIOCHEMICAL CHANGES

One of the most fundamental changes in the lumbar spine occurs in the nuclei pulposi. With ageing, the concentration of proteoglycans in the nucleus pulposus decreases.[45,209,502] In early adult life, proteoglycans amount to about 65% of the dry weight of the nucleus (Ch. 2) but by the age of 60, they constitute only about 30%.[45] Those proteoglycans that persist are smaller in size,[12,79] and have a smaller molecular weight.[98,539]

Apart from these gross changes, the composition of the proteoglycans also changes. While the keratan sulphate content of the disc remains fairly constant, the concentration of chondroitin sulphate falls, and this results in a rise in the keratan sulphate/chondroitin sulphate (KS/CS) ratio.[13,209,399,400,539]

The other major change in the nucleus pulposus is an increase in its collagen content,[252] and an increase in collagen-proteoglycan binding.[12] The collagen content of the anulus fibrosus also increases,[73] but the concentration of elastic fibres in the anulus drops, from 13% at the age of 26 to about 8% at the age of 62.[277]

The collagen of the intervertebral disc not only increases in quantity but also changes in nature. The fibril diameter of collagen in the nucleus pulposus increases,[40,229,401,402] such that the type II collagen of the nucleus starts to resemble the type I collagen of the anulus fibrosus. Reciprocally, the average fibril diameter in the anulus fibrosusdecreases.[229] Consequently, there is less distinction between the collagen of the nucleus pulposus and the anulus fibrosus.

The concentration of non-collagenous proteins in the nucleus pulposus increases,[53,126,197,398,517] and ageing is characterised by the appearance of certain distinctive non-collagenous proteins.[517] However, because the function of non-collagenous proteins is not known (Ch. 2), the significance of changes in these proteins remains obscure. In contrast, the changes in collagen, proteoglycans and elastic fibres have major biomechanical effects on the disc.

Because chondroitin sulphate is the major source of ionic radicals that bind water to proteoglycans (Ch. 2), it is tempting to expect that the change in the KS/CS ratio would result in a decrease in the water-binding capacity and the water content of the nucleus pulposus. Indeed, the water content of the nucleus does decrease with age.[252] At birth, the water content of the nucleus pulposus is about 88%, and this drops to about 65% to 72% by the age of 75 years.[209,453] However, most of this dehydration occurs during childhood and adolscence, and the water content of the nucleus pulposus decreases by only about 6% from early adult life to old age.[534]

Sophisticated biochemical studies indicate that it is not simply the loss of proteoglycans or the change in KS/CS ratio that decreases water-binding in the nucleus. Rather, the increased collagen and increased collagen-proteoglycan binding leaves fewer polar groups of the proteoglycans available to bind water,[252] and the decrease in water-binding capacity of the nucleus is a function of the complex way in which the ionic interactions between proteoglycans and proteins are altered.[79,98]

Regardless of the actual mechanism, the lumbar intervertebral discs become drier with age, and with the increase in collagen and the loss of elastin, they become more fibrous and less resilient. The increased collagen and increased collagen-proteoglycan binding renders the discs stiffer, i.e. more resistant to deformation, and their decreased water-binding capacity renders them less able to recover from creep deformation (Ch. 5). The clinical effect of these changes is expressed as changes in the mobility of the lumbar spine, and these are described in a later section below.

A recent study of the collagen in the anulus fibrosus reveals that the changes which occur are related not only to age but also to location.[73] While the collagen content of the anulus in general increases with age, there is a significant increase in the amount of type I collagen in the outermost laminae of the posterior quadrant of the anulus, and a reciprocal decrease in type II collagen. This suggests that some of the changes in collagen are not generalised age changes but are active metabolic responses to changes in the internal stresses of the anulus.[73]

STRUCTURAL CHANGES IN THE INTERVERTEBRAL DISCS

Macroscopically, as the intervertebral disc becomes more fibrous, the distinction between nucleus pulposus and anulus fibrosus becomes less apparent. The two regions coalesce, and the nucleus pulposus appears to be encroached by the anulus fibrosus.[551] After middle life, the nucleus pulposus becomes progressively solider, drier and more granular.[551]

As the nucleus pulposus dries out and becomes more fibrous, it is less able to exert fluid pressure.[314,558] Thus, the nucleus is less able to transmit weight directly, and less able to exert radial pressure on the anulus fibrosus (c.f. Ch. 2). A greater share of any vertical load is, therefore, borne by the anulus fibrosus. Consequently, the anulus fibrosus is subject to greater stresses, and undergoes changes reflecting the increasing and different strains it suffers.

With age, the collagen lamellae of the anulus may become increasingly fibrillated,[230,451] and cracks and cavities may develop[250] that may enlarge to become clefts and overt fissures.[551] Such changes are not necessarily due to externally applied injuries to the spine, but can simply be due to repeated minor insults sustained by the overloaded anulus fibrosus during trunk movements in the course of activities of daily living.

Thinning of the intervertebral discs has previously been considered one of the signs of pathological ageing of the lumbar spine,[320,478,551] but large-scale post-mortem studies have now refuted this notion. The dimensions of the lumbar intervertebral discs increase with age. Between the 2nd and 7th decades, the antero-posterior diameter of the lumbar discs *increases* by about 10% in females and 2% in males,[534] and there is about a 10% increase in the height of most discs.[534] As well, the upper and lower surfaces of the discs increase in convexity,[534] a change which occurs at the expense of the shape of the vertebral bodies (see below).

Maintenance of disc height is the 'normal' feature of ageing, and any loss of trunk stature with age is the result of decreases in vertebral body height.[150,151,396,535] Overt disc narrowing invites the consideration of some process other than ageing, and this is considered in Chapter 14.

CHANGES IN THE VERTEBRAL END-PLATE

In the newborn, the vertebral end-plate is part of the growth plate of the vertebral body. Towards the intervertebral disc, the articular region of the end-plate is formed by fibrocartilage, while on the vertebral body side, columns of proliferating cells extend into the ossifying vertebral body (Ch. 11). By the age of 10–15 years, the articular region of the end-plate becomes relatively thicker, while the growth zone decreases in thickness and proliferating cells become fewer in number.[51] As vertebral growth slows during the 17th–20th years, the vertebral end-plate is gradually sealed off from the vertebral body by the development of the subchondral bone plate, and after the age of 20, only the articular region of the original growth plate persists.[51] Betwen the ages of 20 and 65, the end-plate becomes thinner[51] and cell death occurs in the superficial layers of the cartilage.[451]

In the subchondral bone of the end-plate, vascular channels are gradually occluded[51] resulting in a decrease in the permeability of the end-plate region for nutrients to the disc. This impaired nutrition may be one of the factors that cause the biochemical changes in the nucleus pulposus, but it seems to come too late in life to be the fundamental cause.

With age, the apparent strength of the vertebral end-plate decreases,[443,558] but because the strength of the end-plate depends on the strength of the underlying vertebral body, this change is better considered together with the other changes that affect the vertebral body.

CHANGES IN THE VERTEBRAL BODY

With age, there is an overall decrease in bone density in the lumbar vertebral bodies,[150,151,536] and a decrease in bone strength.[470,558] These changes in density and strength correlate with changes in the size and pattern of trabeculae in the vertebral body.

Vertical trabeculae are slowly absorbed, although those that persist are said to be thickened.[34] On the other hand, horizontal trabeculae are absorbed and not replaced.[34,536] Consequently, ageing of the vertebral bodies is characterised by the loss of horizontal trabeculae[34,536] and this is most marked in the central portion of the vertebral body (that part overlying the nucleus pulposus).

The loss of horizontal trabeculae removes their bracing effect on the vertical trabeculae (see Ch. 1), and the load-bearing capacity of the central portion of the vertebral body decreases. Overall, with weakening of the trabecular system, a greater proportion of the compressive load on vertebral bodies is borne by cortical bone. Over the age of 40, the trabecular bone bears only 35% of the load.[470,558] However, cortical bone fails at only 2% deformation, whereas trabecular bone tolerates 9.5% deformation before failing.[558] Consequently, with greater reliance on cortical bone, the vertebral body becomes less resistant to deformation and injury.

Lacking support from the underlying bone, the vertebral end-plates deform by microfracture[227] and gradually bow into the vertebral body, imparting a concave shape to the superior and inferior surfaces of the vertebral body.[534,536] Moreover, the central portion of the vertebral end-plate is rendered more liable to fracture in the face of excessive compressive loads applied to the disc, and with increasing age microfractures can be found in the end-plates and vertical trabeculae of vertebral bodies.[76,102,292,477,550,561]

Fractures in the vertebral end-plates may be large enough to allow nuclear material to extrude into the vertebral body, forming so-called **Schmorl's nodes.** Schmorl's nodes, however, are more a feature of the lower thoracic and thoracolumbar spines and have a low incidence below the level of L2.[243,244] Per se, they are not symptomatic, nor are they related to age. Their incidence is greatest in adolescence and they do not increase in frequency with age.[243,244] Nevertheless, smaller protrusions of disc material into the vertebral bodies are not without significance and this is described in Chapter 14.

CHANGES IN THE ZYGAPOPHYSIAL JOINTS

The subchondral bone of the lumbar zygapophysial joints increases in thickness during growth and reaches a maximum between the ages of 20 and 50 years.[514,515] Thereafter, it gradually gets thinner.[514,533] The articular cartilage, on the other hand, steadily increases in thickness with age, but exhibits certain focal changes that start in the fourth decade and which can be related to the stresses applied to these joints.

In the anteromedial third of curved zygapophysial joints, the cartilage exhibits cell hypertrophy (particularly in the midzone layer) which progresses to vertical fibrillation of the cartilage associated with sclerosis of the subchondral bone plate.[515] At any stage, these changes are more advanced in the concave, superior articular process than in the inferior articular process. It is the anteromedial, or backward-facing portion of this facet that resists the forward shear stresses applied to the intervertebral joint during flexion movements and weight-bearing (Chs 2,5 and 7), and it can be surmised that the fibrillation that develops with age in this region reflects the repeated stresses incurred in the course of normal activities of daily living.[513,515,533] Severe or repeated pressures may result in erosion and focal thinning of the cartilage, while other regions may exhibit swelling that accounts for the general increase in thickness of the articular cartilage.[513,533] Where cartilage is lost, fibro-fatty intra-articular inclusions may increase in size to fill the space vacated by the cartilage.[515]

The posterior section of the joint characteristically exhibits a different kind of splitting of cartilage, parallel to the joint surface. A split piece of cartilage may remain attached to the joint capsule and form a false intra-articular meniscoid.[515]

Cell hypertrophy is almost universal in the fourth decade, and minor fibrillation is common in the fourth and fifth decades. Older joints exhibit gross thickening and irregularity of the calcified zone of cartilage and increased collagen in the superficial layers. The cells are fewer and with smaller nuclei. The changes in cartilage are more severe in the polar regions of the joint than at its centre. In older joints the distinction between changes in the anteromedial and posterior portions of the joint are lost.[515]

Other features exhibited by the joints are the development of osteophytes and 'wrap-around bumpers'. Osteophytes develop along the attachment sites of the joint capsule and ligamentum flavum to the superior articular process. Wrap-around bumpers are extensions of the edges of the articular cartilage curving around the dorsal aspect of the inferior articular process. Presumably, as a result of repeated stresses at these sites during rotatory movements, the articular cartilage spreads out to cover and protect the edges of the bony articular process.

CHANGES IN MOVEMENTS

The biochemical and structural changes in the joints of the lumbar spine have an inevitable effect on the mechanical properties, and therefore movements, of the spine. Older lumbar spines show a greater amount of creep and hysteresis, and a greater 'set' after creep deformation,[531] but they show a decreased range of motion. Progressive decrease in range of motion with age has been demonstrated in cadavers,[243,245,511,532] and in living subjects using both clinical[511] and radiographic[243,245,505] methods, and is evident in the ranges of motion both of the entire lumbar spine[511,532] and of individual intervertebral joints.[243,245,505]

Young children strikingly show the greatest lumbar mobility. At various segmental levels they are between 50%–300% more mobile than middle-aged subjects.[505,511] Mobility decreases considerably by adolescence, and beyond the age of 30, there is a gradual but definite decrease in mobility.[243,245,505,511]

Because 'release' experiments show that removing the posterior ligaments and zygapophysial joints does not greatly increase the range of flexion in older cadavers,[532] it appears that increased stiffness in the intervertebral discs is the principal cause of the reduction in mobility that develops with ageing. This can be readily ascribed to the dehydration and fibrosis of older intervertebral discs.

The greater hysteresis seen in older spines is probably due to the decreased water-binding capacity of their intervertebral discs.[531] Less able to attract water, these discs take longer to resume their original configuration and structure after deformation.

SPONDYLOSIS AND DEGENERATIVE JOINT DISEASE

It has been customary to describe certain changes in the intervertebral discs and zygapophysial joints as features of a disease. In the case of the intervertebral discs the disease has been 'spondylosis', and in the cases of the zygapophysial joints it has been called 'osteoarthrosis' or 'degenerative joint disease'.

The cardinal features of spondylosis are said to be the development of osteophytes (bony spurs) along the junction of vertebral bodies and their intervertebral discs.[147,464,521] However, when viewed in the context of other changes that occur with ageing, it is evident that the features of spondylosis are not those of some aggressive disease that seemingly attacks the body, but are the natural consequences of the stresses applied to the spine throughout life. Whether they should be called 'degenerative changes' or 'age changes' may appear simply a matter of semantics, but the development of osteophytes can be viewed as a reactive and adaptive change that seeks to compensate for biomechanical aberrations. The process is active and purposeful, and does not warrant the description as a degenerative process.

As the nucleus pulposus dries out, the intervertebral disc becomes less resilient and stiffer, and the anulus fibrosus bears more of the loads applied to the disc. To sustain greater loads the disc and the vertebral bodies adapt, and the pattern of adaptation depends on the nature and direction of the particular stress being compensated.

Excessive compression can result in the ossification of the terminal ends of the collagen fibres of the anulus fibrosus. This can occur focally, along the anterior and posterior margins of the disc where compressive strains are concentrated during extension and flexion movements and postures. A more prolific development of osteophytes can occur around the entire margin of the vertebral body in response to excessive vertical load-bearing. This phenomenon can be viewed as if the vertebral body is trying to expand its articular surface area. By distributing axial loads over a wider area, the vertebral body lessens the stress applied to the anulus fibrosus during weight-bearing.

Interpreted in this way, the development of osteophytes is only a natural response to the altered mechanics of the lumbar spine in turn due to more fundamental biochemical changes in the intervertebral disc. Consequently, spondylosis should not be viewed as a disease, but an expected morphological change with age.

Similarly, osteoarthrosis is not a disease, but an expression of the morphological consequences of stresses applied to the zygapophysial joints during life. The changes are concentrated at regions subject to the greatest and most repeated stresses. Adaptive changes occur when the stressed tissues are capable of remodelling and opposing the applied stresses, but in the face of severe or repeated stresses, destructive features may develop.

Perhaps the most crucial argument against viewing spondylosis and spinal osteoarthrosis as diseases is that they are so irregularly (if not infrequently) associated with symptoms and disability. The incidence of spondylosis and osteoarthrosis is just as great in patients with symptoms as in patients without symptoms.[321,353,521]

This raises the great paradox in the field of spinal pain, namely that while some patients with spondylosis or osteoarthrosis may present with pain, there are others with the same age changes that do not have pain, and many patients with pain do not have a trace of spondylosis or osteoarthrosis. Consequently, spondylosis or osteoarthrosis cannot legitimately be viewed as a pathological diagnosis. Some other, or additional factor must be the cause of pain, and the resolution of this problem is addressed in the final two chapters.

13. Lumbar spinal pain

Low-back pain is the most common complaint in physical medicine and one of the most costly complaints in medicine in general, yet it remains poorly understood and poorly managed. The reason why back pain is such a problem in clinical practice is that traditionally it has been addressed with limited, almost partisan viewpoints.

Historically, investigators have sought to determine a singular cause for low-back pain, in the expectation that all patients will have this one cause. Moreover, there has been the expectation that low-back pain should be easy to diagnose; that a particular set of symptoms and signs must indicate a particular cause. However, no single cause has been found to be the answer, and no simple clinical test reveals the answer. Consequently, low-back pain has been shrouded in controversy as one school of thought battles to have its views prevail over other schools of thought.

What has compromised the evolution of thought on lumbar pain syndromes has been the tendency simply to infer that a particular mechanism or cause is responsible for a particular syndrome, without actually proving it to be so. Indeed, theories generated in this way, even if incorrect, seem to gain the respectability of a 'rule' or 'dogma', if they are reiterated strongly and often enough, and sometimes become so 'sacred' as to be exempt from challenge. Yet, in some instances, new facts or correct logic expose the limitations or errors in concepts evolved in this way.

As far as possible, concepts should be based on scientific fact, and it is the purpose of this chapter to collate those facts and experimental observations that are relevant to the comprehension of the mechanism of lumbar pain syndromes, providing a rational basis for their interpretation, while at the same time challenging or dispelling certain common misconceptions that are no longer tenable.

THE TYPES OF LUMBAR PAIN

Not all pain in the lumbar region is necessarily due to disorders of the lumbar spine. Lumbar pain may be due to visceral or vascular disease in the abdomen or pelvis, and for this reason, the assessment of lumbar pain must include an assessment of these possibilities. However, it is not the purpose of this chapter to explore the field of visceral and vascular disease. Lumbar pain may also be a presentation of sacro-iliac or other pelvic musculoskeletal problems, but again these disorders are beyond the scope of this chapter. The intention is to explore specifically pain syndromes stemming from disorders of the lumbar spine.

On physiological grounds, two fundamental types of lumbar pain syndrome can be identified. The first are those pain syndromes in which the pain stems directly from one of the musculoskeletal structures of the lumbar spine, and these syndromes are described below under the heading of 'somatic pain'. The second type are those syndromes in which the pain is caused by disorders of the spinal nerves or the spinal nerve roots, and these are described under the heading of 'radicular pain'.

SOMATIC PAIN

For any structure to be a source of pain, it must

be connected to the nervous system and, conversely, any structure that has a nerve supply is potentially a source of pain. Thus, on anatomical grounds, any of the structures in the lumbar spine that receives a nerve supply can become a source of lumbar pain if it is afflicted by an appropriate disease or disorder.

As described in Chapter 9, the structures in the lumbar spine that receive a nerve supply are the zygapophysial joints, the ligaments of the posterior elements, the para-vertebral muscles, the dura mater, the anterior and posterior longitudinal ligaments and the intervertebral discs. At one time or another, each of these structures has been incriminated as a source of low-back pain, although largely on the basis of opinion or just circumstantial evidence, and it has taken some 45 years to collect the necessary experimental evidence that vindicates these incriminations.

In 1938 and 1939, Kellgren[288,289] demonstrated that low-back pain could be induced by noxious stimulation of the lumbar back muscles and interspinous ligaments while, reciprocally, Steindler and Luck[494] had shown that certain forms of low-back pain syndromes could be relieved, at least temporarily, by anaesthetising these same structures. Although the term 'facet syndrome' was introduced in 1933,[196] it is only since the mid-1970s that it has been shown that experimental stimulation of lumbar zygapophysial joints could cause low-back pain in normal volunteers,[363,381] and that back pain stemming from these joints could be relieved by radiologically controlled blocks of the joints themselves,[87-90,123,134,160,333,374,458] or their nerve supply.[413,428,488]

Two lines of evidence revealed that the intervertebral discs could be a source of back pain. Operating on patients under local anaesthetic, Wiberg[562] showed that pressing on the posterior anulus fibrosus could evoke low-back pain. Later, after the introduction of discography as a diagnostic procedure, it was recognised that back pain could be reproduced by injections of contrast medium into lumbar intervertebral discs.[246,332,442] Subsequent experience with provocation discography has confirmed that injection of contrast medium, or even just normal saline, into intervertebral discs can evoke back pain, even if the disc is structurally intact and myelographically normal.[96,423,564]

The dura mater has been shown to be capable of causing back pain in two types of clinical experiment. First, it was shown that back pain could be evoked by traction on the dural sleeves of lumbar nerve roots by pulling on sutures threaded through the dura at operation for laminectomy.[489] Secondly, it has been shown that chemical irritation of the dura, in the form of injections of hypertonic saline, can evoke back pain.[142] The notion of dural pain has been vindicated by recent neurosurgical studies in which patients were relieved of their back pain by selective sectioning of the nerves innervating the dural sleeve of a symptomatic nerve root.[110,111]

There is, therefore, a wealth of clinical experimental data confirming that the ligaments, muscles, joints, discs and dura mater of the lumbar spine are all capable of being a source of back pain. Of the innervated structures of the lumbar spine, only the epidural blood vessels and the vertebral bodies have not been subjected to experimental study to determine whether they too can be a source of pain. Circumstantial evidence, however, is conducive to the notion that distension of epidural veins can cause pain;[54] but while it is presumed that the pain of spinal osteoporosis arises from the vertebral bodies, there have been no formal experimental studies of low-back pain stemming from bone.

Given that various structures in the lumbar spine have been shown to be capable of producing low-back pain, it is important to realise that in each case, the mechanism involved is the stimulation of nerve endings in the affected structure. Lumbar nerve root compression is in no way involved. Thus, to distinguish these forms of low-back pain from root compression syndromes, the term **somatic pain** can be used. This term implies an origin for the pain from one or other of the somatic tissues of the lumbar spine.

The possible causes of somatic lumbar pain would be any pathological process that stimulates the nociceptive nerve endings in one or other of the pain-sensitive structures of the lumbar spine. In this respect, there are only two known mechanisms by which nerve endings may be stimulated: chemical or mechanical irritation.

Chemical irritation occurs in inflammatory diseases or follows tissue damage. While it is very difficult to validate experimentally, the mechanism seems to involve the direct stimulation of nerve endings by chemicals, such as hydrogen and potassium ions, or proteolytic enzymes, that are liberated from inflammatory cells or damaged tissue cells. Mechanical irritation, on the other hand, involves the stretching of connective tissue, without the involvement of any chemical mediators. Exactly how mechanical irritation causes pain remains obscure, but a plausible explanation is that when an array of collagen fibres (in a ligament, joint capsule, or periosteum) is placed under tension, it deforms and closes the available space between individual collagen fibres. Nerve endings, or perhaps nerve fibres, within the array would then be stimulated by being squeezed between the encroaching collagen fibres.

The pathology of somatic lumbar pain is described further in Chapter 14. However, because of its relative novelty, and controversial nature, it is worth elaborating on the concept of primary disc pain. In contradistinction to pain caused by the compression of spinal nerves by herniated intervertebral discs, primary disc pain is pain that stems directly from the disc itself, and it is caused by the stimulation of the nerve endings within the anulus fibrosus (Ch. 9). Pathological processes theoretically responsible for this stimulation include excessive mechanical strain of the anulus, chemical irritation as a result of inflammation following trauma to the anulus, and involvement of the anulus in the chemical degrading processes that occur in disc degeneration (see Ch. 13).

Logical deduction reveals that not every pathological process that affects a disc will necessarily be painful, since only the peripheral anulus is innervated. Disc pain will occur only if a pain-producing process affects the innervated periphery of the disc. Processes like disc degradation, or degeneration, that are restricted to the nucleus or central portions of the anulus, have no access to the nerve supply of the disc, and therefore cannot directly cause pain. Thus, even a severely degenerated disc may remain painless. However, should centrally located processes extend to the innervated periphery, as in a radial fissure,[164] or if the peripheral anulus itself is primarily damaged, as in a torsional strain[162,164,170] (see Ch. 14), then nerve endings may be affected. If enough are stimulated, pain may ensue. On the other hand. a healthy and innervated portion of an anulus could become painful if, as a result of disease in other portions of the disc, it is called upon to bear a greater mechanical load, and thereby is secondarily subjected to excessive strain. Variations and permutations like these explain why discs, apparently affected by similar disease processes, may be inconsistently painful or painless.

SOMATIC REFERRED PAIN

Referred pain is pain perceived in a region topographically displaced from the region of the source of the pain. In lumbar pain syndromes, pain is primarily generated by lesions in the lumbar spine but referred pain may be perceived in the buttocks and lower limbs, or sometimes in the groin or abdominal wall. The term 'somatic referred pain' is used to emphasise the skeletal or 'somatic' origin for this form of pain, and to distinguish it from radicular pain and referred pain caused by visceral or vascular disease.

Virtually any source of local lumbar or lumbosacral pain is also capable of producing somatic referred pain. The mechanism appears to be that afferent impulses from the lumbar spine activate neurons in the central nervous system which also happen to receive afferents from the lower limbs, buttocks, or groin. Stimulation of such central nervous system neurons, by impulses from the lumbar spine, results in the perception of pain arising from all the tissues subtended by these neurons. Thus, the patient complains of pain in the lower limbs as well as the back, even though there is no signal actually emanating from the limbs.

Experimental and clinical studies

The evidence for such a mechanism stems from several experimental and clinical studies. Kellgren[288,289] showed that low-back pain, experimentally induced by stimulating interspinous ligaments and back muscles, could be accompanied by referred pain in the lower limbs. These observations were later corroborated by other investigators.[175,256] More recently, it has been shown that in addition to back pain, experimental noxious stimulation of lumbar zygapophysial joints can cause referred pain in various regions of the lower limbs, buttocks and groin.[363,381] Traction of the dura mater has been shown to produce buttock and thigh pain,[489] and it has been reported, though not formally studied, that in some patients disc stimulation can reproduce not only their back pain but their referred pain as well.[96,251,423,485,564]

Complementing these experimental observations are the reports that anaesthetising intervertebral discs,[423] or anaesthetising[87–90,160,333,338,363,374,381,458,494] or denervating[57,458,488] zygapophysial joints, in appropriately selected patients, relieves not only their local pain but also their lower limb pain.

The critical feature of these various studies is that the stimuli used to evoke referred pain, or the anaesthetics used to relieve it, were delivered directly to somatic elements of the lumbar spine. Nerve roots were not stimulated or anaesthetised. The mechanism for the referred pain, therefore, must lie beyond the nerve roots, and the only possible site is in the central nervous system.

Apparent segmental distribution

An over-emphasised aspect of somatic referred pain is its apparent segmental distribution. Early investigators sought to establish charts of the segmental pattern of pain referral in the anticipation that the axial origin of referred pain could be diagnosed on the basis of its peripheral distribution, just as dermatomes are used to diagnose the segmental level of a root compression or spinal cord injury.[175,253,289] However, it is now evident that the fields of referred pain from particular segments overlap greatly within a given individual and the patterns exhibited by different individuals vary considerably.[57] These irregularities preclude the use of charts of so-called sclerotomes for any legitimate diagnostic purpose. Such charts serve only to illustrate that lumbar pain may be referred into the lower limbs, but not to constant locations.

In this context, it is sometimes maintained that somatic referred pain does not extend beyond the knee, and that pain distal to the knee must be radicular in origin. However, while it is true that somatic referred pain most commonly is distributed in the region of the buttock,[160,253,367,381] it nevertheless can extend as far as the foot.[175,289,381] Indeed, there is even some evidence that the distance of referral into the lower limb is proportional to the intensity of the stimulus to the spine.[381]

An important, though overlooked, legacy of the experimental studies on somatic referred pain relates to its quality. All the studies showed that the referred pain was deep and aching in quality, and was hard to localise. This contrasts with the sharper, lancinating nature of radicular pain, and putatively may be used to distinguish somatic referred pain from radicular pain.[60]

RADICULAR PAIN

The concept of 'sciatica' stems from the coincidental similarity between the distribution of some forms of referred pain and the course of the sciatic nerve. Consequently sciatica was originally ascribed to intrinsic disease of the sciatic nerve. Later it was ascribed to muscular compression, and eventually to compression of the lumbosacral nerve roots by disorders of the vertebral column, which is the prevailing contemporary view.

These notions on the causation of sciatica, however, were based only on inference or circumstantial evidence. For example, because arthritic changes could be demonstrated radiologically in patients with sciatic pain, the cause was deemed to be compression of the L5 spinal nerve by lumbosacral 'arthritis'.[115,565] Later, this notion was superceded by the revelation that herniated intervertebral discs could compress lumbosacral nerve roots.[377] The 'compressive' causes of sciatica, however, were introduced without it being demonstrated that root compression could cause pain.

Early investigators were probably drawn to their conclusions by the observations that most of their patients had weakness or numbness in association with their sciatic pain. Because weakness and numbness are features of nerve compression, it was understandably attractive to ascribe the pain to the same cause and mechanism. Moreover, these conclusions were made, and the nerve root compression theory established, before the earliest experiments on somatic referred pain.[288,289] Consequently, nerve root compression became the senior and dominant explanation for referred pain in the lower limb.

In certain respects, it is surprising that nerve root compression was sustained as the mechanism for referred pain, for it is known that compression of nerves elsewhere in the body does not cause pain.[179] Indeed, this paradox led to criticisms of the nerve root compression theory.[290] However, subsequent clinical and laboratory experiments have helped resolve this paradox, albeit at the expense of raising new enigmas.

Experimental compression of nerve roots

MacNab[350] reported that experimental compression of normal nerve roots, using catheters inserted into intervertebral foramina, evoked paraesthesiae and numbness, but did not cause pain. On the other hand, Smyth and Wright[489] demonstrated that pulling on nerve roots previously affected by disc herniation did evoke sciatic pain. Thus, clinically damaged nerve roots are capable of generating pain, but normal nerve roots are not.

These clinical observations have been corroborated by animal experiments which showed that activity in nociceptive afferent fibres could be elicited by mechanical stimulation of previously damaged nerve roots, but not by stimulation of normal nerve roots.[260,261,337] The questions raised by these experiments are how do normal and damaged roots differ, and how soon after a compressive lesion is a normal root sufficiently damaged to become painful? These questions remained unanswered.

Another observation from these same animal experiments[260,261,337] is that nociceptive activity can be elicited by stimulation of dorsal root ganglia, irrespective of whether they are normal or damaged. Thus, dorsal root ganglia are apparently more susceptible to mechanical stimulation than axons, and pain may occur if the ganglion rather than the root itself is compressed. This

difference may explain why apparent compression of nerve roots is capable of producing pain when compression of nerve trunks is not. Compression of the cell bodies in the dorsal root ganglia seems to be the critical difference.

Other issues aside, there is no doubt that under the appropriate circumstances, compression of dorsal root ganglia, or compression of previously damaged nerve roots can cause pain, but an unfortunate legacy of the concept of sciatica is the tendency, in some circles, to interpret all forms of pain in the lower limb as due to nerve root compression. This is not justified.

The clinical experiments of Smyth and Wright[489] showed that traction on nerve roots produced only a particular form of pain. It was lancinating or shooting in quality, and was felt along a relatively narrow band 'no more than one and a half inches wide'.[489] This neuralgic type of pain is the only type of pain that has been shown to be produced by root compression. Therefore, only this form of pain can legitimately be called 'sciatica' and ascribed to root compression. In contrast, somatic referred pain is static, aching in quality and hard to localise, and should be recognised as a different entity.

This distinction has been verified in recent clinical experiments in which electrodes were used to electrically stimulate various somatic structures and nerve roots.[367] Stimulation of the supraspinous and interspinous ligaments, zygapophysial joints, back muscles, extradural tissues, the posterior longitudinal ligament, and the intervertebral disc produced referred pain to the buttock and posterior or lateral thigh, which was dull and poorly localised. In contrast, stimulation of nerve roots gave a sharper, well-localised pain, commonly with an element of paraesthesia, radiating to or below the ankle.[367]

Other irregularities

There are two further irregularities concerning the concepts of sciatica and nerve root compression. First, there is no known mechanism whereby a compressive lesion can selectively affect only nociceptive axons, i.e. without also affecting large diameter afferent fibres that convey touch and other sensations. Therefore, there is no mechanism whereby root compression can cause pain without causing other neurological abnormalities as well. Thus, for root compression to be deemed the cause, radicular pain must be accompanied by other features of nerve compression: numbness, weakness, or paraesthesiae. In the absence of such accompanying features, it is very difficult to maintain that root compression is the cause of any pain. Pain in the lower limb in the absence of objective neurological signs is most likely to be somatic referred pain.

The second irregularity relates to back pain. All the experimental studies on radicular pain emphasise that root compression causes pain in the lower limb. Thus, although radicular pain may feel as if it starts in the back and radiates into the lower limb, there is no evidence that root compression can, or should, cause isolated low-back pain. It is implausible that a compressive lesion could stimulate only those afferents in a root that come from the lumbar spine, and spare those that come from the lower limb. Isolated low-back pain suggests a somatic lesion, and the pain should not be dismissed as due to nerve root compression when no evidence of compression exists.

PATHOLOGY OF NERVE ROOT COMPRESSION

The pathology of nerve root compression is a simple exercise in applied anatomy. In the radicular canals the nerve roots are ensheathed by pia, arachnoid and dura mater. They are surrounded by epidural fat, and are related to a vertebral body, its pedicle and lamina, and the ligamentum flavum (Chapter 9). In the intervertebral foramina the nerve roots and spinal nerve are related to the ligamentum flavum, the zygapophysial joint, the pedicles above and below, the back of a vertebral body, and an intervertebral disc. Space-occupying lesions of any of these structures can become a cause of nerve root compression.

The rarer causes of nerve root compression include cysts of the nerve root sheath,[94,205,506] ganglion or synovial cyst of the zygapophysial joint,[215,271,284,465] un-united epiphysis of the zygapophysial joint,[449] cyst of the ligamentum flavum,[219] and tumours of the epidural fat, vertebral bodies and pedicles, nerve root sheaths, and of the nerve roots themselves.[147]

More commonly, the roots are affected by the age changes of the lumbar spine, notably by osteophytes from the zygapophysial joints.[149] Such osteophytes may occur focally over one set of roots, or may be part of the more disseminated process of spinal stenosis.[30,138,148,300,546,548] However, the most common cause of nerve root compression is intervertebral disc herniation, and this phenomenon is described further in Chapter 14.

What remains incompletely resolved is how nerve root compression causes symptoms. Objective neurological signs are readily understood, for mechanical compression simply blocks conduction in the affected axons, and the nature of the signs depends on the type of axon affected. Conduction block in motor fibres causes weakness in a myotomal distribution, while conduction block in sensory axons causes paraesthesiae and numbness in a dermatomal distribution. Radicular pain remains the enigma.

As described above, simple compression of normal nerve roots does not cause pain, but pain does occur in previously damaged roots. What appears to be the significant factor is not the compression, but the development of intra-neural or perineural inflammation, or nerve root ischaemia.

In non-inflammatory lesions, inflammation may result from repeated traction of the nerve root over the space-occupying lesion.[523] Otherwise, lesions may themselves be inflammatory in nature, and the nerve roots inevitably become involved in this inflammation regardless of whether or not they are significantly compressed. This is most evident in the case of disc herniation.

Another form of nerve root inflammation is vascular oedema. Because the radicular veins and arteries are embedded within the spinal nerve roots, any space-occupying lesion that compresses the nerve roots must simultaneously compress their blood vessels. The nerve roots are particularly susceptible to the consequences of vascular compression, particularly venous compression, because they lack lymphatics.[384] Consequently, there are no alternative channels whereby normal or exudated extra-cellular fluid can leave the roots.

Intra-neural and perineural oedema can interfere with nerve conduction by exerting pressure on axons. In the case of venous obstruction by space-occupying lesions, the pressure from oedema would be additional to any pressure already exerted on the axons directly by the lesion. Alternatively, space-occupying lesions insufficiently large to cause symptoms alone, could feasibly result in symptoms if they compressed the radicular veins and caused intra-neural oedema. Indeed, it has been stated that, on morphological grounds, any space-occupying lesion would result in nerve root ischaemia or congestion before any gross mechanical compression of the nerve roots.[128]

Nerve root ischaemia may also be the result of long-standing oedema or chronic inflammation. Oedema fluid or inflammatory exudate tends to organise, i.e. convert to fibrous tissue. Thus, in due course, oedematous or inflamed nerve roots can become embedded in fibrous tissue.[384] This tissue can exert either or both of two effects on the nerve roots. It may constrict axons directly, or it may constrict their blood supply, by effectively strangling either the radicular veins or the radicular arteries.

Because of these multiple possibilities and variations, the pathophysiology of nerve root compression is not a simple process. Whereas mechanical compression of axons may be a factor, it is not the only process, and may not be the significant factor. Vascular compression is an obligatory simultaneous process which can cause further axonal compression as a result of oedema, or can render the nerve root ischaemic. Similarly, mechanical irritation of the nerve roots may evoke a sterile inflammatory response. Although the precise mechanism whereby radicular pain is generated still remains to be demonstrated, it seems likely that the ischaemic and inflammatory processes involved in nerve root compression will prove to be the key factors, rather than simple mechanical compression of the roots.

COMBINED STATES

It is evident that back pain and referred pain may be caused by a variety of disorders and mechanisms, but it is critical to realise that a patient's complaints may not be due to a single disorder or a single mechanism. Several disorders may co-exist and different mechanisms may be co-active.

The simplest examples are the co-existence of zygapophysial disorders and disc disorders at the same segmental level, or at different levels; each disorder contributing separately to the patient's overall complaint. A more complex example relates to nerve root compression syndromes.

The cardinal features of nerve root compression are the objective neurological signs of weakness or numbness. In the presence of such signs, accompanied by the lancinating pain which is characteristic of radicular pain, the syndrome may legitimately be ascribed to nerve root compression. However, nerve root compression may only be part of a patient's complaint. Local somatic and somatic referred pain may occur in addition to the symptoms of nerve root compression. In such cases the most likely source, or sources, of the somatic pain are the structures immediately adjacent to the compressed root.

The closest relation of a nerve root is its dural sleeve, and it is obvious that any lesion that might compress a root must first affect its dural sleeve. Given that the dura is pain-sensitive,[142,489] it becomes a potent possible source of low-back pain, and even referred pain,[489] that can occur alone, or be superimposed on any radicular pain. However, the mechanism involved is distinctly different from that of any radicular pain, for dural pain is caused by the stimulation of nerve endings in the dural sleeve; not by nerve compression.

Since the dura is mechano-sensitive,[489] traction of the dura over a space-occupying lesion, like a herniated disc, could be the possible cause of dural pain. The dura is also chemo-sensitive,[142] so an additional or alternative process could be chemical irritation of the dura. With regard to the latter, it has been demonstrated that disc material contains potent inflammatory chemicals,[361,362] and when disc material ruptures into the epidural space, it seems to elicit an auto-immune inflammatory reaction that can affect not only the roots but the dura as well[191,194,195,384] (see Ch. 14). The dural sleeve can remain symptomatic even after succesful 'disc' surgery. Such pain can be diagnosed by selective epidural blocks with local anaesthetic, and treated by denervating the dural sleeve.[110,111]

The other two possible sources of pain concurrent with root compression are the adjacent disc and zygapophysial joint. Regardless of any herniation that compresses a root, an intervertebral disc itself may be an intrinsic source of pain; the pain being mechanical in origin, caused by strain of the anulus fibrosus of the diseased disc. In such cases, treating the nerve root compression may relieve the objective neurological signs and any radicular pain, but the discogenic pain may continue unless it too is treated.

A zygapophysial joint may compress or traumatise the underlying roots by developing osteophytes,[149] but a degenerative zygapophysial joint may also be independently painful, causing both local and referred somatic pain. Thus, while resecting the osteophytes may decompress the roots, it may not relieve the intrinsic low-back pain and referred pain stemming from the diseased joint. This concept has particular ramifications in the interpretation of spinal stenosis, where not all the symptoms are necessarily due to the overt nerve root compression. The back pain and referred pain could be due to the osteoarthrosis of the zygapophysial joints.

PATTERNS OF LUMBAR PAIN

It might be expected that different causes of lumbar pain should be distinguishable from one another on the basis of differences in the distribution and behaviour of symptoms. Frustratingly, however, this is not so. Because different structures in the lumbar spine share a similar segmental nerve supply, and because different disorders share similar mechanisms, no single disorder has a characteristic distribution of local or referred pain.

Zygapophysial pain

With respect to zygapophysial joint disorders, experimental studies have shown that local and referred pain patterns from joints at different levels vary considerably in different individuals, and even in a given individual they overlap greatly.[57,363,381] Furthermore, the incidence of other clinical features in zygapophysial syndromes, including various aggravating factors, is insufficiently different from their incidence in other syndromes. Fairbank et al[160] performed diagnostic joint blocks on patients presenting with back pain and referred pain, and analysed the differences between those who responded and those who did not. Although certain features did occur more commonly in responders, they also occurred so frequently in non-responders that no clinical feature could be identified that could be held to be indicative or pathognomonic of zygapophysial joint pain.

Radicular pain

Although the quality of radicular pain is distinctive, its distribution is not. Radicular pain from a particular nerve root does not follow a constant distribution. In general, L5 radicular pain radiates to the dorsum of the foot and hallux, while S1 pain radiates to the heel or lateral border of the foot.[184,367] However, radicular pain does not always extend into the foot,[410] and in the leg it is usually impossible to distinguish between L5 and S1 pain.[367,489] Both L5 and S1 radicular pain can be felt in the back of the leg, and the pattern can vary with the intensity with which the root is stimulated.[367,489]

DIAGNOSIS

Notwithstanding the variations described above, the diagnosis of nerve root compression by lumbar disc herniation can be made clinically with a known reliability. The sensitivity of clinical examination in the diagnosis of this disorder is about 77%.[303] This means that using clinical features alone 77% of actual disc herniations are accurately detected, but some 23% of cases are misdiagnosed, either in that the herniation is diagnosed at the wrong level, or that some condition other than disc herniation has caused the nerve root compression. Other studies[310] suggest that the sensitivity of clinical examination may only be about 58%, meaning that up to 42% of cases are misdiagnosed.

On the other hand, the specificity of clinical examination for the diagnosis of disc herniation is 90%,[303] meaning that 90% of cases said to have disc herniation, actually do so; but even then, this figure indicates that some 10% of cases prove to be due to some other cause, like zygapophysial osteophytes, spinal stenosis and epidural varices.[303] Electromyography and myelography have sensitivities and specificities similar to those of clinical examination,[152,303] so even on the basis of these investigations a false positive diagnosis of disc herniation is made in some 10% of patients.

Other forms of pain, like disc pain and muscular pain syndromes have not been studied in this same rigorous way. Consequently, there is no scientific evidence that permits any claim that certain pain patterns are characteristic of these syndromes. The only diagnosis that has withstood scientific scrutiny is that of nerve compression by disc herniation. Unfortunately, disc herniation accounts for fewer than 30%[256] and perhaps as few as 5%[183,496] of patients presenting with back pain,[183] and it is little consolation that this condition can be so readily diagnosed. The remaining low-back pain syndromes cannot be reliably diagnosed simply on clinical grounds. Their diagnosis relies on investigations outside the realm of symptomatic and conventional physical examination.

In this regard, plain radiography has little value as a diagnostic tool in low-back pain,[423] while electromyography, myelography and CT scanning are of relevance only in nerve root compression syndromes. For conditions in which pain alone is the complaint, and there are no objective neurological signs indicative of nerve root compression, other investigations are required.

The mainstay for the diagnosis of lumbar pain, in the absence of neurological signs, are diagnostic blocks and provocation radiology. These techniques are based on the principles that if a structure is the cause of pain, then stressing that structure should reproduce the pain, and anaesthetising the structure should relieve the pain. Thus, zygapophysial joints suspected of being the source of pain can be infiltrated with local anaesthetic,[61,87–90] and relief of pain implicates the injected joint as the source. Similarly, interver-tebral discs can be injected with saline or contrast medium to reproduce pain, or with local anaesthetic to relieve pain.[423] Radicular pain and dural pain can be diagnosed by infiltrating the root thought to be responsible, with local anaesthetic.[110,111,312,504,543]

In all of these procedures, failure to provoke or relieve the pain excludes the investigated structure as the source of pain, whereupon other structures or other segmental levels in the lumbar spine may be investigated, until the responsible site is identified. Although subject to certain technical limitations,[423,460] and although they do not reveal the actual cause of pain, these techniques are the only available means of objectively establishing at least the anatomical location of the cause of pain. The cause of the pain remains a matter of informed deduction, and this issue is explored in Chapter 14.

14. Pathology of mechanical lumbar back pain

The lumbar spine can be afflicted by a great variety of pathological conditions. These include congenital malformations, fractures, infectious and neoplastic diseases, inflammatory, metabolic and various miscellaneous disorders. In some of these conditions the lumbar spine may be the primary focus of the disease; in others it may be affected either as part of the vertebral column in generalised spinal disease, or as part of the skeletal system in generalised bone disease or systemic, inflammatory or metabolic disease. However, it is not the intention of this chapter to explore the full spectrum of spinal pathology. This is exhaustively covered in major textbooks of spinal radiology and surgery.[147,474] However, it is a feature of traditional textbooks on the spine to favour the surgical and more exotic pathology of the lumbar spine, at the expense of more common disorders.

By far the majority of troublesome complaints of low-back pain appear to be mechanical in origin, in that the pain appears to have been brought on by some mechanical event, and is aggravated by movements. There is no single cause for such complaints, but the spectrum of possible disorders that underlie mechanical back pain can be derived by considering the structures of the lumbar spine that receive a nerve supply and are therefore able to be a **source** of pain; and how these structures might be injured, rendering them able to be a **cause** of pain.

Such an exercise constitutes a review of most of the preceding chapters of this book. Chapters 1 to 4 and 8 describe the structural components of the lumbar spine and their normal functions. Chapter 9 describes their innervation and Chapter 13 describes how various structures can be a

source of pain. Chapters 6 and 7 and the latter part of Chapter 8 outline the principles of biomechanics and how they apply to normal function. Deriving the pathology of mechanical back pain simply becomes a matter of marshalling this information and considering how excessive forces applied to the lumbar spine could injure the several structures known to be possible sources of low-back pain. This can be done systematically by considering the possible effects of excessive forces applied in each of the standard directions or movements of the lumbar spine: flexion, extension, rotation and compression.

FLEXION

The lumbar spine is well designed to sustain flexion. It is braced against flexion moments by the intervertebral discs, the zygapophysial joints, the posterior ligamentous system and the back muscles (Chs 2–4, 7 and 8). However, in the face of excessive external forces, one or other of these restraining elements may fail and sustain injury.

The interspinous ligaments are the weakest of the posterior elements that resist flexion (Ch. 8) and could be expected to fail first and most often. Indeed, the interspinous ligaments are found frequently to be 'degenerated' in their middle portion (Ch. 4), presumably as the result of previous injury.[466] However, clinical reports of injured interspinous ligaments being a source of back pain are few and are now dated.[494] Either because the diagnosis is no longer fashionable, or because the condition is rarely symptomatic, no contemporary clinical studies have invoked the interspinous ligaments as a significant source of back pain following flexion injury, nor has any evidence of interspinous ligament injury been demonstrated in vivo, either by biopsy or by imaging.

Zygapophysial joint sprains or sprains of the thoracolumbar fascia presumably could occur as a result of excessive flexion, but evidence of such injuries has not been reported in the clinical literature. Some investigators have raised the proposition that compartment syndromes of the back muscles could occur; the notion being that following exertion or spasm, the back muscles swell and strain the overlying thoracolumbar fascia thereby causing pain.[86,437] However, clinical investigations have not shown this condition to be particularly common or easily diagnosed.[499]

Sprains of the anulus fibrosus due to flexion injury are not likely to occur in isolation for the anulus lies close to the axis of sagittal rotation. Structures located more posteriorly, operating on longer moment arms, are more likely to fail before the anulus does. Anular sprains in flexion would thus ordinarily occur only in combination with other injuries.

The disc as a whole is remarkably resistant to flexion injury. Provided it is healthy and intact, the anulus fibrosus protects the disc from herniation. Experiments have shown that it is very difficult to produce herniation by flexion. Only if the spine is hyperflexed, beyond the ranges typically undertaken in activities of daily living, does herniation occur, and then only in a minority of specimens.[10] Even in partially herniated discs it is difficult to complete the herniation by repeated loading in compression and flexion.[8]

Muscle sprain would appear to be the most likely and most common lesion sustained in flexion. The back muscles as a whole are the largest of the posterior structures that resist flexion and could be expected to withstand larger flexion loads than the posterior ligaments. However, as described in Chapter 8, the back muscles consist of individual, segmental strands. Thus, it is possible that individual strands might suffer injury while the rest of the muscle is substantially spared. A sprained muscle could therefore exhibit areas of focal injury that become symptomatic and tender.

Experiments have shown that under strain muscles characteristically fail near their myotendinous junction.[189,190,405] Because the back muscles are polysegmental, myotendinous junctions occur throughout the back. Myotendinous junctions of the longissimus thoracis pars lumborum and the iliocostalis lumborum pars lumborum occur towards the lumbar transverse processes. However, if injured these sites lie too deeply to be reliably detected by clinical examination. On the other hand, the costalattachments of iliocostalis lumborum and the iliac attachments of longissimus through the lumbar intermuscular aponeurosis are relatively superficial and accessible to palpation. These sites are frequently tender in patients with what appear to be acute muscle sprains of the back (Fig. 14.1).

Trigger points are said to be a common cause of back pain, although enigmatically, research reports actually documenting the incidence of trigger points in the lumbar back muscles are few, with most contemporary authors quoting the one original report of such conditions.[522] The aetiology of trigger points is still speculative,[486] but it may be that they represent acute or recurrent sprain of individual strands of one of the back muscles. This would explain their linear, fusiform shape and orientation. Otherwise, it may be that trigger points as strictly defined[486] are not common in the back muscles, and what are misrepresented as trigger points are no more than areas of tender, sprained muscles.[44,161,268,334]

A common clinical presentation is that of acute locked back: a patient undertakes flexion but is then unable to straighten up because of pain; remaining flexed is inconvenient but becomes the least painful posture. The pathology of acute locked back is unknown, but two theories have been elaborated on.

One explanation pertains to meniscus extrapment (Fig. 14.2). It is proposed that upon flexion one of the fibro-adipose meniscoids of a zygapophysial joint (Ch. 3) is drawn out of the joint but upon attempted extension the meniscoid fails to re-enter the joint cavity; instead it impacts against the edge of the articular cartilage, and in this location it buckles and acts as a space-occupying lesion under the capsule, causing pain by distending the capsule.[63] Maintaining flexion is comfortable because this disengages the mensicoid. Treatment by manipulation becomes

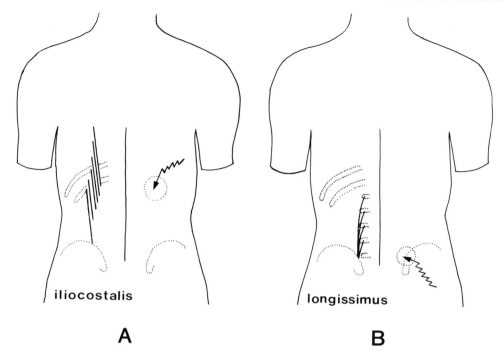

Fig. 14.1 Typical locations of tenderness in relatively superficial back muscles following sprains of their myotendinous junctions. **A**: Tenderness in the iliocostalis lumborum pars thoracis, near the costal attachments of its fascicles. **B**: Tenderness in the longissimus thoracis pars lumborum where its fibres form the lumbar intermuscular aponeurosis.

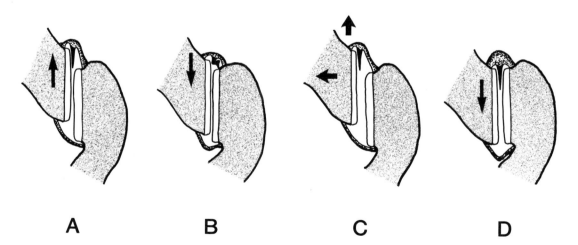

Fig. 14.2 The theory of meniscus extrapment. **A**: Upon flexion, the inferior articular process of a zygapophysial joint moves upwards taking a meniscoid with it. **B**: Upon attempted extension, the inferior articular process returns towards its neutral position, but the meniscoid, instead of re-entering the joint cavity, impacts against the edge of the articular cartilage, and buckles forming a space-occupying 'lesion' under the capsule. Pain occurs as a result of capsular tension and extension is inhibited.
C: Manipulation of the joint involving gapping and flexion reduces the impaction and opens the joint to encourage re-entry of the meniscoid into the joint space (**D**).

logical. Passive flexion of the segment reduces the impaction and rotation gaps the joint, encouraging the meniscoid to re-enter the joint cavity (Fig. 14.2).

An alternative explanation is that upon flexion a fragment of nuclear material displaces along an incomplete radial fissure in the anulus fibrosus and lodges deep to the outer fibres of the anulus. Here it acts as an intradiscal space-occupying lesion. Upon attempted extension the satellite nucleus cannot re-enter the central nucleus and is compressed. Under compression it attempts to expand radially and stretches the anulus fibrosus thereby causing pain.[63] Maintaining flexion is comfortable because this decompresses the satellite nucleus. Reduction of the lesion might be possible by manipulation involving flexion, lateral flexion and extension, aiming to force the satellite back into the nucleus or to disperse it between the lamellae of the anulus fibrosus.

EXTENSION

At large, extension injuries are relatively uncommon because extension is not a movement frequently undertaken in activities of daily living. It is, however, a frequent movement amongst some sports people, and extension injuries may underlie some of the back complaints reported by such individuals.

Extension is limited by bony contact (Ch. 7). Lesions may develop if this contact is sudden and severe or repeated. Contactbetween spinous processes may result in periostitis at the site of contact: a condition known as Baastrup's disease[36] or 'kissing spine' (Fig. 14.3A). This condition may be diagnosed on the basis of discrete interspinous tenderness with relief of pain upon injecting the affected site with local anaesthetic. Clinical studies, however, suggest that the significance of this condition may be overrated; it is not necessarily the source of pain in the affected segment. In one study, only 11 out of 64 patients with this condition responded to surgical excision of the lesion.[48]

When extension is limited by impaction of an inferior articular process against the lamina below (Ch. 7), the inferior capsule may be caught between the bones,[9] or periostitis may develop at the contact point[220] (Fig. 14.3B). Periosteal erosion at these sites has been demonstrated at post-mortem,[230,551] but the condition has not been reported or shown to be painful in living subjects.

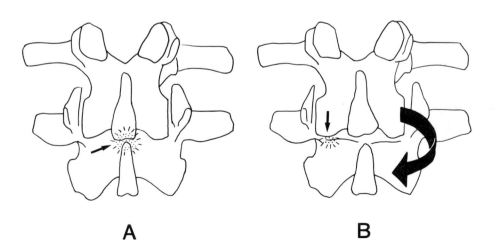

A   **B**

Fig. 14.3 Extension injuries of the lumbar spine. **A**: If extension is limited by impaction of spinous processes, periosteal irritation of the tips of the spinous processes might become a source of pain. **B**: If extension is limited by impaction of an inferior articular process, irritation of the periosteum of the lamina might become painful. Otherwise, if extension is limited by bony contact, any remaining extension force is accommodated by the segment rotating backwards about the impacted articular processes, causing strain of the contralateral zygapophysial joint.

Biomechanical studies reveal another lesion that can occur in extension. In the face of excessive extension forces, extension is initially arrested by impaction of an inferior articular process. Further extension becomes impossible because of the bony contact, but the remaining energy of the extension force must somehow be dissipated. The segment absorbs this energy by rotating backwards around the impacted inferior articular process (Fig. 14.3B). This strains the contralateral zygapophysial joint. If the extension force is large, this latter joint fails by rupturing or avulsing its capsule.[572]

ROTATION

Axial rotation strains the anulus fibrosus in torsion, but the anulus is ordinarily protected from injury by the zygapophysial joints. Zygapophysial impaction occurs before the fibres of the anulus fibrosus undergo more than 4% strain (Ch. 7). However, further rotation can occur about a new axis located through the impacted joint (Ch. 7). This results in the contralateral joint being drawn backwards, and in a lateral shear force being exerted on the anulus fibrosus (Fig. 14.4). In the face of excessive rotatory forces any of the elements resisting axial rotation may fail.

The impacted zygapophysial joint may suffer fractures of the subchondral bone of either the inferior or superior articular facet, or fractures of the entire articular process. The pars interarticularis may fracture. The contralateral zygapophysial joint may suffer tears of its capsule or fracture avulsion of the capsule. The nucleus pulposus is unaffected, but the anulus fibrosus may be injured. The characteristic lesion suffered by the anulus fibrosus under torsion is a circumferential tear (Fig. 14.4).

Circumferential tears of the anulus occur in the more peripheral fibres of the anulus over the posterolateral corner of the disc. These fibres are located furthest from the axis of rotation, and are tightly curved as they wrap around the disc. Consequently, torsional stresses exerted on the anulus are concentrated in this region.[167,172] These tears lie in the innervated, 'ligamentous' portion of the anulus and would produce symptoms analogous to those of a sprained ligament.

In pure axial rotation, the anulus fibrosus is ordinarily protected from excess torsional strain by the zygapophysial joints (Ch. 7), and would be injured only if the one or other of the impacting articular processes was competely fractured. However, the likelihood of torsional injury to the anulus fibrosus increases if axial rotation is undertaken in conjunction with flexion.

The safe limit for strain of a collagen fibre before it starts to be injured is about 4% (Ch. 6). If some of this strain is taken up by flexion, less remains available to accommodate subsequent rotation. Flexion of a lumbar joint therefore reduces its safe capacity for rotation to less than 3°. Beyond this range, fibres of the posterolateral anulus become liable to injury. Moreover, during flexion the inferior articular processes move upwards, and less articular surface remains in contact with the superior articular process to resist rotation. The protection of the anulus fibrosus provided by the zygapophysial joints is thus reduced. Consequently, the combination of flexion and rotation of the lumbar spine renders the anulus fibrosus vulnerable to torsional injury.

The various lesions described above have all been produced experimentally in biomechanical studies of cadaveric specimens of lumbar joints subject to torsion.[7,162,164,165,168,170,317,500] They have also been detected in post-mortem studies of victims of traumatic death such as motor vehicle accidents;[516,537] so it is reasonable to assume that such lesions could occur in patients who have sustained rotation or flexion-rotation injuries.

There is no way of predicting which structure would be injured by forceful rotation. The lesion could lie in the anulus fibrosus, the impacted zygapophysial joint, the pars interarticularis, or in some combination of any of these sites. Which structure fails is determined by its relative weakness and the strength of others. Individuals with a relatively weak articular process may sustain fracture of that process; but in those with robust articular processes the torsional stress may be transferred to the anulus fibrosus or the opposite zygapophysial joint.

Clinically, the various lesions would be indistinguishable; all would present with a similar history, similar clinical features and similar ag-

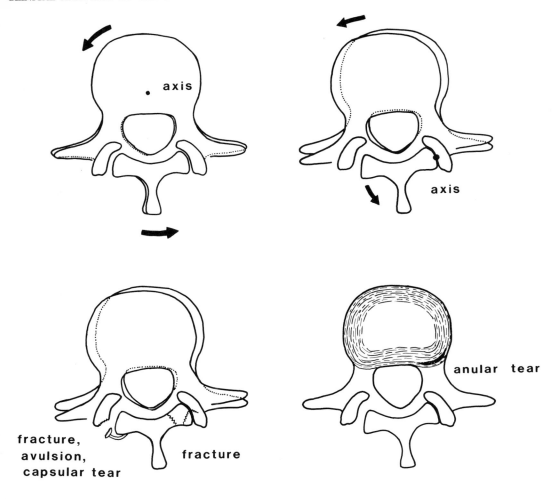

Fig. 14.4 Rotation injuries of the lumbar spine. Axial rotation of a lumbar segment is initially limited by impaction of a zygapophysial joint, but further rotation may occur about a new axis in the impacted joint, resulting in the disc being exposed to a lateral shear force and the contralateral zygapophysial joint swinging backwards. The impacted zygapophysial joint may suffer fractures of its articular processes or of the pars interarticularis. The contralateral joint may suffer fracture avulsions or tears of its capsule. The anulus fibrosus of the intervertebral disc may suffer peripheral, circumferential tears.

gravating factors. There would be a history of flexion-rotation precipitating the pain; back pain would be present, with or without referred pain; and the pain would be aggravated largely by rotation and to various extents by other lumbar movements; antalgic muscle spasm might be present; but there would be no reliable signs that would indicate the site of the lesion.

Small fractures of the lumbar zygapophysial joints can be seen if stereoradiography is used,[273,487] but it is noteworthy that none of the torsional lesions found in post-mortem studies of lumbar zygapophysial joints was evident on plain radiography.[516,537] Resolution of the exact source of pain resulting from torsional injuries can be achieved only by the judicious application of high-resolution imaging techniques and the use of zygapophysial joint blocks, discography and the newly developed technique of CT anulography.

Until recently, clinical evidence of torsional injury to the anulus fibrosus had been lacking.

However, it has now been shown that a symptomatic anulus fibrosus can be demonstrated by injecting local anaesthetic to abolish pain stemming from a putatively injured portion of the anulus fibrosus. Concurrent injection of contrast medium allows a subsequent CT scan to demonstrate the crescentic spread of local anaesthetic restricted to the anulus fibrosus in the zone affected by circumferential tears.[177,178] This procedure enables the existence of a lesion in the anulus to be demonstrated in vivo, where hitherto it had only been demonstrated at post-mortem or in biomechanical experiments on cadavers.

COMPRESSION

Perhaps contrary to popular or traditional belief, intervertebral discs do not herniate if compressed. Even if channels are experimentally cut into the anulus fibrosus and the disc is compressed, it is difficult, if not impossible to cause the nucleus to herniate through the artificial channel.[74,358,552] It appears that a normal nucleus is intrinsically cohesive. For disc herniation to occur not only must there be a defect in the anulus fibrosus, but also the nucleus must be somehow altered, to render it expressable.

When compressed, lumbar discs characteristically fail by fracture of the vertebral end-plate. This is most evident from biomechanical studies,[8,10,76,265,276,443,472] but is also evident in discographic studies of patients with acute back pain following compression injuries.[364]

Ordinarily, discs should not fail in the course of activities of daily living. They are well designed to sustain compressive loads. However, failure of the end-plate could occur in the face of excessive axial loads incurred by a fall into a standing or sitting position or during heavy lifting when the back muscles exert a large compressive load on the disc.

Because the back muscles are orientated substantially parallel to the lumbar vertebral column, their force of contraction is experienced as a compressive load on the lumbar spine (Ch. 8). This load is of the order of 4000 N[372] in average individuals.

In the case of lifting, one would expect that the body is designed such that its own muscles could not break its own bones. In the case of trained weight-lifters, this appears to be so, for as they increase muscular strength, their vertebrae become conditioned; they adapt to the loads to which they are being exposed during training, and become more robust than normal.[213]

However, one can envisage an untrained individual undertaking unaccustomed lifting for which their vertebrae are not optimally designed, e.g. the 'occasional' gardener pulling on a stubborn tree root; lifting heavy objects when 'moving house' for the first time; starting a new job requiring heavylifting without prior conditioning. Under these conditions, the back muscles may be strong enough and can be exerted in an effort to provide the necessary power, but without conditioning the vertebrae may not be appropriately strong, and the risk of end-plate fracture pertains. In this context, 'conditioning' and 'training' pertains not to 'correct lifting techniques' but to training that strengthens vertebrae rendering them less susceptible to failure under compression.

The normal strength of lumbar vertebrae varies considerably, and is related to sex, body mass and age.[265] In most individuals the strength of the vertebrae is such as to be able to withstand in excess of the load ordinarily exerted by the back muscles. However, the lower end of the normal range for the strength of lumbar vertebrae is within the range of compression loads exerted by the back muscles.[265] Thus, in susceptible individuals with relatively weak bones, undertaking inordinate exertion of their back muscles could result in end-plate fractures.

The significance of end-plate fractures was first highlighted by Farfan and his colleagues[162,164,168,172] who suggested that end-plate fractures could set in train a series of processes that resulted in a variety of changes in the disc. This suggestion has increasingly attracted favour, attention and circumstantial evidence.

There is no reason for an end-plate fracture to be symptomatic in the first instance; the lesion is not painful because the end-plate is not innervated. An individual may therefore remain oblivious to having sustained an end-plate fracture unless and until they suffer the consequences of the lesion.

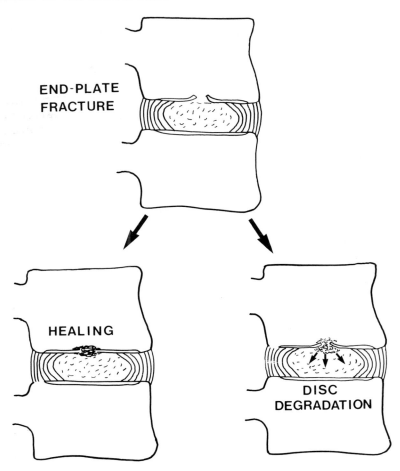

Fig. 14.5 Compression injury of an intervertebral joint. Excessive compression force may result in fracture of a vertebral end-plate. This lesion may heal and be of no consequence, but on the other hand it may initiate a process of disc degradation affecting the nucleus pulposus near the fracture site but gradually extending into the rest of the nucleus.

On the one hand, an end-plate fracture may heal and the individual may suffer no ill-effects (Fig. 14.5). On the other hand, a variety of changes may result if healing is not complete or is abnormal.

Originally, it was proposed that an end-plate fracture could evoke an inflammatory repair response that if unrestricted, could extend beyond the fracture site and invade the nucleus pulposus.[162,164,168,172] This view is consistent with the presence within the nucleus pulposus of endogenous autolytic enzymes,[359,375,398,399,480] and is further consistent with the recent detection of inflammatory cells in the anulus fibrosus of painful discs.[274] The degradative enzymes, normally present in the disc, are ordinarily inhibited by proteinase inhibitors,[375] but this inhibition is critically dependent on factors such as pH. The slightest drop in pH may be enough to activate endogenous proteolytic enzymes in the disc,[375] and an end-plate fracture may be enough of a disturbance to initiate degradation of the nucleus pulposus.

A bolder interpretation is that following an end-plate fracture the nucleus pulposus elicits an auto-immune response. The proteins of the nucleus pulposus are never exposed to the body's immune system, for at no time in its development does the nucleus pulposus have a blood supply. In the presence of an end-plate fracture, the nucleus pulposus is exposed for the first time to the circulation within the vertebral spongiosa. If recognised as non-self, the nuclear material will elicit an immune response.

This phenomenon is analogous to the condition of sympathetic ophthalmia in which, following a penetrating injury to the eye, the vitreous humour is exposed to the body's immune system and becomes antigenic; so much so that the opposite uninjured eye becomes susceptible to auto-immune attack. No studies have yet demonstrated an immune response to nuclear material in the vertebral spongiosa, but the antigenic properties of herniated material in the vertebral canal are well known.[55,143,191,194,195,365] It is a simple deduction that if nuclear material can elicit an inflammatory immune response in the vertebral canal, it should also do so in the vertebral spongiosa. Some circumstantial evidence of this effect is available in that in patients with compression injuries in whom nuclear material actually herniates into the spongiosa it elicits an inflammatory response evident on bone scan.[364]

Regardless of whether the mechanism is auto-immune or simply unrestricted inflammatory repair, the consequences to the nucleus pulposus are the same. The nucleus pulposus undergoes progressive, relentless degradation of its matrix (Fig. 14.5).

Nuclear 'degradation' may appear synonomous with disc 'degeneration', and indeed other authors have implicated the same biochemical processes described above as the explanation for disc degeneration.[375] However, they view this as an idiopathic phenomenon, and do not relate it to end-plate fracture. In the present context, nuclear 'degradation' is not intended to mean 'degeneration'. 'Degeneration' is an emotive term, conjuring images of inevitable decay and destruction, yet many of the pathological changes said to characterise disc degeneration are little more than normal age changes (Ch. 12). In contrast, nuclear degradation is a process, initiated by an end-plate fracture, that progressively de-

stroys the nucleus pulposus. It is an active consequence of trauma; not a passive consequence of age.

When degradation is restricted to the nucleus pulposus, proteolysis and deaggregation of the nuclear matrix result in a progressive loss of water-binding capacity and a deterioration of nuclear function. Less able to bind water, the nucleus is less able to sustain pressures, and greater loads must be borne by the anulus fibrosus. In time, the anulus buckles under this load and the disc loses height, which compromises the functions of all joints in the affected segment (Fig. 14.6). As a result, reactive changes occur in the form of osteophyte formation in the zygapophysial joints and in the anulus fibrosus. This state, characterised by osteophytes and disc narrowing, has been recognised clinically and described as 'isolated disc resorption'[103,545] which becomes symptomatic if nerve roots are compromised by canal stenosis or foraminal stenosis.

In Chapter 12 it was explained that disc narrowing is not a consequence of age; discs retain their height with age.[534] A different explanation is required for disc narrowing, especially if it occurs at only one out of five lumbar segments. The explanation lies in disc narrowing being a consequence of nuclear degradation following end-plate fracture; but disc narrowing and isolated disc resorption is only one possible end-stage of disc degradation. It occurs when the anulus fibrosus remains intact circumferentially but when nuclear degradation and dehydration are severe. In contrast, the water-binding capacity of the nucleus may not be so severely affected by nuclear degradation, whereupon the disc relatively retains its height.

In time, nuclear degradation extends peripherally to erode the anulus fibrosus, typically along radial fissures (Fig. 14.6). This condition of the disc is known as 'internal disc disruption'.[105] The essence of this condition is that the pathological changes are restricted to the centre of the disc. There are no external manifestations of the disease in the form of disc bulge, herniation or loss of disc height. It is an inflammatory condition that involves degradation of the nuclear matrix and progressive erosion of the anulus fibrosus, typically along radial fissures (Fig. 14.6).

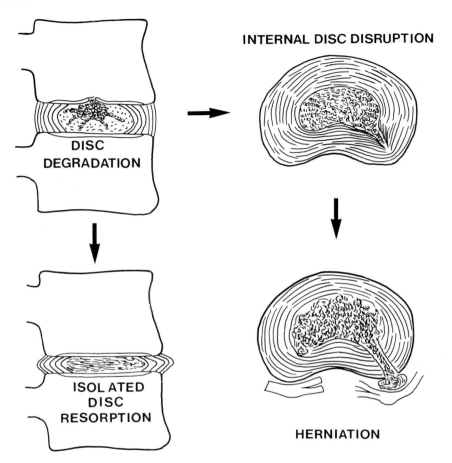

Fig. 14.6 Disc degradation and internal disc disruption. Disc degradation spreads to involve all of the nucleus pulposus. If the anulus fibrosus remains relatively intact, the disc narrows because of the loss in water-binding capacity of the nucleus, resulting in the condition of isolated disc resorption. On the other hand, disc degradation may spread radially into the anulus fibrosus causing a fissure. The external appearance of the disc remains normal; the pathological process remains wholly within the disc, and the condition of the disc is described as internal disc disruption. If the remaining fibres of the anulus fibrosus are breached, nuclear herniation may follow internal disc disruption.

Ultimately, it is possible for internal disc disruption to progress to disc herniation (Fig. 14.6). This occurs if the inflammatory degradation extends along a radial fissure for the entire thickness of the anulus. The conditions for disc herniation are thereby set; a defect has been produced in the anulus fibrosus and the nucleus pulposus has been denatured into a form that is expressable. In such a disc, compression loading during normal flexion may be sufficient to herniate the nucleus.

However, although the clinical presentation of disc prolapse is clear and dramatic, the emphasis laid on this lesion in clinical circles outweighs its relative prevalence. In the laboratory, disc prolapse is difficult to produce, even in partially herniated discs,[8] and epidemiologically disc prolapse accounts for fewer than 5% of presentations of low-back pain.[183,380] Some other lesion must underlie the remaining cases, and one explanation is that internal disc disruption can become painful well before and in the absence of nuclear herniation.

Internal disc disruption can become symptomatic as a result of mechanical or chemical irritation of the nerve endings in the anulus fibrosus. A normal anulus fibrosus consists of some 10 layers of collagen which collectively share the loads normally borne by the anulus fibrosus in the course of activities of daily living. If any layers of collagen are lost in the course of a disease, the normal load borne by the anulus fibrosus must be sustained by the remaining, intact fibres; the relative stress imparted on these remaining fibres during normal activities must therefore increase. If a few of the inner layers of the anulus are eroded by internal disc disruption, the remaining intact fibres may well be able to sustain the increased relative stress. However, with further erosion a critical stage will be reached when the increased stress on the intact fibres exceeds their normal capacity. A stage can therefore be reached in internal disruption when the outer fibres of the anulus fibrosus are insufficient in number to withstand normal, everyday loads without excessively straining. Since these are also the innervated layers of the anulus, pain in the form of 'ligament strain' will result.

The critical feature of this mechanism of mechanical pain from the disc is that the source of pain is not directly affected by any disease process. The internal disc disruption is located centrally, but it is the unaffected, intact, outer fibres of the anulus fibrosus that become symptomatic.

A chemical mechanism for pain can operate if the inflammatory process of internal disc disruption reaches the innervated outer third of the anulus fibrosus. While the process is restricted to the nucleus or inner third of the anulus, inflammatory chemicals have no access to nerve endings, and there is no basis for chemical pain, but when radial fissures extend into the outer third, inflammatory chemicals are brought into the vicinity of the nerve endings, and chemical pain can operate.

Chemical stimulation provides the basis for constant pain unrelated to activities; internal disc disruption thereby effectively constitutes a condition analagous to a painful, sterile abscess. However, inflammatory chemicals also have the capacity to sensitise nerve endings rendering them more susceptible to mechanical stimulation, whereupon a patient with internal disc disruption could suffer not only unremitting pain unrelated

to activity, generated by chemical irritation of nerves in the anulus fibrosus, but also pain aggravated by activity that strains the anulus, representing mechanical pain superimposed on the chemically mediated pain.

On theoretical grounds, the clinical picture of internal disc disruption would be pain at rest, aggravated by any activity that stresses the disc, but without any other physical signs. Notably, there would be no neurological signs because the disease is located centrally within the disc and has no external manifestations. For similar reasons, plain radiography, CT scans and myelography would be normal for the disc does not bulge or deform.

The attraction of this model of disc pathology is that it provides an explanation for a common clinical picture while also unifying many pathological and clinical observations. It provides a reason for a disc to be abnormal — internal disc disruption is the consequence of an end-plate fracture and is therefore an acquired traumatic disorder; it unifies isolated disc resorption and disc herniation as certain end stages of internal disc disruption, and explains that disc herniation cannot be an acute injury but is but one consequence of a pre-existing disorder, internal disruption; but most attractively it provides an explanation for pain in patients presumably with a disc lesion but with no signs of a herniation and in whom conventional investigations of the disc prove paradoxically normal.

For logistic reasons it is difficult to validate this model directly. Ethically one cannot experimentally induce end-plate fractures in volunteers to follow their progression; nor can one aspire to follow the natural history of this proposed disease because end-plate fractures are silent and there is no cue to indicate when serial investigations should start. However, the most satisfying evidence for this model comes from the fact that, notwithstanding arguments as to its cause, internal disc disruption does occur and can be demonstrated in vivo.

The internal features of a disc can be demonstrated if a CT scan is performed shortly after discography. This provides an axial view of the disc which demonstrates the radial extent of any spread of contrast medium injected into the nu-

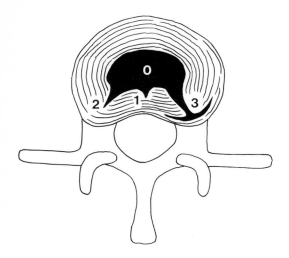

Fig. 14.7 Grades of internal disc disruption (based on Vanharanta et al[544]). Grade '0': the disruption, if any, is confined to the nucleus pulposus. Grade '1': disruption extends into the inner third of the anulus fibrosus. Grade '2': disruption extends as far as the inner two-thirds of the anulus. Grade '3': disruption extends into the outer third of the anulus fibrosus, and may spread circumferentially between the lamina of collagen.

cleus pulposus. Meanwhile, the provocation phase of the discography provides information as to whether the disc is symptomatic or not.

On theoretical grounds one would expect that if contrast medium were restricted to the nucleus pulposus or the inner third of the anulus fibrosus the disc should be asymptomatic. Discs in which internal disruption extended half-way through the anulus fibrosus may or may not be symptomatic, depending on whether nerve endings extended that far into the anulus and whether the integrity of the outer half of the anulus was enough for it to tolerate normal mechanical stresses. However, if radial fissures reached the outer third of the anulus fibrosus, the disc would be expected to become symptomatic, for not only could inflammatory chemicals reach the innervated portion of the anulus fibrosus but also, so little of the anulus would remain intact that it would be subjected to excessive strains in the course of normal activities. These correlations between symptoms and pathological changes are borne out by CT discography.

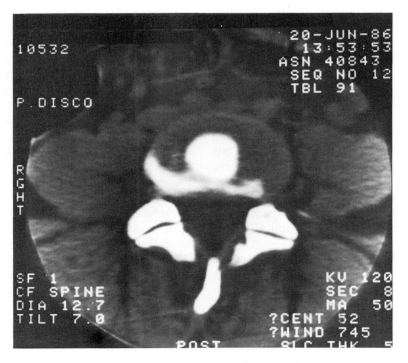

Fig. 14.8 A CT discogram of a disc showing grade '3' internal disc disruption; the contrast medium spreads from the nucleus into the outer third of the anulus fibrosus, and spreads circumferentially around the anulus. The outer perimeter of the disc is intact; there is no herniation or disc bulge. This disc was symptomatic. (Courtesy of Dr C. Aprill.)

In a study of 91 patients, Vanharanta et al[544] classified their CT discograms into four grades; '0' if contrast medium remained centrally in the nucleus; '1' if it extended into the inner third of the anulus fibrosus; '2' if it reached the middle third; and '3' if it extended into the outer third (Fig. 14.7). Grade 0 and grade 1 discs were rarely symptomatic, but the vast majority of grade 3 discs were associated with exact or similar reproduction of the patient's back pain, with grade 2 discs exhibiting an intermediate incidence of symptom reproduction (Fig. 14.8). These correlations are fully consistent with what would be expected on the basis of the innervation of the disc and the effects of internal disc disruption, and they constitute the first time in the history of back pain research where there has been a strong correlation between symptoms and demonstrable morphological changes.

Although the actual mechanism by which internal disc disruption develops may be argued, there can be no question that its features are demonstrable by CT discography and that there is a strong correlation between the demonstrable changes and disc pain. CT discography, therefore, constitutes the mainstay for confirming a diagnosis of internal disc disruption. However, discography is at best unpleasant and not without risks, and CT discography is tedious and expensive. It would therefore be attractive to have an alternative means of establishing the diagnosis.

Magnetic resonance imaging (MRI) has the prospect of providing this alternative, preferable means. A characteristic of internal disc disruption is degradation of the nuclear matrix with loss of water-binding capacity. T2-weighted images on MRI correlate with water density. One can therefore expect that internal disc disruption should be evident on T2 images in the form of decreased signal intensity (darkening) from the nucleus. Preliminary studies suggest a 90% correlation between severe darkening of the disc on T2 images and discogenic pain as determined by provocation discography.[577] Understandably, larger studies would still be required to establish false positive and false negative rates for this correlation, but it appears promising that if MRI technology is further developed it may provide a safe and rapid means of identifying internal disc disruption, and perhaps even tracing its development and natural history.

Appendix: Identification of the lumbar vertebrae

A skill practised by some anatomists is the ability to identify individual bones, and students of Anatomy are sometimes asked in examinations to identify individual bones. While the identification of large bones like the femur and humerus may be easy, to identify the individual lumbar vertebrae seems a daunting challenge. Specifically, the vertebrae seem so alike.

The ability to identify bones has little intrinsic value, except in forensic osteology. Therefore, it may seem pointless to expect students to learn how to identify individual lumbar vertebrae. However, the practice (and examination) of this skill has a certain implicit value. It determines if the student understands the functions of the bone in question, and how it is designed to subserve these functions. The exercise of identifying bones is made pointless only if some routine is mindlessly memorised simply to pass a possible examination question. However, if the bone is used to prompt a revision of its functions, then the exercise can be done with insight and purpose, and consequently becomes rewarding and easier. Moreover, if superficially similar bones have different functions or biomechanical needs, then subtle differences in structure can be sought and discovered, whereby individual bones can be recognised.

Having studied the structure of the lumbar vertebrae (Ch. 1), the nature of their joints and ligaments (Ch. 2–4), and the form of the intact lumbar spine (Ch. 5), it is possible to review the detailed structure of the lumbar vertebrae and highlight the differences that correlate with the different functions of individual vertebrae. Some of the differences are present in only one vertebra. Others are part of a series of differences seen throughout the lumbar spine. Accordingly both the structure of individual vertebrae and the structure of the entire lumbar spine should be considered.

The most individual lumbar vertebra is the fifth. Its characteristic feature is the thickness of its transverse processes and their attachment along the whole length of the pedicles as far as the vertebral body. Examining this feature serves to remind the student of the attachment of the powerful ilio-lumbar ligaments to the L5 transverse processes, and their role in restraining the L5 vertebra. In turn, this is a reminder of the problem that L5 faces in staying in place on top of the sloping sacrum.

There are no absolute features that enable the other four lumbar vertebrae to be distinguished, but there are relative differences that reflect trends evident along the lumbar spine. First, as a general rule, the lengths of the upper four transverse processes vary in a reasonably constant pattern. From above downwards, they increase in length and then decrease such that the L3 transverse process is usually the longest, and the transverse processes of L1 and L4 are usually the shortest. The reason for this difference is still obscure, but the long length of the L3 transverse processes seems to correlate with the central location of the L3 vertebra in the lumbar lordosis, and its long transverse process probably provide a necessary extra, mechanical advantage for the muscles that act on them.

The other serial change in the lumbar spine is the orientation of the zygapophysial joints. Sagittally orientated joints are a feature of upper lumbar levels, while joints orientated closer to 45° are more characteristic of lower levels. Examining this feature serves as a reminder of the compound role of the zygapophysial joints in resisting forward displacement and rotation, and the need at lower lumbar levels for stabilisation against forward displacement.

From above downwards, the vertebral bodies tend to be slightly larger, and their transverse dimension tends to be relatively longer in proportion to their antero-posterior dimension. This correlates with the increasing load that lower vertebrae have to bear.

A structural idiosyncrasy of the lumbar vertebrae is that if four-sided figures are constructed to include in their angles the four articular processes of each vertebra, different shapes are revealed.[174] For the upper two lumbar vertebrae, a trapezium is constructed. The L3 vertebra forms an upright rectangle. The L4 vertebra forms a square, and the L5 vertebra forms a parallelogram with its longer sides aligned horizontally (Fig. A.1).

By examining these various features a student should be able to identify individual lumbar vertebrae to within, at least, one segment. The L5 vertebra is readily recognised. L4 will tend to have inferior articular processes orientated towards 45°, and will have short transverse processes and a relatively wider body. Its four articular processes will fall inside a square. L3 should have inferior articular processes with intermediate orientations, but most often close to 45°. Its transverse processes will be long, and its articular processes will fall inside a rectangle. The L1 and L2 vertebrae remain with more sagittally orientated articular facets and articular processes that fall within trapezia. The only feature that may distinguish L1 from L2 is a better development of the mamillary and accessory processes on L1 and its shorter transverse processes. Apart from this, however, the upper two lumbar vertebrae maybe indistinguishable.

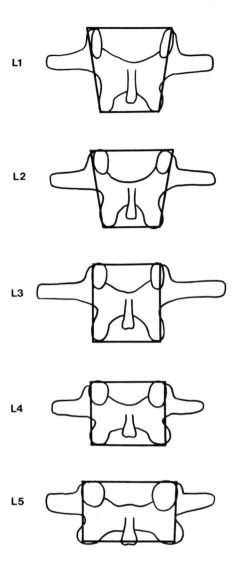

Fig. A.1 Identification of individual lumbar vertebrae. By constructing four sided figures around the tips of the articular processes of the lumbar vertebrae, distinguishing features are revealed. The figures formed around the upper two lumbar vertebrae are trapezia; that around L3 is an upright rectangle; that around L4 is a square; and that around L5 is a horizontal rectangle.

References

1. Abrahams M 1967 Mechanical behaviour of tendon in vitro. A preliminary report. Med Biol Engin 5: 433–443
2. Abrahams V C 1977 The physiology of neck muscles; their role in head movement and maintenance of posture. Can J Physiol Pharmacol 55: 332–338
3. Abrahams V C 1981 Sensory and motor specialization in some muscles of the neck. TINS 4: 24–27
4. Adams M 1989 Letter to the editor. Spine 14: 1272
5. Adams M A, Dolan P, Hutton W C 1988 The lumbar spine in backward bending. Spine 13: 1019–1026
6. Adams M A, Hutton W C 1980 The effect of posture on the role of the apophyseal joints in resisting intervertebral compression force. J Bone Joint Surg (Br) 62B: 358–362
7. Adams M A, Hutton W C 1981 The relevance of torsion to the mechanical derangement of the lumbar spine. Spine 6: 241–248
8. Adams M A, Hutton W C 1985 Gradual disc prolapse. Spine 10: 524–531
9. Adams M A, Hutton W C 1983 The mechanical function of the lumbar apophyseal joints. Spine 8: 327–330
10. Adams M A, Hutton W C 1982 Prolapsed intervertebral disc. A hyperflexion injury. Spine 7: 184–191
11. Adams M A, Hutton W C, Stott J R R 1980 The resistance to flexion of the lumbar intervertebral joint. Spine 5: 245–253
12. Adams P, Muir H 1976 Qualitative changes with age of human lumbar disks. Ann Rheum Dis 35: 289–296
13. Adams P, Eyre D R, Muir H 1977 Biochemical aspects of development and ageing of human lumbar intervertebral discs. Rheumatol Rehab 16: 22–29
14. Allbrook D 1957 Movements of the lumbar spinal column. J Bone Joint Surg (Br) 39B: 339–345
15. Allen C E L 1948 Muscle action potentials used in the study of dynamic anatomy. Br J Phys Med 11: 66–73
16. Anderson J 1980 Pathogenesis of back pain. In: Grahame R, Anderson J A D (eds) Low Back Pain, Volume 2. Eden Press, Westmount, ch 4, p 23–32.
17. Andersson G B J 1983 Loads on the lumbar spine: in vivo measurements and biomechanical analyses. In: Winter D A, Norman R W, Wells R P, Hayes K C, Patla A E (eds) Biomechanics IX-B, International Series on Biomechanics. Human Kinetics, Champaign, p 32–37
18. Andersson B J G, Ortengren R 1974 Myoelectric activity during sitting. Scand J Rehab Med Suppl 3: 73–90
19. Andersson B J G, Ortengren R 1974 Lumbar disc pressure and myoelectric back muscle activity during sitting. II. Studies of an office chair. Scand J Rehab Med 6: 115–121
20. Andersson B J G, Jonsson B, Ortengren R 1974 Myoelectric activity in individual lumbar erector spinae muscles in sitting: a study with surface and wire electrodes. Scand J Rehab Med Suppl 3: 91–108
21. Andersson G B J, Ortengren R, Herberts P 1977 Quantitative electromyographic studies of back muscle activity related to posture and loading. Orthop Clin North Am 8: 85–96
22. Andersson G B J, Ortengren R, Nachemson A 1976 Quantitative studies of back loads in lifting. Spine 1: 178–184
23. Andersson G B J, Ortengren R, Nachemson A 1977 Intradiscal pressure, intra-abdominal pressure and myoelectric back muscle activity related to posture and loading. Clin Orthop 129: 156–164
24. Andersson G B J, Ortengren R, Nachemson A 1978 Quantitative studies of the back in different working postures. Scand J Rehab Med Suppl 6: 173–181
25. Andersson B J G, Ortengren R, Nachemson A, Elfstrom G 1974 Lumbar disc pressure and myoelectric activity during sitting. I. Studies on an experimental chair. Scand J Rehab Med 6: 104–114
26. Andersson B J G, Ortengren R, Nachemson A, Elfstrom G 1974 Lumbar disc pressure and myoelectric back muscle activity during sitting. IV. Studies on a car driver's seat. Scand J Rehab Med 6: 128–133
27. Andersson B J G, Ortengren R, Nachemson A L, Elfstrom G, Broman H 1975 The sitting posture: an electromyographic and discometric study. Orthop Clin North Am 6: 105–120
28. Arcamano J P, Karas S 1982 Congenital absence of the lumbosacral articular process. Skeletal Radiol 8: 133–134
29. Armstrong J R 1965 Lumbar Disc Lesions, 3rd edn. Livingstone, Edinburgh, p 13
30. Arnoldi C C, Brodsky A E, Cauchoix J, Crock H V, Dommisse G F, Edgar M A, Gargano F P, Jacobson R E, Kirkaldy-Willis W H, Kurihara A, Langenskiold

A, Macnab I, MacIvor G W D, Newman P H, Paine K W E, Russin L A, Sheldon J, Tile M, Urist M R, Wilson W E, Wiltse L L 1976 Lumbar spinal stenosis. Clin Orthop 115: 4–5

31. Asmussen E, Klausen K 1962 Form and function of the erect human spine. Clin Orthop 25: 55–63
32. Aspden R M 1987 Intra-abdominal pressure and its role in spinal mechanics. Clin Biomech 2: 168–174
33. Aspden R M 1989 The spine as an arch. A new mathematical model. Spine 14: 266–274
34. Atkinson P J 1967 Variations in trabecular structure of vertebrae with age. Calcif Tissue Res 1: 24–32
35. Auteroche P 1983 Innervation of the zygapophseal joints of the lumbar spine. Anat Clin 5: 17–28
36. Baastrup C I 1933 Proc. Spin. vert. Lumb. und einige zwischen diesen leigende Gelenkbildungen mit pathologischen Prozessen in dieser Region. Fortschritee auf den Gebiete der Rontgenstrahlen 48: 430–435
37. Badgley C E 1941 The articular facets in relation to low-back pain and sciatic radiation. J Bone Joint Surg 23: 481–496
38. Bagnall K M, Harris P F, Jones P R M 1977 A radiographic study of the human fetal spine 2. The sequence of development of ossification centres in the vertebral column. J Anat 124: 791–802
39. Bagnall K M, Harris P F, Jones P R M 1984 A radiographic study of variations of the human fetal spine. Anat Rec 208: 265–270
40. Bailey A J, Herbert C M, Jayson M I V 1976 Collagen of the intervertebral disc. In: Jayson M I V (ed) The Lumbar Spine and Backache. Grune & Stratton, New York, ch 12, p 327–340
41. Bailey W 1937 Anomalies and fractures of the vertebral articular processes. JAMA 108: 266–270
42. Bartelink D L 1957 The role of abdominal pressure in relieving the pressure on the lumbar intervertebral discs. J Bone Joint Surg (Br) 39B: 718–725
43. Bastide G, Zadeh J, Lefebvre D 1989 Are the 'little muscles' what we think they are? Surg Radiol Anat 11: 255–256
44. Bauwens P, Coyer A B 1955 The multifidus triangle syndrome as a cause of recurrent low-back pain. Br Med J 2: 1306–1307
45. Beard H K, Stevens R L 1980 Biochemical changes in the intervertebral disc. In: Jayson M I V (ed) The Lumbar Spine and Backache, 2nd edn. Pitman, London, ch 14, p 407–436
46. Bearn J G 1961 The significance of the activity of the abdominal muscles in weight lifting. Acta Anat 45: 83–89
47. Beers G J, Carter A P, McNary W F 1984 Vertical foramina in the lumbosacral region: CT appearance. Am J Roentgenol 143: 1027–1029
48. Beks J W F 1989 Kissing spines: fact or fancy? Acta Neurochir 100: 134–135
49. Benini A 1979 Das klein Gelenk der lenden Wirbelsaule. Fortschr Med 97: 2103–2106
50. Benson D R, Schultz A B, Dewald R L 1976 Roentgenographic evaluation of vertebral rotation. J Bone Joint Surg 58A: 1125–1129
51. Bernick S, Cailliet R 1982 Vertebral end-plate changes with aging of human vertebrae. Spine 7: 97–102
52. Bick E M, Copel J W 1950 Longitudinal growth of the human vertebrae. J Bone Joint Surg (Am) 32A: 803–814
53. Blakely P R, Happey F, Naylor A, Turner R L 1962 Protein in the nucleus pulposus of the intervertebral disc. Nature 195: 73
54. Boas R A 1980 Post-surgical low back pain. In Peck C, Wallace M (eds) Problems in Pain. Pergamon, Sydney, p 188–191
55. Bobechko W T, Hirsch C 1965 Autoimmune response to nucleus pulposus in the rabbit. J Bone Joint Surg (Br) 47B: 574–580
56. Bogduk N 1980 A reappraisal of the anatomy of the human lumbar erector spinae. J Anat 131: 525–540
57. Bogduk N 1980 Lumbar dorsal ramus syndrome. Med J Aust 2: 537–541
58. Bogduk N 1981 The lumbar mamillo-accessory ligament. Its anatomical and neurosurgical significance. Spine 6: 162–167
59. Bogduk N 1983 The innervation of the lumbar spine. Spine 8: 286–293
60. Bogduk N 1984 The rationale for patterns of neck and back pain. Patient Management 13: 17–28
61. Bogduk N 1988 Back pain: zygapophysial blocks and epidural steroids. In: Cousins M J, Bridenbaugh P O (eds) Neural Blockade in Clinical Anesthesia and Pain Management, 2nd edn. Lippincott, Philadelphia, ch 27.3, p 935–954
62. Bogduk N, Engel R 1984 The menisci of the lumbar zygapophyseal joints. A review of their anatomy and clinical significance. Spine 9: 454–460
63. Bogduk N, Jull G 1985 The theoretical pathology of acute locked back: a basis for manipulative therapy. Man Med 1: 78–82
64. Bogduk N, Macintosh J 1984 The applied anatomy of the thoracolumbar fascia. Spine 9: 164–170
65. Bogduk N, Tynan W, Wilson A S 1981 The nerve supply to the human lumbar intervertebral discs. J Anat 132: 39–56
66. Bogduk N, Wilson A S, Tynan W 1982 The human lumbar dorsal rami. J Anat 134: 383–397
67. Bose K, Balasubramaniam P 1984 Nerve root canals of the lumbar spine. Spine 9: 16–18
68. Bouchard J M, Copty M, Langelier R 1978 Preoperative diagnosis of conjoined roots anomaly with herniated lumbar disks. Surg Neurol 10: 229–231
69. Bradley K C 1951 Observations on the surgical anatomy of the thoracolumbar sympathetic system. Aust NZ J Surg 20: 171–177
70. Bradley K C 1974 The anatomy of backache. Aust NZ J Surg 44: 227–232
71. Brailsford J F 1929 Deformities of the lumbosacral region of the spine. Br J Surg 16: 562–627
72. Brandner M F 1970 Normal values of the vertebral body and intervertebral disc index during growth. Am J Roentgenol 110: 618–627
73. Brickley-Parsons D, Glimcher M J 1984 Is the chemistry of collagen in intervertebral discs an expression of Wolff's law? A study of the human lumbar spine. Spine 9: 148–163
74. Brinckmann P 1986 Injury of the annulus fibrosus and disc protrusions: an in vitro investigation on human lumbar discs. Spine 11: 149–153
75. Broberg K B 1983 On the mechanical behaviour of intervertebral discs. Spine 8: 151–165

76. Brown T, Hansen R J, Yorra A J 1957 Some mechanical tests on the lumbosacral spine with particular reference to the intervertebral discs. J Bone Joint Surg (Am) 39A: 1135–1164

77. Buckwalter J A, Cooper R R, Maynard J A 1976 Elastic fibers in human intervertebral disks. J Bone Joint Surg (Am) 58A: 73–76

78. Buckwalter J A, Pedrini-Mille, Pedrini V, Tudisco C 1985 Proteoglycans of human infant intervertebral discs. J Bone Joint Surg (Am) 67A: 284–294

79. Bushell G R, Ghosh P, Taylor T F K, Akeson W H 1977 Proteoglycan chemistry of the intervertebral disks. Clin Orthop 129: 115–123

80. Caffey J 1972 Pediatric X-ray Diagnosis, 6th edn. Year Book Medical Publishers, Chicago.

81. Calvo L J 1957 Observations on the growth of the female adolescent spine and its relation to scoliosis. Clin Orthop 10: 40–46

82. Cannon B W, Hunter S E, Picaza J A 1962 Nerve root anomalies in lumbar disc surgery. J Neurosurg 19: 208–214

83. Carlsoo S 1961 The static muscle load in different work positions: an electromyographic study. Ergonomics 4: 193–211

84. Carlsoo S 1964 Influence of frontal and dorsal loads on muscle activity and on the weight distribution in the feet. Acta Orthop Scand 34: 299–309

85. Carpenter E B 1961 Normal and abnormal growth of the spine. Clin Orthop 21: 49–55

86. Carr D, Gilbertson L, Frymoyer J, Krag M, Pope M 1985 Lumbar paraspinal compartment syndrome: a case report with physiologic and anatomic studies. Spine 10: 816–820

87. Carrera G F 1979 Lumbar facet arthrography and injection in low back pain. Wis Med J 78: 35–37

88. Carrera G F 1980 Lumbar facet joint injection in low back pain and sciatica. Description of technique. Radiology 137: 661–664

89. Carrera G F 1980 Lumbar facet joint injection in low back pain and sciatica. Preliminary results. Radiology 137: 665–667

90. Carrera G F, Williams A L 1984 Current concepts in evaluation of the lumbar facet joints. CRC Crit Rev Diagn Imag 21: 85–104

91. Cave A J E 1937 The innervation and morphology of the cervical intertransverse muscles. J Anat 71: 497–515

92. Chow D H K, Luk K D K, Leong J C Y, Woo C W 1989 Torsional stability of the lumbosacral junction: significance of the iliolumbar ligament. Spine 14: 611–615

93. Clayson S J, Newman I M, Debevec D F, Anger R W, Showlund H V, Kottke F J 1962 Evaluation of mobility of hip and lumbar vertebrae of normal young women. Arch Phys Med Rehab 43: 1–8

94. Cloward R B 1968 Congenital spinal extradural cysts. Ann Surg 168: 851–864

95. Cohen J, Currarino G, Neuhauser E B D 1956 A significant variant in the ossification centers of the vertebral bodies. Am J Roentgenol 76: 469–475

96. Collis J S, Gardner W J 1962 Lumbar discography — an analysis of 1,000 cases. J Neurosurg 19: 452–461

97. Comper W D, Laurent T C 1978 Physiological function of connective tissue polysaccharides. Physiol Rev 58: 255–315

98. Comper W D, Preston B N 1974 Model connective tissue systems. A study of the polyion-mobile ion and of excluded volume interactions of proteoglycans. Biochem J 143: 1–9

99. Cooper S, Danial P M 1963 Muscles spindles in man, their morphology in the lumbricals and the deep muscles of the neck. Brain 86: 563–594

100. Cossette J W, Farfan H F, Robertson G H, Wells R V 1971 The instantaneous center of rotation of the third lumbar intervertebral joint. J Biomech 4: 149–153

101. Coventry M B 1969 Anatomy of the intervertebral disk. Clin Orthop 67: 9–15

102. Coventry M B, Ghormley R K, Kernohan J W 1945 The intervertebral disc: its microscopic anatomy and pathology. Part I. Anatomy, development and physiology. J Bone Joint Surg 27: 105–112

103. Crock H V 1970 A reappraisal of intervertebral disc lesions. Med J Aust 1: 983–989 and supplementary pages i–ii

104. Crock H V 1981 Normal and pathological anatomy of the lumbar spinal nerve root canals. J Bone Joint Surg (Br) 63B: 487–490

105. Crock H V 1986 Internal disc disruption: a challenge to disc prolapse 50 years on. Spine 11: 650–653

106. Crock H V, Goldwasser M 1984 Anatomic studies of the circulation in the region of the vertebral end-plate in adult greyhound dogs. Spine 9: 702–706

107. Crock H V, Crock M C 1988 A technique for decompression of the lumbar spinal canal. Neuro-orthopaedics 5: 96–99

108. Crock H V, Yoshizawa H 1976 The blood supply of the lumbar vertebral column. Clin Orthop 115: 6–21

109. Crock H V, Yoshizawa H, Kame S 1973 Observations on the venous drainage of the human vertebral body. J Bone Joint Surg (Br) 55B: 528–533

110. Cuatico W, Parker J C, Pappert E, Pilsl S 1988 An anatomical and clinical investigation of spinal meningeal nerves. Acta Neurochir 90: 139–143

111. Cuatico W, Parker J C 1989 Further observations on spinal meningeal nerves and their role in pain production. Acta Neurochir 101: 126–128

112. Cyron B M, Hutton W C 1979 Variations in the amount and distribution of cortical bone across the partes interarticulares of L5. A predisposing factor in spondylolysis? Spine 4: 163–167

113. Cyron B M, Hutton W C 1980 Articular tropism and stability of the lumbar spine. Spine 5: 168–172

114. Cyron B M, Hutton W C 1981 The tensile strength of the capsular ligaments of the apophyseal joints. J Anat 132: 145–150

115. Danforth M S, Wilson P D 1925 The anatomy of the lumbosacral region in relation to sciatic pain. J Bone Joint Surg 7: 109–160

116. d'Avella D, Mingrino S 1979 Microsurgical anatomy of lumbosacral spinal roots. J Neurosurg 51: 819–823

117. Davis P R 1959 Posture of the trunk during the lifting of weights. Br Med J 1: 87–89

118. Davis P R 1981 The use of intra-abdominal pressure in evaluating stresses on the lumbar spine. Spine 6: 90–92

119. Davis P R, Stubbs D A 1977 Safe levels of manual forces for young males (1). Appl Ergon 8: 141–150

120. Davis P R, Troup J D G 1964 Pressures in the trunk cavities when pulling, pushing and lifting. Ergonomics 7: 465–474

121. De Boeck M, De Smedy E, Potvliege R 1982 Computed tomography in the evaluation of a congenital absent lumbar pedicle. Skeletal Radiol 8: 197–199

122. Delmas A, Ndjaga-Mba M, Vannareth T 1970 Le cartilage articulaire de L4-L5 et L5-S1. Comptes Rendus de l'Association des Anatomistes 147: 230–234

123. Destouet J M, Gilula L A, Murphy W A, Monsees B 1982 Lumbar facet joint injection: indication, technique, clinical correlation and preliminary results. Radiology 145: 321–325

124. De Vries H A 1965 Muscle tonus in postural muscles. Am J Phys Med 44: 275–291

125. Diamant J, Keller A, Baer E, Lit M, Arridge R G C 1972 Collagen ultrastructure and its relation to mechanical properties as a function of ageing. Proc Roy Soc, Series B 180: 293–315

126. Dickson I R, Happey F, Pearson C H, Naylor A, Turner R L 1967 Variations in the protein components of human intervertebral disk with age. Nature 215: 52–53

127. Dommisse G F 1975 The Arteries and Veins of the Human Spinal Cord from Birth. Churchill-Livingstone, Edinburgh

128. Dommisse G F 1975 Morphological aspects of the lumbar spine and lumbosacral regions. Orthop Clin North Am 6: 163–175

129. Dommisse G F, Grobler L 1976 Arteries and veins of the lumbar nerve roots and cauda equina. Clin Orthop 115: 22–29

130. Donisch E W, Basmajian J V 1972 Electromyography of deep back muscles in man. Am J Anat 133: 25–36

131. Donisch E W Trapp W 1971 The cartilage endplate of the human vertebral column (some considerations of postnatal development). Anat Rec 169: 705–716

132. Dorr W M 1958 Uber die Anatomie der Wirbelgelenke. Arch Orthop Unfall-Chir 50: 222–234

133. Dorr W M 1962 Nochmals zu den Menisci in den Wirbelbogengelenken. Z Orthop 96: 457–461

134. Dory M A 1981 Arthrography of the lumbar facet joints. Radiology 140: 23–27

135. Dunham W F 1949 Ankylosing spondylitis: measurement of hip and spinal movements Br J Phys Med 12: 126–129

136. Dunlop R B, Adams M A, Hutton W C 1984 Disc space narrowing and the lumbar facet joints. J Bone Joint Surg (Br) 66B: 706–710

137. Edgar M A, Nundy S 1964 Innervation of the spinal dura mater. J Neurol Neurosurg Psychiatry 29: 530–534

138. Ehni G 1962 Significance of the small lumbar spinal canal: cauda equina compression syndromes due to spondylosis. J Neurosurg 31: 490–494
Ehrenhaft J C 1943 Development of the vertebral column as related to certain congenital and pathological changes. Surg Gynec Obstet 76: 282–292

140. Eisenstein S 1980 The trefoil configuration of the lumbar vertebral canal. J Bone Joint Surg (Br) 62B: 73–77

141. El-Bohy A A, Yang K H, King A I 1989 Experimental verification of facet load transmission by direct measurement of facet lamina contact pressure. J Biomech 22: 931–941

142. El Mahdi M A, Latif F Y A, Janko M 1981 The spinal nerve root innervation, and a new concept of the clinicopathological interrelations in back pain and sciatica. Neurochirurgia 24: 137–141

143. Elves M W, Bucknill T, Sullivan M F 1975 In vitro inhibition of leucocyte migration in patients with intervertebral disc lesions. Orthop Clin North Am 6: 59–65

144. Elward J F 1939 Motion in the vertebral column. Am J Roentgenol 42: 91–99

145. Emminger E 1972 Les articulations interapophysaires et leurs structures meniscoides vues sous l'angle de la pathologie. Ann Med Phys 15: 219–238

146. Engel R, Bogduk N 1982 The menisci of the lumbar zygapophyseal joints. J Anat 135: 795–809

147. Epstein B S 1976 The Spine. A Radiological Text and Atlas, 4th edn. Lea & Febiger, Philadelphia

148. Epstein J A, Epstein B S, Levine L 1962 Nerve root compression associated with narrowing of the lumbar spinal canal. J Neurol Neurosurg Psychiatry 25: 165–176

149. Epstein J A, Epstein B S, Levine L S, Carras R, Rosenthall A D, Sumner P 1973 Lumbar nerve root compression at the intervertebral foramina caused by arthritis of the posterior facets. J Neurosurg 39: 362–369

150. Ericksen M F 1974 Ageing changes in the shape of the human lumbar vertebrae. Am J Phys Anthropol 41: 477

151. Ericksen M F 1975 Some aspects of ageing in the lumbar spine. Am J Phys Anthropol 45: 575–580

152. Espersen J O, Kosteljanetz M, Halabut H, Miletic T 1984 Predictive value of radiculography in patients with lumbago-sciatica. A prospective study (Part II). Acta Neurochir 73: 213–221

153. Ethelberg S, Rishede J 1952 Malformation of lumbar spinal nerve roots and sheaths in the causation of low backache and sciatica. J Bone Joint Surg (Br) 34B: 442–446

154. Evans F G, Lissner H R 1959 Biomechanical studies on the the lumbar spine and pelvis. J Bone Joint Surg (Am) 41A: 278–290

155. Eyre D 1988 Collagens of the disc. In: Ghosh P (ed) The biology of the Intervertebral Disc, Volume I. CRC Press, Boca Raton, ch 7, p 171–188

156. Eyre D, Muir H 1976 Type I and Type II collagen in intervertebral disk. Interchanging radial distribution in annulus fibrosus. Biochem J 157: 267–270

157. Eyre D, Muir H 1977 Quantitative analysis of types I and II collagen in human intervertebral discs at various ages. Biochimica et Biophysica Acta 492: 29–42

158. Eyring E J 1969 The biochemistry and physiology of the intervertebral disk. Clin Orthop 67: 16–28

159. Fairbank J C T, O'Brien J P 1980 The abdominal cavity and thoracolumbar fascia as stabilisers of the lumbar spine in patients with low back pain. Volume 2, Engineering Aspects of the Spine. Mechanical Engineering Publications, London, p 83–88

160. Fairbank J C T, Park W M, McCall I W, O'Brien J

P 1981 Apophyseal injections of local anaesthetic as a diagnostic aid in primary low-back pain syndromes. Spine 6: 598–605

161. Fairbank J C T, O'Brien J P 1983 The iliac crest syndrome: a treatable cause of low-back pain. Spine 8: 220–224

162. Farfan H F 1973 Mechanical Disorders of the Low Back. Lea & Febiger, Philadelphia

163. Farfan H F 1975 Muscular mechanism of the lumbar spine and the position of power and efficiency. Orthop Clin North Am 6: 135–144

164. Farfan H F 1977 A reorientation in the surgical approach to degenerative lumbar intervertebral joint disease. Orthop Clin North Am 8: 9–21

165. Farfan H F 1978 The biomechanical advantage of lordosis and hip extension for upright activity. Man as compared with other anthropoids. Spine 3: 336–342

166. Farfan H F, Gracovetsky S 1983 The abdominal mechanism. Paper presented at the International Society for the Study of the Lumbar Spine Meeting, Paris, 1981

167. Farfan H F, Gracovetsky S 1984 The nature of instability. Spine 9: 714–719

168. Farfan H F, Kirkaldy-Willis W H 1981 The present status of spinal fusion in the treatment of lumbar intervertebral joint disorders. Clin Orthop 158: 198–214

169. Farfan H F, Sullivan J D 1967 The relation of facet orientation to intervertebral disc failure. Can J Surg 10: 179–185

170. Farfan H F, Cossette J W, Robertson G H, Wells R V, Kraus H 1970 The effects of torsion on the lumbar intervertebral joints: the role of torsion in the production of disc degeneration. J Bone Joint Surg (Am) 52A: 468–497

171. Farfan H F, Gracovetsky S, Helleur C 1983 The role of mathematical models in the assessment of task in the workplace. In: Winter D A, Norman R W, Wells R P, Hayes K C, Patla A E (eds) Biomechanics IX-B, International Series on Biomechanics. Human Kinetics, Champaign, p 38–43

172. Farfan H F, Huberdeau R M, Dubow H I 1972 Lumbar intervertebral disc degeneration. The influence of geometrical features on the pattern of disc degeneration — a post mortem study. J Bone Joint Surg (Am) 54A: 492–510

173. Farmer H L 1936 Accessory articular processes in the lumbar spine. Am J Roentgenol 36: 763–767

174. Fawcett E 1932 A note on the identification of the lumbar vertebrae of man. J Anat 66: 384–386

175. Feinstein B, Langton J N K, Jameson R M, Schiller F 1954 Experiments on pain referred from deep structures. J Bone Joint Surg (Am) 36A: 981–997

176. Fernand R, Fox D E 1985 Evaluation of lumbar lordosis. A prospective and retrospective study. Spine 10: 799–803

177. Finch P M, Khangure M S 1990 Analgesic discography and magnetic resonance imaging (MRI). Pain Suppl 5: S285

178. Finch P 1990 Analgesic discography in the diagnosis of spinal pain. Paper presented at "Spinal Pain": precision diagnosis and treatment, Official Sattelite Meeting of the VIth World Congress on Pain, Perth, April 8–10. Meeting Abstracts p 8

179. Fisher C M 1984 Pain states: a neurological commentary. Clin Neurosurg 31: 32–53

180. Floyd W F, Silver P H S 1951 Function of erectores spinae in flexion of the trunk. Lancet 1: 133–134

181. Floyd W F, Silver P H S 1955 The function of the erectores spinae muscles in certain movements and postures in man. J Physiol 129: 184–203

182. Francois R J 1975 Ligament insertions into the human lumbar vertebral body. Acta Anat 91: 467–480

183. Friberg S 1954 Lumbar disc degeneration in the problem of lumbago sciatica. Bull Hosp Joint Dis 15: 1–20

184. Friis M L, Gulliksen G C, Rasmussen P, Husby J 1977 Pain and spinal root compression. Acta Neurochirurgica 39: 241–249

185. Froning E C, Frohman B 1968 Motion of the lumbosacral spine after laminectomy and spine fusion. J Bone Joint Surg (Am) 50A: 897–918

186. Frymoyer J W, Frymoyer W W, Pope M H 1979 The mechanical and kinematic analysis of the lumbar spine in normal living human subjects in vivo. J Biomech 12: 165–172

187. Fulton W S, Kalbfleisch W K 1934 Accessory articular processes of the lumbar vertebrae. Ach Surg 29: 42–48

188. Galante J O 1967 Tensile properties of the human lumbar annulus fibrosus. Acta Orthop Scand Suppl 100: 1–91

189. Garrett W E, Saffrean M R, Seaber A V, Glisson R R, Ribbeck B M 1987 Biomechanical comparison of stimulated and non-stimulated skeletal muscle pulled to failure. Am J Sports Med 15: 448–454

190. Garrett W E, Nikolaou P K, Ribbeck B M, Glisson R R, Seaber A V 1988 The effect of muscle architecture on the biomechanical failure properties of skeletal muscle under passive tension. Am J of Sports Med 16: 7–12

191. Gertzbein S D 1977 Degenerative disk disease of the lumbar spine: immunological implications. Clin Orthop 129: 68–71

192. Gertzbein S D, Seligman J, Holtby R, Chan K W, Ogston N, Kapasouri A, Tile M 1986 Centrode characteristics of the lumbar spine as a function of segmental instability. Clin Orthop 208: 48–51

193. Gertzbein S D, Seligman J, Holtby R, Chan K H, Kapasouri A, Tile M, Cruickshank B 1985 Centrode patterns and segmental instability in degenerative disc disease. Spine 10: 257–261

194. Gertzbein S D, Tait J H, Devlin S R 1977 The stimulation of lymphocytes by nucleus puplosus in patients with degenerative disk disease of the lumbar spine. Clin Orthop 123: 149–154

195. Gertzbein S D, Tile M, Gross A, Falk R 1975 Autoimmunity in degenerative disc disease of the lumbar spine. Orthop Clin North Am 6: 67–73

196. Ghormley R K 1933 Low back pain with special reference to the articular facets with presentation of an operative procedure. JAMA 10: 1773–1177

197. Ghosh P, Bushell G K, Taylor T F K, Akeson W H 1977 Collagen, elastin, and non-collagenous protein of the intervertebral disk. Clin Orthop 129: 123–132

198. Gianturco C 1944 A roentgen analysis of the motion of the lower lumbar vertebrae. Am J Roentgenol 52: 261–267

199. Gilad I, Nissan M 1985 Sagittal evaluation of

elemental geometrical dimensions of human vertebrae. J Anat 143: 115–120

200. Giles L G F 1988 Human lumbar zygapophyseal joint inferior recess synovial folds: a light microscope examination. Anat Rec 220: 117–124

201. Giles L G F, Harvey A R 1987 Immunohistochemical demonstration of nociceptors in the capsule and synovial folds of human zygapophysial joints. Br J Rheumatol 26: 362–364

202. Giles L G F, Taylor J R 1982 Inter-articular synovial protrusions. Bull Hosp Joint Dis 42: 248–255

203. Giles L G F, Taylor J R 1987 Innervation of lumbar zygapophyseal joint synovial folds. Acta Orthop Scand 58: 43–46

204. Giles L G F, Taylor J R, Cockson A 1986 Human zygapophyseal joint synovial folds. Acta Anat 126: 110–114

205. Glasauer F E 1966 Lumbar extradural cysts. J Neurosurg 25: 567–570

206. Golding J S R 1952 Electromyography of the erector spinae in low back pain. Postgrad Med J 28: 401–406

207. Golub B S, Silverman B 1969 Transforaminal ligaments of the lumbar spine. J Bone Joint Surg (Am) 51A: 947–956

208. Gooding C A, Neuhauser E B D 1965 Growth and development of the vertebral body in the presence and absence of normal stress. Am J Roentgenol 93: 388–394

209. Gower W E, Pedrini V 1969 Age related variation in protein polysaccharides from human nucleus pulposus, annulus fibrosus and costal cartilage. J Bone Joint Surg (Am) 51A: 1154–1162

210. Gracovetsky S, Farfan H F, Helleur C 1985 The abdominal mechanism. Spine 10: 317–324

211. Gracovetsky S, Farfan H F, Lamy C 1977 A mathematical model of the lumbar spine using an optimal system to control muscles and ligaments. Orthop Clin North Am 8: 135–153

212. Gracovetsky S, Farfan H F, Lamy C 1981 The mechanism of the lumbar spine. Spine 6: 249–262

213. Granhed H, Johnson R, Hansson T 1987 The loads on the lumbar spine during extreme weight lifting. Spine 12: 146–149

214. Gregersen G, Lucas D B 1967 An in vivo study of the axial rotation of the human thoracolumbar spine. J Bone Joint Surg (Am) 49A: 247–262

215. Gritzka T L, Taylor T K F 1970 A ganglion arising from a lumbar articular facet associated with low back pain and sciatica. Report of a case. J Bone Joint Surg 52B: 528–531

216. Groen G, Baljet B, Drukker J 1988 The innervation of the spinal dura mater: anatomy and clinical implications. Acta Neurochir 92: 39–46

217. Groen G, Baljet B, Drukker J 1990 Nerves and nerve plexuses of the human vertebral column. Am J Anat 188: 282–296

218. Guntz E 1933–34 Die Erkrankungen der Zwischenwirbelgelenke. Arch Orthop Unfall-Chir 34: 333–355

219. Haase J 1972 Extradural cyst of ligamentum flavum L4 — a case. Acta Orthop Scand 43: 32–38

220. Hadley L A 1935 Subluxation of the apophyseal articulations with bony impingement as a cause of back pain. Am J Roentgenol 33: 209–213

221. Hadley L A 1956 Secondary ossification centers and the intra-articular ossicle. Am J Roentgenol 76: 1095–1101

222. Hadley L A 1961 Anatomico-roentgenographic studies of the posterior spinal articulations. Am J Roentgenol 86: 270–276

223. Hadley L A 1964 Anatomico-Roentgenographic Studies of the Spine. Thomas, Springfield

224. Hakim N S, King A I 1976 Static and dynamic facet loads. Proceedings of the Twentieth Stapp Car Crash Conference p 607–639

225. Ham A W, Cormack D H 1979 Histology, 8th edn. Lippincott, Philadelphia, p 373

226. Hamilton W J, Boyd J D, Mossman H W 1962 Human Embryology, 3rd edn. Heffer, Cambridge

227. Hansson T, Roos B 1981 Microcalluses of the trabeculae in lumbar vertebrae and their relation to the bone mineral content. Spine 6: 375–380

228. Hansson T, Bigos S, Beecher P, Wortley M 1985 The lumbar lordosis in acute and chronic low-back pain. Spine 10: 154–155

229. Happey F 1976 A biophysical study of the human intervertebral disc. In: Jayson M I V (ed) The Lumbar Spine and Back Pain. Grune & Stratton, New York, ch 13, p 293–316

230. Harris R I, MacNab I 1954 Structural changes in the lumbar intervertebral discs. Their relationship to low back pain and sciatica. J Bone Joint Surg (Br) 36B: 304–322

231. Hasner E, Schalintzek M, Snorrason E 1952 Roentgenological exmanination of the function of the lumbar spine. Acta Radiol 37: 141–149

232. Hasue M, Kikuchi S, Sakuyama Y, Ito T 1983 Anatomic study of the interrelation between lumbosacral nerve roots and their surrounding tissues. Spine 8: 50–58

233. Hellems H K, Keates T E 1971 Measurement of the normal lumbosacral angle. Am J Roentgenol 113: 642–645

234. Hemborg B, Moritz, Hamberg J, Lowing, H, Akesson I 1983 Intra-abdominal pressure and trunk muscle activity during lifting — effect of abdominal muscle training in healthy subjects. Scand J Rehab Med 15: 183–196

235. Hemborg B, Moritz U 1985 Intra-abdominal pressure and trunk muscle activity during lifting II: chronic low-back patients. Scand J Rehab Med 17: 5–13

236. Hemborg B, Moritz U, Hamberg J, Holmstrom E, Lowing H, Akesson I 1985 Intra-abdominal pressure and trunk muscle activity during lifting III: effects of abdominal muscle training in chronic low-back patients. Scand J Rehab Med 17: 15–24

237. Herbert C M, Lindberg K A, Jayson M I V, Bailey A J 1975 Changes in the collagen of human intervertebral discs during ageing and degenerative disc disease. J Mol Med 1: 79–91

238. Heylings D J A 1978 Supraspinous and interspinous ligaments of the human spine. J Anat 125: 127–131

239. Hickey D S, Hukins S W L 1980 X-ray diffraction studies of the arrangement of collagen fibres in human fetal intervertebral disc. J Anat 131: 81–90

240. Hickey D S, Hukins D W L 1980 Relation between the structure of the annulus fibrosus and the function and failure of the intervertebral disc. Spine 5: 100–116

241. Hickey D S, Hukins D W L 1981 Collagen fibril diameters and elastic fibres in the annulus fibrosus of human fetal intervertebral disc. J Anat 133: 351–357

242. Hickey D S, Hukins D W L 1982 Aging changes in the macromolecular organization of the intervertebral disc. An X-ray diffraction and electron microscopic study. Spine 7: 234–242

243. Hilton R C 1980 Systematic studies of spinal mobility and Schorml's nodes. In: Jayson M I V (ed) The Lumbar Spine and Back Pain, 2nd edn. Pitman, London, ch 5, p 115–134

244. Hilton R C, Ball J, Benn R T 1976 Vertebral end-plate lesions (Schmorl's nodes) in the dorsolumbar spine. Ann Rheum Dis 35: 127–132

245. Hilton R C, Ball J, Benn R T 1979 In-vitro mobility of the lumbar spine. Ann Rheum Dis 38: 378–383

246. Hirsch C 1949 An attempt to diagnose the level of a disc lesion clinically by disc puncture. Acta Orthop Scand 18: 132–140

247. Hirsch C 1955 The reaction of the intervertebral discs to compression forces. J Bone Joint Surg (Am) 37A: 1188–1196

248. Hirsch C, Lewin T 1968 Lumbosacral synovial joints in flexion-extension. Acta Orthop Scand 39: 303–311

249. Hirsch C, Nachemson A 1954 New observations on mechanical behaviour of lumbar discs. Acta Orthop Scand 23: 254–283

250. Hirsch C, Schajowicz F 1952 Studies on structural changes in the lumbar annulus fibrosus. Acta Orthop Scand 22: 184–189

251. Hirsch C, Ingelmark B E, Miller M 1963 The anatomical basis for low back pain. Acta Orthop Scand 33: 1–17

252. Hirsch C, Paulson S, Sylven B, Snellman O 1953 Biophysical and physiological investigation on cartilage and other mesenchymal tissues; characteristics of human nuclei pulposi during aging. Acta Orthop Scand 22: 175–183

253. Hockaday J M, Whitty C W M 1967 Patterns of referred pain in the normal subject. Brain 90: 481–496

254. Holm S, Nachemson A 1983 Variations in the nutrition of the canine intervertebral disc induced by motion. Spine 8: 866–874

255. Holm S, Maroudas A, Urban J P G, Selstam G, Nachemson A 1981 Nutrition of the intervertebral disc: solute transport and metabolism. Connect Tiss Res 8: 101–119

256. Horal J 1969 The clinical appearance of low back disorders in the city of Gothenburg Sweden. Acta Orthop Scand Suppl 118

257. Horst M, Brinckmann P 1981 Measurement of the distribution of axial stress on the end-plate of the vertebral body. Spine 6: 217–232

258. Horwitz T, Smith R M 1940 An anatomical, pathological and roentgenological study of the intervertebral joints of the lumbar spine and of the sacroiliac joints. Am J Roentgenol 43: 173–186

259. Hovelacque A 1927 Anatomie des Nerfs Craniens et Rachidiens et du Systeme Grande Sympathique. Doin, Paris

260. Howe J F 1979 A neurophysiological basis for the radicular pain of nerve root compression. In: Bonica J J, Liebeskind J C, Albe-Fessard D G (eds) Advances in Pain Research and Therapy, Volume 3. Raven Press, New York, p 647–657

261. Howe J F, Loeser J D, Calvin W H 1977 Mechanosensitivity of dorsal root ganglia and chronically injured axons: a physiological basis for the radicular pain of nerve root compression. Pain 3: 25–41

262. Hukins D W L 1988 Disc structure and function. In: Ghosh P (ed) The biology of the intervertebral disc, Volume 1 C R C Press, Boca Raton, ch 1, p 1–37

263. Hukins D W L, Aspden R M, Hickey D S 1990 Thoracolumbar fascia can increase the efficiency of the erector spinae muscles. Clin Biomech 5: 30–34

264. Huson A 1967 Les articulations intervertebrales chez le foetus humain. Comptes Rendus de l'Association des Anatomistes 52: 676–683

265. Hutton W C, Adams M A 1982 Can the lumbar spine be crushed in heavy lifting? Spine 7: 586–590

266. Hutton W C, Stott J R R, Cyron B M 1977 Is spondylolysis a fatigue fracture? Spine 2: 202–209

267. Ikari C 1954 A study of the mechanism of low-back pain. The neurohistological examination of the disease. J Bone Joint Surg (Am) 36A: 195

268. Ingpen M L, Burry H C 1970 A lumbo-sacral strain syndrome. Ann Phys Med 10: 270–274

269. Inoue H, Takeda T 1975 Three-dimensional observation of collagem framework of lumbar intervertebral discs. Acta Orthop Scand 46: 949–956

270. Inoue H 1981 Three dimensional architecture of lumbar intervertebral discs. Spine 6: 138–146

271. Jackson D E, Atlas S W, Mani J R, Norman D 1989 Intraspinal synovial cysts: MR imaging. Radiology 170: 527–530

272. Jackson H C, Winkelmann R K, Bickel W H 1966 Nerve endings in the human lumbar spinal column and related structures. J Bone Joint Surg (Am) 48A: 1272–1281

273. Jacoby R K, Sims-Williams H, Jayson M I V, Baddeley H 1976 Radiographic stereoplotting: a new technique and its application to the study of the spine. Ann Rheum Dis 35: 168–170

274. Jaffray D, O'Brien J P 1986 Isolated intervertebral disc resorption: a source of mechanical and inflammatory back pain? Spine 11: 397–401

275. Jayson M I V, Barks J S 1973 Structural changes in the intervertebral disc. Ann Rheum Dis 32: 10–15

276. Jayson M I V, Herbert C M, Barks J S 1973 Intervertebral discs: nuclear morphology and bursting pressures. Ann Rheum Dis 32: 308–315

277. Johnson E F, Berryman H, Mitchell R, Wood W B 1985 Elastic fibres in the anulus fibrosus of the human lumbar intervertebral disc. A preliminary report. J Anat 143: 57–63

278. Johnson E F, Chetty K, Moore I M, Stewart A, Jones W 1982 The distribution and arrangement of elastic fibres in the IVD of the adult human. J Anat 135: 301–309

279. Johnston H M 1908 The cutaneous branches of the posterior primary divisions of the spinal nerves, and their distribution in the skin. J Anat Physiol 43: 80–91

280. Jonck L M, Van Niekerk J M 1961 A roentgenological study of the motion of the lumbar spine of te Bantu. S Afr J Lab Clin Med 2: 67–71

281. Jonsson B 1970 The functions of the individual muscles in the lumbar part of the spinae muscle. Electromyography 10: 5–21
282. Joseph J, McColl I 1961 Electromyography of muscles of posture: posterior vertebral muscles in males. J Physiol 157: 33–37
283. Jung A, Brunschwig A 1932 Recherches histologiques des articulations des corps vertebraux. Presse Med 40: 316–317
284. Kao C C, Uihein A, Bichel W H, Soule E H 1968 Lumbar intraspinal extradural ganglion. J Neurosurg 29: 168–172
285. Kazarian L 1972 Dynamic response characteristics of the human lumbar vertebral column. Acta Orthop Scand Suppl 146: 1–86
286. Kazarian L E 1975 Creep characteristics of the human spinal column. Orthop Clin North Am 6: 3–18
287. Keim H A, Keagy R D 1967 Congenital absence of lumbar articular facets. J Bone Joint Surg (Am) 49A: 523–526
288. Kellgren J H 1938 Observations on referred pain arising from muscle. Clin Sci 3: 175–190
289. Kellgren J H 1939 On the distribution of pain arising from deep somatic structures with charts of segmental pain areas. Clin Sci 4: 35–46
290. Kelly M 1956 Is pain due to pressure on nerves? Neurology 6: 32–36
291. Keon-Cohen B 1968 Abnormal arrangements of the lower lumbar and first sacral nerve roots within the spinal canal. J Bone Joint Surg (Br) 50B: 261–266
292. Keyes D C, Compere E L 1932 The normal and pathological physiology of nucleus pulposus of the intervertebral disc. J Bone Joint Surg 14: 897–938
293. Kimmel D L 1960 Innervation of spinal dura mater and dura mater of the posterior cranial fossa. Neurology 10: 800–809
294. King A B 1955 Back pain due to loose facets of the lower lumbar vertebrae. Bull Johns Hopk Hosp 97: 271–283
295. King A E, Vulcan A P 1971 Elastic deformation characteristics of the spine. J Biomech 4: 413–429
296. Kingsley J S 1925 The Vertebrate Skeleton. Murray, London, p 22
297. Kippers V, Parker A W 1984 Posture related to myoelectric silence of erectores spinae during trunk flexion. Spine 7: 740–745
298. Kippers V, Parker A W 1985 Electromyographic studies of erectores spinae: symmetrical postures and sagittal trunk motion. Aust J Physiother 31: 95–105
299. Kirby M C, Sikoryn T A, Hukins D W L, Aspden R M 1989 Structure and mechanical properties of the longitudinal ligaments and ligamentum flavum of the spine. J Biomed Eng 11: 192–196
300. Kirkaldy-Willis W H, Wedge J H, Yong-Hing K, Reilly L 1978 Pathology and pathogenesis of lumbar spondylosis and stensosis. Spine 3: 319–328
301. Klausen K 1965 The form and function of the loaded human spine. Acta Physiol Scand 65: 176–190
302. Klinghoffer L K, Muedock M M, Hermal M B 1975 Congenital absence of lumbar articular facets. Clin Orthop 106: 151–154
303. Knuttson B 1961 Comparative value of electromyography, myelography and clinico-neurological examination in diagnosis of lumbar root compression syndrome. Acta Orthop Scand Suppl 49
304. Knuttson F 1961 Growth and differentiation of the post-natal vertebrae. Acta Radiol 55: 401–408
305. Koreska J, Robertson D, Mills R H 1977 Biomechanics of the lumbar spine and its clinical significance. Orthop Clin North Am 8: 121–123
306. Korkala O, Gronblad M, Liesi P, Karaharju E 1985 Immunohistochemical demonstration of nociceptors in the ligamentous structures of the lumbar spine. Spine 10: 156–157
307. Kos J 1969 Contribution a l'etude de l'anatomie et de la vascularisation des articulations intervertebrales. Bull Ass Anat 142: 1088–1105
308. Kos J, Wolf J 1972 Les menisques intervertebraux et leur role possible dans les blocages vertebraux. Ann Med Phys 15: 203–218
309. Kos J, Wolf J 1972 Die 'Menisci' der Zwischenwirbelgelenke und ihre mogliche Rolle bei Wirbelblockierung. Man Med 10: 105–114
310. Kosteljanetz, M Espersen J O, Halaburt H, Miletic T 1984 Predictive value of clinical and surgical findings in patients with lumbago-sciatica. A prospective study (Part I). Acta Neurochir 73: 67–76
311. Kraemer J, Kolditz D, Gowin R 1985 Water and electrolyte content of human intervertebral discs under variable load. Spine 10: 69–71
312. Krempen J F, Smith B S, DeFreest L J 1975 Selective nerve root infiltration for the evaluation of sciatica. Orthop Clin North Am 6: 311–315
313. Krenz J, Troup J D G 1973 The structure of the pars interarticularis of the lower lumbar vertebrae and its relation to the etiology of spondylolysis. J Bone Joint Surg (Br) 55B: 735–741
314. Kulak R F, Belytschko T B, Schultz A B, Galante J O 1976 Non-linear behaviour of the human intervertebral disc under axial load. J Biomech 9: 377–386
315. Kumar S, Davis P R 1973 Lumbar vertebral innervation and intra-abdominal pressure. J Anat 114: 47–53
316. Lamb D W 1979 The neurology of spinal pain. Phys Ther 59: 971–973
317. Lamy C, Kraus H, Farfan H F 1975 The strength of the neural arch and the etiology of spondylosis. Orthop Clin North Am 6: 215–231
318. Larsen J L 1985 The posterior surface of the lumbar vertebral bodies — part 1. Spine 10: 50–58
319. Larsen J L 1985 The posterior surface of the lumbar vertebral bodies — part 2: an anatomic investigation concerning the curvatures in the horizontal plane. Spine 10: 901–906
320. Lawrence J S 1969 Disc degeneration, its frequency and relationship to symptoms. Ann Rheum Dis 28: 121–138
321. Lawrence J S, Bremner J M, Bier F 1966 Osteoarthrosis: prevalence in the population and relationship between symptoms and X-ray changes. Ann Rheum Dis 25: 1–24
322. Lazorthes G, Poulhes J, Espagno J 1947 Etude sur les nerfs sinu-vertebraux lombaires. Le nerf de Roofe, existe-t-il? Comptes Rendus de l'Association des Anatomistes 34: 317–320
323. Lazorthes G, Juskiewenski S 1964 Etude

comparative des branches posterieures des nerfs dorsaux et lombaires et leurs rapports avec les articulations interapophysaires vertebrales. Bulletin de l'Association des Anatomistes, 49e Reunion, 1025–1033

324. Le Double A F 1912 Traite des variations de la colonne vertebral de l'homme. Vigot Freres, Paris, p 271–274

325. Leighton J R 1967 The Leighton flexometer and flexibility test. J Assoc Phys Ment Rehab 20: 86–93

326. Leong J C Y, Luk K D K, Chow D H K, Woo C W 1987 The biomechanical functions of the iliolumbar ligament in maintaining stability of the lumbosacral junction. Spine 12: 669–674

327. Leskinen T P J, Stalhammar H R, Kuorinka I A A, Troup J D G 1983 Hip torque, lumbosacral compression, and intraabdominal pressure in lifting and lowering tasks. In: Winter D A, Norman R W, Wells R P, Hayes K C, Patla A E (eds) Biomechanics IX-B, International Series on Biomechanics. Human Kinetics, Champaign, p 55–59

328. Lewin T 1964 Osteoarthritis in lumbar synovial joints. Acta Orthop Scand Suppl 73

329. Lewin T, Moffet B, Viidik A 1962 The morphology of the lumbar synovial intervertebral joints. Acta Morphol Neerlando-Scandinav 4: 299–319

330. Lin H S, Liu Y K, Adams K H 1978 Mechanical response of the lumbar intervertebral joint under physiological (complex) loading. J Bone Joint Surg (Am) 60A: 41–54

331. Lindahl O 1966 Determination of the sagittal mobility of the lumbar spine — a clinical method. Acta Orthop Scand 37: 341–354

332. Lindblom K 1950 Technique and results in myelography and disc puncture. Acta Radiol 34: 321–330

333. Lippit A B 1984 The facet joint and its role in spine pain. Spine 9: 746–750

334. Livingstone W K 1941 Back disabilities due to strain of the multifidus muscle. West J Surg 49: 259–263

335. Loebl W Y 1967 Measurement of spinal posture and range of spinal movement. Ann Phys Med 9: 103–110

336. Loebl W Y 1973 Regional rotation of the spine. Rheumatol Rehab 12: 223

337. Loeser J D 1985 Pain due to nerve injury. Spine 10: 232–235

338. Lora J, Long D M 1976 So-called facet denervation in the management of intractable back pain. Spine 1: 121–126

339. Lorenz M, Patwardhan A, Vanderby R 1983 Load-bearing characteristics of lumbar facets in normal and surgically altered spinal segments. Spine 8: 122–130

340. Louis R 1978 Topographic relationships of the vertebral column, spinal cord, and nerve roots. Anat Clin 1: 3–12

341. Louyot P 1976 Propos sur le tubercle accessoire de l'apophyse costiforme lombaire. J Radiol Electrol 57: 905–906

342. Luk K D K, Ho H C, Leong J C Y 1986 The iliolumbar ligament. A study of its anatomy, development and clinical significance. J Bone Joint Surg (Br) 68B: 197–200

343. Lutz G 1967 Die Entwicklung der kleinen Wirbelgelenke. Z Orth 104: 19–28

344. Lynch M C, Taylor J F 1986 Facet joint injection for low back pain. J Bone Joint Surg (Br) 68B: 138–141

345. Macintosh J E, Bogduk N 1986 The biomechanics of the lumbar multifidus. Clin Biomech 1: 205–213

346. Macintosh J E, Bogduk N 1986 The morphology of the lumbar erector spinae. Spine 12: 658–668

347. Macintosh J E, Bogduk N, Gracovetsky S 1987 The biomechanics of the thoracolumbar fascia. Clin Biomech 2: 78–83

348. Macintosh J E, Valencia F, Bogduk N, Munro R R 1986 The morphology of the lumbar multifidus muscles. Clin Biomech 1: 196–204

349. Macleod S, Hendry G M A 1982 Congenital absence of a lumbar pedicle. Pediatr Radiol 12: 207–210

350. MacNab I 1972 The mechanism of spondylogenic pain. In: Hirsch C, Zotterman Y (eds) Cervical Pain. Pergamon, Oxford, p 89–95

351. MacNab I 1977 Backache. Williams & Wilkins, Baltimore, p 4–7

352. Macrae I F, Wright V 1969 Measurement of back movement. Ann Rheum Dis 28: 584–589

353. Magora A, Schwartz A 1876 Relation between the low back pain syndrome and x-ray findings. 1. Degenerative osteoarthritis. Scand J Rehab Med 8: 115–125

354. Maigne J Y, Lazareth J P, Surville H G, Maigne R 1989 The lateral cutaneous branches of the dorsal rami of the thoraco-lumbar junction. Surg Radiol Anat 11: 289–293

355. Malinsky J 1959 The ontogenetic development of nerve terminations in the intervertebral discs of man. Acta Anat 38: 96–113

356. Marchi G F 1963 Le articolazioni intervertebrali. La Clinica Ortopedica 15: 26–33

357. Markolf K L 1972 Deformation of the thoracolumbar intervertebral joints in response to external loads. J Bone Joint Surg (Am) 54A: 511–533

358. Markolf K L, Morris J M 1974 The structural components of the intervertebral disc. J Bone Joint Surg (Am) 56A: 675–687

359. Maroudas A 1988 Nutrition and metabolism of the intervertebral disc. In : Ghosh P (ed) The biology of the Intervertebral Disc, Volume II. CRC Press, Boca Raton, ch 9, p 1–37

360. Maroudas A, Nachemson A, Stockwell R, Urban J 1975 Some factors involved in the nutrition of the intervertebral disc. J Anat 120: 113–130

361. Marshal L L, Trethewie E R 1973 Chemical irritation of nerve-root in disc prolapse. Lancet 2: 320

362. Marshall L L, Trethewie E R, Curtain C C 1977 Chemical radiculitis. A clinical, physiological and immunological study. Clin Orthop 129: 61–67

363. McCall I W, Park W M, O'Brien J P 1979 Induced pain referral from posterior lumbar elements in normal subjects. Spine 4: 441–446

364. McCall I W, Park W M, O'Brien J P, Seal V 1985 Acute traumatic intraosseous disc herniation. Spine 10: 134–137

365. McCarron R F, Wimpee M W, Hudkins P G, Laros G S 1987 The inflammatory effect of nucleus pulposus: a possible element in the pathogenesis of low-back pain. Spine 12: 760–764

366. McCulloch J A 1983 Congenital anomalies of the lumbosacral spine. In: Genanat H K (ed) Spine Update 1984. Radiology Research and Education Foundation, San Francisco, ch 6, p 43–49

367. McCulloch J A, Waddell G 1980 Variation of the lumbosacral myotomes with bony segmental anomalies. J Bone Joint Surg (Br) 62B: 475–480

368. McDevitt C A 1988 Proteoglycans of the intervertebral disc. In: Ghosh P (ed) The biology of the Intervertebral Disc, Volume 1. CRC Press, Boca Raton, ch 6, p 151–170

369. McElverry R T 1956 Anomalies of the lumbar spinal cord and roots. Clin Orthop 8: 61–64

370. McGill S M, Norman R W 1988 Potential of lumbodorsal fascia forces to generate back extension moments during squat lifts. J Biomed Eng 10: 312–318

371. McMurrich J P 1919 The Development of the Human Body, 6th edn. Blakiston, Philadelphia, p 167

372. McNeill T, Warwick D, Andersson G, Schultz A 1980 Trunk strengths in attempted flexion, extension, and lateral bending in healthy subjects and patients with low-back disorders. Spine 5: 529–538

373. Meachim G, Cornah M S 1970 Fine structure of juvenile human nucleus pulposus. J Anat 107: 337–350

374. Mehta M, Sluijter M E 1979 The treatment of chronic back pain. Anaesthesia 34: 768–775

375. Melrose J, Ghosh P 1988 The noncollagenous proteins of the intervertebral disc. In: Ghosh P (ed) The Biology of the Intervertebral Disc, Volume I. CRC Press, Boca Raton, ch 8, p 189–237

376. Miller J A A, Haderspeck K A, Schultz A B 1983 Posterior element loads in lumbar motion segments. Spine 8: 327–330

377. Mixter W J, Barr J S 1934 Rupture of the intervertebral disc with involvement of the spinal canal. New Engl J Med 211: 210–215

378. Moll J, Wright V 1976 Measurement of spinal movement. In: Jayson M I V (ed) The Lumbar Spine and Back Pain. Grune & Stratton, New York ch 6, p 93–112

379. Moll J M H, Liyanage S P, Wright V 1976 An objective clinical method to measure spinal extension. Rheumatol Phys Med 11: 293–312

380. Mooney V 1987 Where is the pain coming from? Spine 12: 754–759

381. Mooney V, Robertson J 1976 The facet syndrome. Clin Orthop 115: 149–156

382. Morris J M, Benner G, Lucas D B 1962 An electromyographic study of the intrinsic muscles of the back in man. J Anat 96: 509–520

383. Morris J M, Lucas D B, Bresler B 1961 Role of the trunk in stability of the spine. J Bone Joint Surg (Am) 43A: 327–351

384. Murphy R W 1977 Nerve roots and spinal nerves in degenerative disk disease. Clin Orthop 129: 46–60

385. Mykelbust J B, Pintar F, Yoganandan N, Cusick J, Maiman D, Myers T J, Sances A 1988 Tensile strength of spinal ligaments. Spine 13: 526–531

386. Nachemson A 1960 Lumbar intradiscal pressure. Acta Orthop Scand Suppl 43: 1–104

387. Nachemson A 1963 The influence of spinal movements on the lumbar intradiscal pressure and on the tensile stresses in the annulus fibrosus. Acta Orthop Scand 33: 183–207

388. Nachemson A 1966 The load on lumbar disks in different positions of the body. Clin Orthop 45: 107–122

389. Nachemson A L 1976 The lumbar spine. An orthopaedic challenge. Spine 1: 59–71

390. Nachemson A 1980 Lumbar intradiscal pressure. In: Jayson M I V (ed) The Lumbar Spine and Backache, 2nd edn. Pitman, London, ch 12, p 341–358

391. Nachemson A L 1981 Disc pressure measurements Spine 6: 93–97

392. Nachemson A L, Andersson G B J, Schultz A B 1986 Valsalva maneuver Biomechanics. Effects on trunk load of elevated intraabdominal pressure. Spine 11: 476–479

393. Nachemson A L, Evans J H 1968 Some mechanical properties of the third human lumbar interlaminar ligament (ligamentum flavum). J Biomech 1: 211–220

394. Nachemson A L, Elfstrom G 1970 Intravital dynamic pressure measurments in lumbar discs. A study of common movements, manoeuvers and exercises. Scand J Rehabil Med 2 Suppl 1: 1–40

395. Nachemson A, Morris J M 1964 In vivo measurements of intradiscal pressure. J Bone Joint Surg 46: 1077–1092

396. Nachemson A L, Schultz A B, Berkson M H 1979 Mechanical properties of human lumbar spinal segments. Spine 4: 1–8

397. Naffziger H C, Inman V, Saunders J B de C M 1938 Lesions of the intervertebral disc and ligamenta flava. Surg Gynec Obstet 66: 288–299

398. Naylor A 1971 The biochemical changes in the human intervertebral disc in degeneration and nuclear prolapse. Orthop Clin North Am 2: 343–358

399. Naylor A 1976 Intervertebral disc prolapse and degeneration. The biochemical and biophysical approach. Spine 1: 108–114

400. Naylor A, Shental R 1976 Biochemical aspects of intervertebral discs in ageing and disease. In: Jayson M I V (ed) The Lumbar Spine and Backache. Grune & Stratton, New York, ch 14, p 317–326

401. Naylor A, Happey F, MacRae T P 1954 The collagenous changes in the intervertebral disc with age and their effect on elasticity Br Med J 2: 570–573

402. Naylor A, Happey F, Turner R L, Shentall R D, West D C, Richardson C 1975 Enzymic and immunological activity in the intervertebral disc. Orthop Clin North Am 6: 51–58

403. Neidre A, MacNab I 1983 Anomalies of the lumbosacral nerve roots. Spine 8: 294–299

404. Nichols B H, Shiflet E L 1933 Ununited anomalous epiphyses of the inferior articular processes of the lumbar vertebrae. J Bone Joint Surg 15: 591–600

405. Nikoloau P K, MacDonald B L, Glisson R R, Seaber A V, Garrett W E 1987 Biomechanical and histological evaluation of muscle after controlled strain injury. Am J Sports Med 15: 9–14

406. Ninghsia Medical College 1978 Anatomical observations on lumbar nerve posterior rami. Chin Med J 4: 492–496

407. Nitz A J, Peck D 1986 Comparison of muscle spindle concentrations in large and small human epaxial muscles acting in parallel combinations. Am Surg 52: 273–277

408. Nomina Anatomica, 6th edn. 1989 Churchill Livingstone, Edinburgh

409. Nordin M, Frankel V H 1980 Biomechanics of collagenous tissues. In: Frankel V H, Nordin M Basic Biomechanics of the Skeletal System. Lea & Febiger, Philadelphia, ch 3, p 87–110

410. Norlen G 1944 On the value of the neurological symptoms in sciatica for the localization of a lumbar disc herniation. Acta Chir Scand Suppl 95: 1–96

411. Noyes F R 1977 Fundamental properties of knee ligaments and alterations induced by immobilization. Clin Orthop 123: 210–242

412. Odgers P N B 1933 The lumbar and lumbosacral diarthrodial joints. J Anat 67: 301–317

413. Ogsbury J S, Simons H, Lehman R A W 1977 Facet 'denervation' in the treatment of low back syndrome. Pain 2: 257–263

414. Okada M 1970 Electromyographic assessment of the muscular load in forward bending postures. J Fac Sci Univ Tokyo 8: 311–336

415. O'Rahilly R, Meyer D B 1979 The timing and sequence of events in the development of the human vertebral column during the embryonic period proper. Anat Embryol 157: 167–176

416. O'Rahilly R, Muller F, Meyer D B 1980 The human vertebral column at the end of the embryonic period proper. J Anat 131: 565–575

417. Ortengren R, Andersson G B J 1977 Electromyographic studies of trunk muscles with special reference to the functional anatomy of the lumbar spine. Spine 2: 44–52

418. Ortengren R, Andersson G, Nachemson A 1978 Lumbar loads in fixed working postures during flexion and rotation. In: Asmussen E, Jorgensen K (eds) Biomechanics VI-B, International Series on Biomechanics, Volume 2B, University Park Press, Baltimore p 159–166

419. Ortengren R, Andersson G B J, Nachemson A L 1981 Studies of relationships between lumbar disc pressure, myoelectric back muscle activity, and intra-abdominal (intragastric) pressure. Spine 6: 98–103

420. Pallie W 1959 The intersegmental anastomoses of posterior spinal rootlets and their significance. J Neurosurg 16: 187–196

421. Panjabi M M 1977 Experimental determination of spinal motion segment behaviour. Orthop Clin North Am 8: 169–180

422. Paris S V 1983 Anatomy as related to function and pain. Orthop Clin North Am 14: 475–489

423. Park W M 1980 The place of radiology in the investigation of low back pain. Clin Rheum Dis 6: 93–132

424. Parke W W, Watanabe R 1985 The intrinsic vasculature of the lumbosacral spinal nerve roots. Spine 10: 508–515

425. Parke W W, Gammell K, Rothman R H 1981 Arterial vascularisation of the cauda equina. J Bone Joint Surg (Am) 63A: 53–62

426. Parkin I G, Harrison G R 1985 The topographical anatomy of the lumbar epidural space. J Anat 141: 211–217

427. Pauly J E 1966 An electromyographic analysis of certain movements and excercises. I. Some deep muscles of the back. Anat Rec 155: 223–234

428. Pawl R P 1974 Results in the treatment of low back syndrome from sensory neurolysis of the lumbar facets (facet rhizotomy) by thermal coagulation. Proc Inst Med Chgo 30: 150–151

429. Peacock A 1951 Observations on the pre-natal development of the intervertebral disc in man. J Anat 85: 260–274

430. Pearcy M J 1985 Stereo-radiography of lumbar spine motion. Acta Orthop Scand Suppl 212: 1–41

431. Pearcy M J, Bogduk N 1988 Instantaneous axes of rotation of the lumbar intervertebral joints. Spine 13: 1033–1041

432. Pearcy M J, Tibrewal S B 1984 Axial rotation and lateral bending in the normal lumbar spine measured by three-dimensional radiography. Spine 9: 582–587

433. Pearcy M, Portek I, Shepherd J 1984 Three-dimensional X-ray analysis of normal movement in the lumbar spine. Spine 9: 294–297

434. Pearcy M J, Portek I, Shepherd J 1985 The effect of low-back pain on lumbar spinal movements measured by three-dimensional X-ray analysis. Spine 10: 150–153

435. Pearson C H, Happey F, Naylor A, Turner R L, Palframan J, Shentall R D 1972 Collagens and associated glycoproteins in the human intervertebral disc. Ann Rheum Dis 31: 45–53

436. Peck D, Buxton D F, Nitz A 1984 A comparison of spindle concentrations in large and small muscles acting in parallel combinations. J Morphol 180: 243–252

437. Peck D, Nicholls P J, Beard C, Allen J R 1986 Are there compartment syndromes in some patients with idiopathic back pain? Spine 11: 468–475

438. Pedersen H E, Blunck C F J, Gardner E 1956 The anatomy of lumbosacral posterior rami and meningeal branches of spinal nerves (sinu-vertebral nerves): with an experimental study of their function. J Bone Joint Surg (Am) 38A: 377–391

439. Pelker R R, Gage J R 1982 The correlation of idiopathic lumbar scoliosis and lumbar lordosis. Clin Orthop 163: 199–201

440. Pellegrini V D, Hardy J H 1983 The absent lumbosacral articular process. A report of three cases and review of the literature. Clin Orthop 175: 197–201

441. Peretti F, Micalef J P, Bourgeon A, Argenson C, Rabischong P 1989 Biomechanics of the lumbar spinal nerve roots and the first sacral root within the intervertebral foramina. Surg Radiol Anat 11: 221–225

442. Perey O 1951 Contrast medium examination of the intervertebral discs of the lower lumbar spine. Acta Orthop Scand 20: 327–391

443. Perey O 1957 Fracture of the vertebral end-plate in the lumbar spine Acta Orthop Scand Suppl 25: 1–101

444. Pheasant H C, Swenson P C 1942 The lumbosacral region. A correlation of the roentgenographic and anatomical observations. J Bone Joint Surg 24: 299–306

445. Poirier P 1912 Myologie. In: Poirier P, Charpy A Traite d'Anatomie Humaine, 3rd edn, Volume 2, Fasc 1. Masson, Paris, p 139–140

446. Pope M H, Bevins T, Wilder D G, Frymoyer J W 1985 The relationship between anthropometric,

postural, muscular, and mobility characteristics of males ages 18–55. Spine 10: 644–648

447. Portnoy H, Morin F 1956 Electromyographic study of the postural muscles in various positions and movements. Am J Physiol 186: 122–126

448. Postacchini F, Urso S, Ferro L 1982 Lumbosacral nerve-root anomalies. J Bone Joint Surg (Am) 64A: 721–729

449. Pou-serradell A, Casademont M 1972 Syndrome del al queue de cheval et presence d'appendices apophysaires vertebraux, ou apophyses articulaires accessoires, dans la region lombaire. Rev Neurol 126: 435–440

450. Prasad P, King A I, Ewing C L 1974 The role of articular facets during +Gz acceleration. J Appl Mech 41: 321–326

451. Pritzker K P H 1977 Aging and degeneration in the lumbar intervertebral discs. Orthop Clin North Am 8: 65–77

452. Pukey P 1935 The physiological oscillation of the length of the body. Acta Orthop Scand 6: 338–347

453. Puschel J 1930 Der Wassergehalt normaler und degenerierter Zwischenwirbelscheiben. Beitr Path Anat 84: 123–130

454. Putti V 1927 New conceptions in the pathogenesis of sciatic pain. Lancet 2: 53–60

455. Rabischong P, Louis R, Vignaud J, Massare C 1978 The intervertebral disc. Anat Clin 1: 55–64

456. Ramsey R H 1966 The anatomy of the ligamenta flava. Clin Orthop 44: 129–140

457. Rask M R 1977 Anomalous lumbosacral nerve roots associated with spondylolisthesis. Surg Neurol 8: 139–140

458. Rashbaum R F 1983 Radiofrequency facet denervation. Orthop Clin North Am 14: 569–575

459. Ratcliffe J F 1980 The arterial anatomy of the adult human vertebral body: a micrarteriographic study. J Anat 131: 57–79

460. Raymond J, Dumas J M 1984 Intra-articular facet blocks: diagnostic test or therapeutic procedure? Radiology 151: 333–356

461. Reichmann S 1971 The postnatal development of form and orientation of the lumbar intervertebral joint surfaces. Z Anat Entwickl-Gesch 133: 102–121

462. Reichmann S, Lewin T 1971 Growth processes in the neural arch. Z Anat Entwickl-Gesch 133: 89–101

463. Rendich R A, Westing S W 1933 Accessory articular process of the lumbar vertebrae and its differentiation from fracture. Am J Roentgenol 29: 156–160

464. Resnick D 1983 Common disorders of the aging lumbar spine: radiographic-pathologic correlation. In: Genanat H K (ed) Spine Update 1984. Radiology Research and Education Foundation, San Francisco, ch 5, p 35–42

465. Reust P, Wendling D, Lagier R, Pageaut G, Reverdin A, Jacquet G, Guidet M, Fallet G H 1988 Degenerative spondylolisthesis, synovial cyst of the zygapophyseal joints, and sciatic syndrome: report of two cases and review of the literature. Arth Rheum 31: 288–294

466. Rissanen P M 1960 The surgical anatomy and pathology of the supraspinous and interspinous ligaments of the lumbar spine with special reference to ligament ruptures. Acta Orthop Scand Suppl 46: 1–100

467. Roaf R 1960 Vertebral growth and its mechanical control. J Bone Joint Surg (Br) 42B: 40–59

468. Roaf R 1960 A study of the mechanics of spinal injuries. J Bone Joint Surg (Br) 42B: 810–823

469. Roberts S, Menage J, Urban P G 1989 Biochemical and structural properties of the cartilage end-plate and its relation to the intervertebral disc. Spine 14: 166–174

470. Rockoff S F, Sweet E, Bleustein J 1969 The relative contribution of trabecular and cortical bone to the strength of human lumbar vertebrae. Calci Tissue Res 3: 163–175

471. Rolander S D 1966 Motion of the lumbar spine with special reference to the stabilising effect of posterior fusion. Acta Orthop Scand Suppl 90

472. Rolander S D, Blair W E 1975 Deformation and fracture of the lumbar vertebral end plate. Orthop Clin North Am 6: 75–81

473. Roofe P G 1940 Innervation of annulus fibrosus and posterior longitudinal ligament. Arch Neurol Psychiatry 44: 100–103

474. Rothman R H, Simeone F A 1975 The Spine. Volumes 1 and 2. Saunders, Philadelphia

475. Santo E 1935 Zur Entwicklungdgeschichte und Histologie der Zwischenscheiben in den kleinen Gelenken. Z Anat Entwickl Gesch 104: 623–634

476. Santo E 1937 Die Zwischenscheiben in den kleinen Gelenken. Anat Anz 83: 223–229

477. Saunders J B deC M, Inman V T 1940 Pathology of the intervertebral disk. Arch Surg 40: 380–416

478. Schmorl G, Junghanns H 1971 The Human Spine in Health and Disease, 2nd American edn. Grune & Stratton, New York, p 18

479. Schulz A, Andersson G B J, Ortengren R, Bjork R, Nordin M 1982 Analysis and quantitative myoelectric measurements of loads on the lumbar spine when holding weights in standing postures. Spine 7: 390–397

480. Sedowfia K A, Tomlinson I W, Weiss J B, Hilton R C, Jayson M I V 1982 Collagenolytic enzyme systems in human intervertebral disc. Spine 7: 213–222

481. Shah J S 1980 Structure, morphology and mechanics of the lumbar spine. In: Jayson M I V (ed) The Lumbar Spine and Backache, 2nd edn. Pitman, London, ch 13, p 359–405

482. Shah J S, Jayson M I V, Hampson W G J 1977 Low tension studies of collagen fibres from ligaments of the human spine. Ann Rheum Dis 36: 139–148

483. Shah J S, Hampson W G J, Jayson M I V 1978 The distribution of surface strain in the cadaveric lumbar spine. J Bone Joint Surg (Br) 60B: 246–251

484. Shellshear J L, Macintosh N W G 1949 The transverse process of the fifth lumbar vertebra. In: Shellshear J L, Macintosh N W G Surveys of Anatomical Fields. Grahame, Sydney, ch 3, p 21–32

485. Simmons E H, Segil C M 1975 An evaluation of discography in the localization of symptomatic levels in discogenic disease of the spine. Clin Orthop 108: 57–69

486. Simons D G 1988 Myofascial pain syndromes: where are we? Where are we going? Arch Phys Med Rehab 69: 207–212

487. Sims-Williams H, Jayson M I V, Baddeley H 1978 Small spinal fractures in back pain patients. Ann Rheum Dis 37: 262–265

488. Sluijter M E, Mehta M 1981 Treatment of chronic back and neck pain by percutaneous thermal lesions. In: Lipton S, Miles J (eds) Persistent Pain. Modern Methods of Treatment, Volume 3. Academic Press, London, p 141–179

489. Smyth M J, Wright V 1959 Sciatica and the intervertebral disc. An experimental study. J Bone Joint Surg (Am) 40A: 1401–1418

490. Souter W A, Taylor T K F 1970 Sulphated acid mucopolysaccharide metabolism in the rabbit intervertebral disc J Bone Joint Surg (Br) 52B: 371–384

491. Southworth J D, Bersack S R 1950 Anomalies of the lumbosacral vertebrae in five hundred and fifty individuals without symptoms referrable to the low back. Am J Roentgenol 64: 624–634

492. Spencer D L, Irwin G S, Miller J A A 1983 Anatomy and significance of fixation of the lumbosacral nerve roots in sciatica. Spine 8: 672–679

493. Splithoff C A 1953 Lumbosacral junction: roentgenographic comparisons of patients with and without backache. JAMA 152: 199–201

494. Steindler A, Luck J V 1938 Differential diagnosis of pain low in the back: allocation of the source of pain by the procain hydrochloride method. JAMA 110: 106–112

495. Stevens F S, Jackson D S, Broady K 1968 Protein of the human intervertebral disc. The association of collagen with a protein fraction having an unusual amino acid composition. Biochim Biophys Acta 160: 435–446

496. Stevens R L, Ryvar R, Robertson W R, O'Brien J P, Beard H K 1982 Biological changes in the annulus fibrosus in patients with low back pain. Spine 7: 223–233

497. Stubbs D A 1981 Trunk stresses in construction and other industrial workers. Spine 6: 83–89

498. Sturrock R D, Wojtulewski J A, Dudley Hart F 1973 Spondylometry in a normal population and in ankylosing spondylitis. Rheumatol Rehab 12: 135–142

499. Styf J, Lysell E 1987 Chronic compartment syndrome in the erector spinae muscle. Spine 12: 680–682

500. Sullivan J D, Farfan H F 1975 the crumpled neural arch. Orthop Clin North Am 6: 199–213

501. Sweetman B J, Anderson A D, Dalton E R 1974 The relationship between little finger mobility, lumbar mobility, straight-leg raising and low back pain. Rheumatol Rehab 13: 161–166

502. Sylven B, Paulson S, Hirsch C, Snellman O 1951 Biophysical and physiological investigations on cartilage and other mesenchymal tissues. J Bone Joint Surg (Am) 33A: 333–230

503. Tager K H 1965 Wirbelmeniskus oder synovial Forsatz. Z Orthop 99: 439–447

504. Tajima T, Furukawa K, Kuramachi E 1980 Selective lumbosacral radiculography and block. Spine 5: 68–77

505. Tanz S S 1953 Motion of the lumbar spine: a roentgenologic study. Am J Roentgenol 69: 399–412

506. Tarlov I M 1970 Spinal perineurial and meningeal cysts. J Neurol Neurosurg Psychiatry 33: 833–843

507. Taylor J R 1972 Persistence of the notochordal canal in vertebrae. J Anat 111: 211—217

508. Taylor J R 1975 Growth of the human intervertebral discs and vertebral bodies. J Anat 120: 49–68

509. Taylor J R 1990 The development and adult structure of lumbar intervertebral discs. J Man Med 5: 43–47

510. Taylor J R, Twomey L T 1979 Innervation of lumbar intervertebral discs. Med J Aust 2: 701–702

511. Taylor J, Twomey L 1980 Sagittal and horizontal plane movement of the human lumbar vertebral column in cadavers and in living. Rheumatol Rehab 19: 223–232

512. Taylor J R, Twomey L T 1984 Sexual dimorphism in human vertebral body shape. J Anat 138: 281–286

513. Taylor J R, Twomey L T 1985 Vertebral column development and its relation to adult pathology. Aust J Physiother 31: 83–88

514. Taylor J R, Twomey L T 1985 Age changes in the subchondral bone of human lumbar apophyseal joints. J Anat 143: 233

515. Taylor J R, Twomey L T 1986 Age changes in lumbar zygapophyseal joints. Spine 11: 739–745

516. Taylor J R, Twomey L T, Corker M 1990 Bone and soft tissue injuries in post-mortem lumbar spines. Paraplegia 28: 119–129

517. Taylor T K F, Little K 1965 Intercellular matrix of the intervertebral disk in ageing and in prolapse. Nature 208: 384–386

518. Tibrewal S B, Pearcy M J, Portek I, Spivey J 1985 A prospective study of lumbar spinal movements before and after discectomy using biplanar radiography. Spine 10: 455–460

519. Tondury G 1940 Beitrag zur Kenntnis der klein Wirbelgelenke. Z Ant Entwickl Gesch 110: 568–575

520. Tondury G 1972 Anatomie fonctionelle des petits articulations du rachis. Ann Med Phys 15: 173–191

521. Torgerson W R, Dotter W E 1976 Comparative roentgenographic study of the asymptomatic and symptomatic lumbar spine. J Bone Joint Surg (Am) 58A: 850–853

522. Travell J, Rinzler S H 1952 The myofascial genesis of pain, Postgrad Med 11: 425–434

523. Triano J J, Luttges M W 1982 Nerve irritation: a possible model for sciatic neuritis. Spine 7: 129–136

524. Troup J D G 1965 Relation of lumbar spine disorders to heavy manual work and lifting. Lancet 1: 857–861

525. Troup J D G 1977 Dynamic factors in the analysis of stoop and crouch lifting methods: a methodological approach to the development of safe materials handling standards. Orthop Clin North Am 8: 201–209

526. Troup J D G 1977 The etiology of spondylolysis. Orthop Clin North Am 8: 57–64

527. Troup J D G 1979 Biomechanics of the vertebral column. Physiotherapy 65: 238–244

528. Troup J D G, Hodd C A, Chapman A E 1967 Measurements of the sagittal mobility of the lumbar spine and hips. Ann Phys Med 9: 308–321

529. Twomey L 1985 Sustained lumbar traction. An experimental study of long spine segments. Spine 10: 146–149

530. Twomey L T, Taylor J R 1979 A description of two new instruments for measuring the ranges of sagittal

and horizontal plane motion in the lumbar region. Aust J Physiother 25: 201–204

531. Twomey L, Taylor J 1982 Flexion creep deformation and hysteresis in the lumbar vertebral column. Spine 7: 116–122

532. Twomey L T, Taylor J R 1983 Sagittal movements of the human lumbar vertebral column: a quantitative study of the role of the posterior vertebral elements. Arch Phys Med Rehab 64: 322–325

533. Twomey L T, Taylor J R 1985 Age changes in the lumbar articular triad. Aust J Physiother 31: 106–112

534. Twomey L, Taylor J 1985 Age changes in lumbar intervertebral discs. Acta Orthop Scand 56: 496–499

535. Twomey L T, Taylor J R 1986 The effects of ageing on the lumbar intervertebral discs. In: Grieve G (ed) Modern Manual Therapy. Churchill Livingstone, Edinburgh, ch 12, p 129–137

536. Twomey L, Taylor J, Furniss B 1983 Age changes in the bone density and structure of the lumbar vertebral column. J Anat 136: 15–25

537. Twomey L T, Taylor J R, Taylor M M 1989 Unsuspected damage to lumbar zygapophyseal (facet) joints after motor-vehicle accidents. Med J Aust 151: 210–217

538. Tyrrell A J, Reilly T, Troup J D G 1985 Circadian variation in stature and the effects of spinal loading. Spine 10: 161–164

539. Urban J, Maroudas A 1980 The chemistry of the intervertebral disc in relation to its physiological function. Clin Rheum Dis 6: 51–76

540. Urban J P G, Holm S, Maroudas A 1978 Diffusion of small solutes into the intervertebral disc. Biorheology 15: 203–223

541. Valencia F P, Munro R R 1985 An electromyographic study of the lumbar multifidus in man. Eltromyogr Clin Neurophysiol 25: 205–221

542. Vallois H V 1926 Arthologie. In: Nicolas A (ed) Poirier and Charpy's Traite d'Anatomie Humaine. Volume 1. Masson, Paris, p 68

543. VanderLinden R G 1984 Subarticular entrapment of the dorsal root ganglion as a cause of sciatic pain. Spine 9: 19–22

544. Vanharanta H, Sachs B L, Spivey M A et al 1987 The relationship of pain provocation to lumbar disc deterioration as seen by CT/discography. Spine 12: 295–298

545. Venner R M, Crock H V 1981 Clinical studies of isolated disc resorption in the lumbar spine. J Bone Joint Surg (Br) 63B: 491–494

546. Verbiest H 1954 A radicular syndrome from developmental narrowing of the lumbar vertebral canal. J Bone Joint Surg (Br) 36B: 230–237

547. Verbiest H 1975 Pathomorphological aspects of developmental lumbar stenosis. Orthop Clin North Am 6: 177–196

548. Verbiest H 1976 Fallacies of the present definition, nomenclature and classification of the stenoses of the lumbar vertebral canal. Spine 1: 217–225

549. Verbout A J 1985 The development of the vertebral column. Adv Anat Embryol Cell Biol 90

550. Vernon-Roberts B, Pirie C J 1973 Healing trabecular microfractures in the bodies of lumbar vertebrae. Ann Rheum Dis 32: 406–412

551. Vernon-Roberts B, Pirie C J 1977 Degenerative changes in the intervertebral discs of the lumbar spine and their sequelae. Rheumatol Rehab 16: 13–21

552. Virgin W J 1951 Experimental investigations into the physical properties of the intervertebral disc. J Bone Joint Surg (Br) 33B: 607–611

553. Vital J M, Lavignolle B, Grenier N, Rouais F, Malgat R, Senegas J 1983 Anatomy of the lumbar radicular canal. Anat Clin 5: 141–151

554. von Lackum H L 1924 The lumbosacral region. An anatomic study and some clinical observations. JAMA 82: 1109–1114

555. Walmsley R 1953 Growth and development of the intervertebral disc. Edinburgh Med J 60: 341–364

556. Warwick R, Williams P L (eds) 1973 Gray's Anatomy, 35 edn. Longman, London

557. White A A 1969 Analysis of the mechanics of the thoracic spine in man. Acta Orthop Scand Suppl 127

558. White A A, Panjabi M M 1978 Clinical Biomechanics of the Spine. Lippincott, Philadelphia.

559. White A A, Panjabi M M 1978 The basic kinematics of the human spine. A review of past and current knowledge. Spine 3: 12–20

560. White A, Handler P, Smith E L 1968 Principles of Biochemistry, 4th edn. McGraw-Hill, New York, ch 38, p 871–886

561. Whitehouse W J, Dyson E D, Jackson C K 1971 The scanning electron microscope in studies of trabecular bone from a human vertebral body. J Anat 108: 481–496

562. Wiberg G 1947 Back pain in relation to the nerve supply of the intervertebral disc. Acta Orthop Scand 19: 211–221

563. Wiles P 1935 Movements of the lumbar vertebra during flexion and extension. Proc R Soc Med 28: 647

564. Wiley J J, MacNab I, Wortzman G 1968 Lumbar discography and its clinical applications. Can J Surg 11: 280–289

565. Williams P C 1932 Reduced lumbosacral joint space. Its relation to sciatic irritation. JAMA 99: 1677–1682

566. Willis T A 1929 An analysis of vertebral anomalies. Am J Surg 6: 163–168

567. Willis T A 1941 Anatomical variations and roentgenographic appearance of the low back in relation to sciatic pain. J Bone Joint Surg 23: 410–416

568. Wiltse L L, Guyer R D, Spencer C W, Glenn W V, Porter I S 1984 Alar transverse process impingement of the L5 spinal nerve: The far-out syndrome. Spine 9: 31–41

569. Winckler G 1948 Les muscles profonds du dos chez l'homme. Arch Anat Histol Embryol 31: 1–58

570. Wolf J 1975 The reversible deformation of the joint cartilage surface and its possible role in joint blockage. Rehabilitacia Suppl 10–11: 30–36

571. Wyke B 1980 The neurology of low back pain. In: Jayson M I V (ed) The lumbar Spine and Back Pain, 2nd edn. Pitman, London, ch 11, p 265–339

572. Yang K H, King A I 1984 Mechanism of facet load transmission as a hypothesis for low-back pain. Spine 9: 557–565

573. Yong-Hing K, Reilly J, Kirkaldy-Willis W H 1976 The ligamentum flavum. Spine 1: 226–234

574. Yoshizawa H, O'Brien J P, Thomas-Smith W, Trumper M 1980 The neuropathology of

intervertebral discs removed for low-back pain. J Path 132: 95–104

575. Yousefzadeh D K, El-Khoury G Y, Lupetin A R 1982 Congenital aplastic-hypolastic lumbar pedicle in infants and young children. Skeletal Radiol 7: 259–265

576. Zaccheo D, Reale E 1956 Contributo alla conoscenza delle articolazioni tra i processi articolari delle vertebre dell'uomo. Archivio di Anatomia 61: 1–46

577. Zindriek M R, Lorenz M A, Noonan C, Mategrano V C 1987 The correlation between MRI, discogram and pain reproduction. Paper presented at the Annual Scientific Meeting of the International Society for the Study of the Lumbar Spine, Rome, 24th–28th May

Index